Clinical Applications of Digital Dental Technology

MW00724021

Clinical Applications of Digital Dental Technology

Edited by

Radi Masri, DDS, MS, PhD
Associate Professor, Department of Endodontics, Prosthodontics, and Operative Dentistry,
School of Dentistry, University of Maryland, Baltimore, Maryland, USA

Carl F. Driscoll, DMD
Professor and Director, Prosthodontic Residency, Department of Endodontics, Prosthodontics, and Operative Surgery,
School of Dentistry, University of Maryland, Baltimore, Maryland, USA

WILEY Blackwell

This edition first published 2015 © 2015 by John Wiley & Sons, Inc.

Editorial offices:
1606 Golden Aspen Drive, Suites 103 and 104, Ames, Iowa 50010, USA
The Atrium, Southern Gate, Chichester, West Sussex, PO19 8SQ, UK
9600 Garsington Road, Oxford, OX4 2DQ, UK

For details of our global editorial offices, for customer services and for information about how to apply for permission to reuse the copyright material in this book please see our website at www.wiley.com/wiley-blackwell.

Authorization to photocopy items for internal or personal use, or the internal or personal use of specific clients, is granted by Blackwell Publishing, provided that the base fee is paid directly to the Copyright Clearance Center, 222 Rosewood Drive, Danvers, MA 01923. For those organizations that have been granted a photocopy license by CCC, a separate system of payments has been arranged. The fee codes for users of the Transactional Reporting Service are ISBN-13: 978-1-1186-5579-5 / 2015.

Designations used by companies to distinguish their products are often claimed as trademarks. All brand names and product names used in this book are trade names, service marks, trademarks or registered trademarks of their respective owners. The publisher is not associated with any product or vendor mentioned in this book.

The contents of this work are intended to further general scientific research, understanding, and discussion only and are not intended and should not be relied upon as recommending or promoting a specific method, diagnosis, or treatment by health science practitioners for any particular patient. The publisher and the author make no representations or warranties with respect to the accuracy or completeness of the contents of this work and specifically disclaim all warranties, including without limitation any implied warranties of fitness for a particular purpose. In view of ongoing research, equipment modifications, changes in governmental regulations, and the constant flow of information relating to the use of medicines, equipment, and devices, the reader is urged to review and evaluate the information provided in the package insert or instructions for each medicine, equipment, or device for, among other things, any changes in the instructions or indication of usage and for added warnings and precautions. Readers should consult with a specialist where appropriate. The fact that an organization or Website is referred to in this work as a citation and/or a potential source of further information does not mean that the author or the publisher endorses the information the organization or Website may provide or recommendations it may make. Further, readers should be aware that Internet Websites listed in this work may have changed or disappeared between when this work was written and when it is read. No warranty may be created or extended by any promotional statements for this work. Neither the publisher nor the author shall be liable for any damages arising herefrom.

Library of Congress Cataloging-in-Publication Data

Clinical applications of digital dental technology / editors, Radi Masri, Carl F. Driscoll.
    p. ; cm.
  Includes bibliographical references and index.
  ISBN 978-1-118-65579-5 (pbk.)
  I. Masri, Radi, 1975- , editor. II. Driscoll, Carl F., editor.
  [DNLM: 1. Radiography, Dental, Digital–methods. 2. Computer-Aided Design. 3. Radiation Dosage.
4. Technology, Dental. WN 230]
  RK309
  617.6'07572–dc23
                                                                          2015007790

A catalogue record for this book is available from the British Library.

Wiley also publishes its books in a variety of electronic formats. Some content that appears in print may not be available in electronic books.

Cover image: [Production Editor to insert]
Cover design by [Production Editor to insert]

Typeset in 9.5/11.5pt Palatino by Laserwords Private Limited, Chennai, India.
Printed and bound in Singapore by Markono Print Media Pte Ltd

1 2015

To family, near, and far.

Contents

Contributors

Nadim Z. Baba, DMD, MSD
Professor, Department of Restorative Dentistry, Loma Linda University School of Dentistry, Loma Linda, CA, USA

Francesca Bonino, DDS
Postgraduate resident, Department of Periodontology, Tufts University School of Dental Medicine, Boston, MA, USA

Jacinto A. Cano Peyro, DDS
Instructor, Department of Prosthodontics & Operative Dentistry, Tufts University School of Dental Medicine, Boston, MA, USA

Carl F. Driscoll, DMD
Professor and Director, Advanced Education in Prosthodontics, Department of Endodontics, Prosthodontics, and Operative Dentistry, School of Dentistry, Maryland, Baltimore, MD, USA

Dennis J. Fasbinder, DDS
Clinical Professor, Department of Cariology, Endodontics, and Restorative Services, University of Michigan School of Dentistry, Ann Arbor, MI, USA

Ashraf F. Fouad, BDS, DDS, MS
Professor and Chair, Department of Endodontics, Prothodontics and Operative Dentistry, School of Dentistry, University of Maryland, Baltimore, MD, USA

Charles J. Goodacre, DDS, MSD
Professor, Restorative Dentistry, Loma Linda University, School of Dentistry, Loma Linda, CA, USA

Gerald T. Grant DMD, MS
Captain, Dental Crops, United States Navy, Service Chief, 3D Medical Applications Center, Department of Radiology, Walter Reed National Military Medical Center, Director of Craniofacial Imaging Research, Naval Postgraduate Dental School, Bethesda, MD, USA

Gary D. Hack
Associate Professor and Director of Clinical Stimulation, Department of Endodontics, Prosthodontics, and Operative Dentistry, School of Dentistry, University of Maryland, Baltimore, MD, USA

Julie Holloway, DDS, MS
Professor and Head, Department of Prosthodontics, The University of Iowa College of Dentistry, Iowa City, IA, USA

Jason Jamali, DDS, MD
Clinical Assistant Professor, Department of Oral and Maxillofacial Surgery, University of Illinois, Chicago, IL, USA

Georgios Kanavakis, DDS, MS
Assistant Professor, Department of Orthodontics and Dentofacial Orthopedics, Tufts University,

School of Dental Medicine, Boston, MA, USA

Mathew T. Kattadiyil, BDS, MDS, MS, FACP
Director, Advanced Specialty Education Program in Prosthodontics, Loma Linda University School of Dentistry, Loma Linda, CA, USA

Joanna Kempler, DDS, MS
Clinical Assistant Professor, Department of Endodontics, Prosthodontics and Operative Dentistry, University of Maryland, Baltimore, MD, USA

Antonia Kolokythas, DDS, MSc
Associate Professor, Program Director, Department of Oral and Maxillofacial Surgery, Multidisciplinary Head and Neck Cancer Clinic, University of Illinois at Chicago, Chicago, IL, USA

Radi Masri, DDS, MS, PhD
Associate Professor, Advanced Education in Prosthodontics, Department of Endodontics, Prosthodontics, and Operative Dentistry, School of Dentistry, Maryland, Baltimore, MD, USA

Michael Miloro, DMD, MD, FACS
Professor and Head, Department of Oral and Maxillofacial Surgery, University of Illinois at Chicago, Chicago, IL, USA

Alexandra Patzelt, DMD, Dr med dent
Visiting Scholar, Department of Periodontics, School of Dentistry, University of Maryland, Baltimore, MD, USA

Sebastian B. M. Patzelt, DMD, Dr med dent
Associate Professor, Department of Prosthetic Dentistry, Center for Dental Medicine, Medical Center – University of Freiburg, Freiburg i. Br., Germany

Jeffery B. Price, DDS, MS
Associate Professor, Director of Oral & Maxillofacial Radiology, Department of Oncology & Diagnostic Sciences, University of Maryland School of Dentistry, Baltimore, MD, USA

Carroll Ann Trotman, BDS, MS, MA
Professor and Chair, Department of Orthodontics, Tufts University School of Dental Medicine, Boston, MA, USA

Hans-Peter Weber, DMD, Dr med dent
Professor and Chair, Department of Prosthodontics and Operative Dentistry, Tufts University School of Dental Medicine, Boston, MA, USA

Foreword

Advances in technology have resulted in the development of diagnostic tools that allow clinicians to gain a better appreciation of patient anatomy that then leads to potential improvements in treatment options. Biomechanical engineering coupled with advanced computer science has provided dentistry with the ability to incorporate three-dimensional imaging into treatment planning and surgical and prosthodontic treatment. Optical scanning of tooth preparations and dental implant positions demonstrates accuracy that is similar to or possibly an improvement upon that seen with traditional methods used to make impressions and create casts.

For example, with this technology, orthodontic treatment can be reevaluated to assess outcomes. Today, orthodontic treatment can be planned and executed differently. With CT scanning on the orthodontic patient, dentists can better understand the boney limitation of a proposed treatment and timing of the treatment and dental implants can be used to create anchorage to move the teeth more easily. Every aspect of dentistry has been affected by digital technology, and in most instances, this has resulted in improvements of clinical treatment.

Restorative Dentistry and Prosthodontics are likely to experience the most dramatic changes relative to the incorporation of digital technology. Three-dimensional imaging provides the clinician with an ability to analyze bone quantity and quality that should lead to more effective development

of surgical guides. Likewise, hard and soft tissue grafting may be anticipated in advance, which will allow improved site development for esthetics and function. Such planning allows more affective provisionalization of the teeth and implants. By digitally understanding the design and tooth position, a provisional prosthesis can be fabricated using a monolithic premade block of acrylic, composite, or hybrid resin, thereby improving the ultimate strength of these prostheses. Dental material science has responded by producing materials that are more esthetic and can best provide a better potential for long-term survival and stability. Dental ceramics now can be milled on machines that can accept ever-improving algorithms to provide the most accurate prosthesis. Today, materials such as lithium disilicate, zirconia, and titanium are easily milled in machines that are self-calibrating and can eliminate the cuttings, so that accuracy is insured. In-office or in-laboratory CAD/CAM equipment is constantly improving, and it is clear that in years to come surgical guides and most types of ceramic restorations will able to be produced accurately and predictably in the office environment. This will change some of the duties of the dental technologist but in no way will compromise the necessity of having these trained and very talented professionals more involved in designing, individualizing color and characterization, correcting marginal discrepancies, and refining the prosthetic occlusions that are required. The dental technologist represents the most important function in delivering a restoration, that of quality control.

The future is exceedingly bright for all involved in the provision of dental care; moreover, the incorporation of digital dental procedures promises to improve care for the most important person in the treatment team, the patient.

The authors should be commended for bringing such valuable information and insight to the profession. At this point, information is what everyone most desire and one can be very proud of all the efforts forward-thinking professionals, engineers, and material scientists are bringing to the table. An honest appraisal of where we are today and what the potential future can be will drive the industry to create better restorative materials and engineered equipment and algorithms to dentistry.

Kenneth Malament

Preface

The evolution of the art and science of dentistry has always been gradual and steady, driven primarily by innovations and new treatment protocols that challenged the conventional wisdom such as the invention of the turbine handpiece and the introduction of dental endosseous implants.

While these innovations were few and far between, the recent explosion in digital technology, software, scanning, and manufacturing capabilities caused an unparalleled revolution leading to a major paradigm shift in all aspects of dentistry. Not only is digital radiography routine practice in dental clinics these days, but virtual planning and computer-aided design and manufacturing are also becoming mainstream. Digital impressions, digitally fabricated dentures, and the virtual patient are no longer science fiction, but are, indeed, a reality.

A new discipline, digital dentistry, has emerged, and the dental field is scrambling to fully integrate it into clinical practice and educational curriculums and as such, a comprehensive textbook that details the digital technology available and describes its indications, contraindications, advantages, disadvantages, limitations, and applications in the various dental fields is sorely needed.

There are a limited number of books and book chapters that address digital radiography, digital surgical treatment planning, and digital photography, but none address *digital dentistry* comprehensively. Although these topics will be addressed in this book, the scope is entirely different. The main focus is the practical application of digital technology in all aspects of dentistry. Available technologies will be discussed and critically evaluated to detail how they are incorporated in daily practice across all specialties. Realizing that technology changes rapidly, developing technologies and those expected to be on the market in the future will also be discussed.

Thus, this book is intended for a broad audience that includes dental students, general practitioners, and specialists of all the dental disciplines including prosthodontists, endodontists, orthodontists, oral and maxillofacial surgeons, periodontists, and oral and maxillofacial radiologists. It is also useful for laboratory technicians, dental assistants and dental hygienists, and anyone interested in recent digital advances in the dental field. We hope that the reader will gain a comprehensive understanding of digital applications in dentistry.

1 Digital Imaging

Jeffery B. Price and Marcel E. Noujeim

Introduction

Imaging, in one form or another, has been available to dentistry since the first intraoral radiographic images were exposed by the German dentist, Otto Walkhoff (Langland *et al.*, 1984), in early 1896, just 14 days after W.C. Roentgen publicly announced his discovery of X-rays (McCoy, 1919; Bushong, 2008). Many landmark improvements have been made over the more than 115-year history of oral radiography.

The first receptors were glass, however, film set the standard for the greater part of the twentieth century until the 1990s, when the development of digital radiography for dental use was commercialized by the Trophy company who released the RVGui system (Mouyen *et al.*, 1989). Other companies such as Kodak, Gendex, Schick, Planmeca, Sirona, and Dexis were also early pioneers of digital radiography.

The adoption of digital radiography by the dental profession has been slow but steady and seems to have been governed, at least partly, by the "diffusion of innovation" theory espoused by Dr. Everett Rogers (Rogers, 2003). His work describes how various technological improvements have been adopted by the end users of technology throughout the second half of the twentieth century and the early twenty-first century. Two of the most important tenets of adoption of technology are the concepts of threshold and critical mass.

Threshold is a trait of a group and refers to the number of individuals in a group who must be using a technology or engaging in an activity before an interested individual will adopt the technology or engage in the activity. Critical mass is another characteristic of a group and occurs at the point in time when enough individuals in the group have adopted an innovation to allow for self-sustaining future growth of adoption of the innovation. As more innovators adopt a technology such as digital radiography, the perceived benefit of the technology becomes greater and greater to ever-increasing numbers of other future adopters until eventually the technology becomes commonplace.

Digital radiography is the most common advanced dental technology that patients experience during diagnostic visits. According to one leading manufacturer in dental radiography, digital radiography is used by 60% of the dentists in the United States (Tokhi, J., 2013, personal communication). If you are still using film, the

Clinical Applications of Digital Dental Technology, First Edition. Edited by Radi Masri and Carl F. Driscoll.
© 2015 John Wiley & Sons, Inc. Published 2015 by John Wiley & Sons, Inc.

question should not be "Should I switch to a digital radiography system?", but instead "Which digital system will most easily integrate into my office?"

This leads to another question, what advantages does digital radiography offer the dental profession as compared to simply continuing with the use of conventional film? What are the reasons that increasing numbers of dentists are choosing digital radiographic systems over conventional film systems? Let us look at them.

Digital versus conventional film radiography

The most common speed class, or sensitivity, of intraoral film has been, and continues to be, D-speed film; the prime example of this film in the US market is Kodak's Ultra-Speed (NCRP, 2012). The amount of radiation dose required to generate a diagnostic image using this film is approximately twice the amount required for Kodak's Insight, an F-speed film. In other words, F-speed film is twice as fast as D-speed film. According to Moyal, who used a randomly selected survey of 340 dental facilities from 40 states found in the 1999 NEXT data, the skin entrance dose of a typical D-speed posterior bitewing is approximately 1.7 mGy (Moyal, 2007). Furthermore, according to the National Council on Radiation Protection and Measurements (NCRP) Report #172, the median skin entrance dose for a D-speed film is approximately 2.2 mGy while the typical E-F-speed film dose is approximately 1.3 mGy and the median skin entrance dose from digital systems is approximately 0.8 mGy (NCRP, 2012). According to NCRP Report #145 and others, it appears that dentists who are using F-speed film tend to overexpose the film and then under develop it; this explains why the radiation dose savings with F-speed film is not as great as it could be because F-speed film is twice as fast as D-speed film (NCRP, 2004; NCRP, 2012). If F-speed film were used per the manufacturers' instructions, the exposure time and/or milliamperage (total mAs) would be half that of D-speed film and the radiation dose would then be half.

Why has there been so much resistance for dentists to move away from D-speed film and embrace digital radiography? First of all, operating a dental office is much like running a fine-tuned production or manufacturing facility; dentists spend years perfecting all the systems needed in a dental office, including the radiography system. Changing the type of imaging system risks upsetting the dentist's capability to generate comprehensive diagnoses; therefore, in order to persuade individual dentists to change, there has to be compelling reasons, and, until recently, most of the dentists in the United States have not been persuaded to make the change to digital radiography. It has taken many years to reach the threshold and the critical mass for the dental profession to make the switch to digital radiography. Moreover, in all likelihood, there are dentists today who will retire from active practice before they switch from film to digital.

There are many reasons to adopt digital radiography: decreased environmental burdens by eliminating developer and fixer chemicals along with silver and iodide bromide chemicals; improved accuracy in image processing; decreased time required to capture and view images, which increases the efficiency of patient treatment; reduced radiation dose to the patient; improved ability to involve the patient in the diagnosis and treatment planning process with co-diagnosis and patient education; and viewing software to dynamically enhance the image (Wenzel, 2006; Wenzel and Møystad, 2010; Farman et al., 2008). However, if dentists are to enjoy these benefits, the radiographic diagnoses for digital systems must be at least as reliably accurate as those obtained with film (Wenzel, 2006).

Two primary cofactors seem to be more important than others in driving more dentists away from D-speed and toward digital radiography – the increased use of computers in the dental office and the reduced radiation doses seen in digital radiography. We will explore these factors further in the next section.

Increased use of computers in the dental office

This book's focus is digital dentistry and later sections will deal with how computers interface with every facet of dentistry. The earliest uses of the computer in dentistry were in the business office and accounting. Over the ensuing years, computer use spread to full-service practice management systems with digital electronic patient charts including digital image management systems. The use of computers in the business operations side of the dental practice allowed dentists to gain experience and confidence in how computers could increase efficiency and reliability in the financial side of their practices. The next step was to allow computers into the clinical arena and use them in patient care. As a component of creating the virtual dental patient, initially, the two most prominent roles were electronic patient records and digital radiography. In the following sections, we will explore the attributes of digital radiography including decreased radiation doses as compared to film; improved operator workflow and efficiency; fewer errors with fewer retakes; wider dynamic range; increased opportunity for co-diagnosis and patient education; improved image storage and retrievability; and communication with other providers (Farman *et al.*, 2008; Wenzel and Møystad, 2010).

Review of basic terminology

Throughout this section, we will be using several terms that may be new to you, especially if you have been using conventional film; therefore, we will include the following discussion of some basic oral radiology terms, both conventional and digital. Conventional intraoral film technology, such as periapical and bitewing imaging, uses a *direct* exposure technique whereby the X-ray photons directly stimulate the silver bromide crystals to create the latent image. Today's *direct digital* X-ray sensor refers most commonly to a complementary metal oxide semiconductor (CMOS) sensor that is directly connected to the computer via a USB port. At the time of the exposure, X-ray photons are detected by cesium iodide or perhaps gadolinium oxide scintillators within the sensor, which then emit light photons; these light photons are then detected within the sensor pixel by pixel, which allows for almost instantaneous image formation on the computer display. Most clinicians view this instantaneous image formation as the most advantageous characteristic of direct digital imaging.

The other choice for digital radiography today is an *indirect digital* technique known as photostimulable phosphor or PSP plates; these plates resemble conventional film in appearance and clinical handling. During exposure, the latent image is captured within energetic phosphor electrons; during processing, the energetic phosphors are stimulated by a red laser light beam; the latent energy stored in the phosphor electrons is released as a green light, which is captured, processed, and finally digitally manipulated by the computer's graphic card into images relayed to the computer's display. The "indirect" term refers to the extra processing step of the plates as compared to the direct method when using the CMOS sensor. The most attractive aspect of PSP may be that the clinical handling of the phosphor plates is exactly like handling film; so, most offices find that the transition to PSP to be very manageable and user-friendly.

Panoramic imaging commonly uses direct digital techniques as well. The panoramic X-ray beam is collimated to a slit; therefore, the direct digital sensor is several pixels wide and continually captures the signal of the remnant X-ray beam as the panoramic X-ray source/sensor assembly continually moves around the patient's head; the path of the source/sensor assembly is the same whether the receptor is an indirect film, PSP, or direct digital system. Clinicians who are using intraoral direct digital receptors generally opt for a direct digital panoramic system to avoid the need to purchase a PSP processor for their panoramic system.

Orthodontists require a cephalometric system and when moving from film to digital, again have two choices: direct digital and indirect digital. The larger flat panel digital receptor systems provide the instantaneous image but are slightly more costly than the indirect PSP systems; however, the direct digital systems obviate the need to purchase and maintain PSP processors. The higher the volume of patients in the office, the quicker is the financial payback for the direct digital X-ray machine.

Image quality comparison between direct and indirect digital radiography

Some dentists will make the decision of which system to purchase based solely on the speed of the system, with the direct digital system being the fastest. There are other factors as well: dentists often ask about image quality. Perhaps the better question to ask may be, "Is there a significant difference between the diagnostic capability of direct and indirect digital radiography systems?" One of the primary diagnostic tasks facing dentists on a daily basis is caries diagnosis, and there are several studies that have evaluated the efficacy of the two systems at this common task. The answer is that there is no difference between the two systems in diagnostic efficacy – either direct digital or indirect digital with PSP plates will diagnose caries equally well, in today's modern systems (Wenzel *et al.*, 2007; Berkhout *et al.*, 2007; Li *et al.*, 2007).

One important consideration to consider when comparing systems is to make sure that the images have the same *bit depth*. Bit depth refers to the numbers of shades of gray used to generate the image and are expressed exponentially in Table 1.1.

The early digital systems had a bit depth of 8 with 256 shades of gray, which may seem fine because the human eye can only detect approximately 20 to 30 shades of gray at any one time in any one image; however, most digital systems today generate images at 12 or even 16 bit depth, that is, images that have 4,096 to 65,536 shades of gray (Russ, 2007). Proper image processing is a skill that must be learned in order to fully utilize all of the information contained in today's digital images. Conventional film systems do not have discrete shades of gray; rather, film systems are analog and have an infinite number of possible shades of gray depending only on the numbers of silver atoms activated in each cluster of silver atoms in the latent image within the silver halide lattice of the film emulsion. Therefore, when comparing systems, ensure that the bit depth of the systems is comparable; and, remember that over time, the higher bit depth systems will require larger computer storage capacities due to the larger file sizes associated with the increased amount of digital information requirements of the larger bit depth images. It is expected that

Table 1.1   Bit depth table that gives the relation of the exponential increase in the number of shades of gray available in images as the bit depth increases.

Bit depth	Expression	Number of shades of gray
1	2^1	2
2	2^2	4
3	2^3	8
4	2^4	16
5	2^5	32
6	2^6	64
7	2^7	128
8	2^8	256
9	2^9	512
10	2^{10}	1024
11	2^{11}	2048
12	2^{12}	4096
13	2^{13}	8192
14	2^{14}	16384
15	2^{15}	32768
16	2^{16}	65536

in the future, most systems will use images of a minimum of 12 bit depth quality and many are already using images of 16 bit depth quality.

Amount of radiation required to use direct and indirect digital radiography

One other factor that dentists should consider when evaluating which system to use is how much radiation is required for each system to generate a diagnostic image. In order to determine the answer to this question, clinicians should be familiar with the term *dynamic range,* which refers to the performance of a radiographic receptor system in relation to the amount of radiation required to produce a desired amount of optical density within the image. The Hurter and Driffield (H&D) characteristic curve chart was initially developed for use with film systems and can also be used with direct digital and indirect digital systems

(Bushong, 2008; Bushberg *et al.*, 2012). The indirect digital system with PSP plates has the widest dynamic range, even wider than film, which means that PSP plates are more sensitive to lower levels of radiation than either conventional film or direct digital CMOS detectors; and, at the upper range of diagnostic exposures, the PSP plates do not experience burnout as quickly as film or direct digital until very high radiation doses are delivered. This means that the PSP system can handle a wider range of radiation dose and still deliver a diagnostic image, which may be a good feature, but for patient safety, this may be a negative feature because dentists may consistently be unaware that the operator of the equipment is delivering higher radiation doses than are necessary simply because their radiographic system has not been calibrated properly (Bushong, 2008; Bushberg *et al.*, 2012; Huda *et al.*, 1997; Hildebolt *et al.*, 2000).

Radiation safety of digital radiography

There are several principles of radiation safety: ALARA, justification, limitation, optimization, and the use of selection criteria. We will briefly review these and then discuss how digital radiography plays a vital role in the improved safety of modern radiography.

The acronym *ALARA* stands for As Low As Reasonably Achievable and, in reality, is very straightforward. In the dental profession, dental auxiliaries and dental professionals are required to use medically accepted radiation safety techniques that keep radiation doses low and that do not cause an undue burden on the operator or clinician. An example from the NCRP Report #145 Section 3.1.4.1.4 states "Image receptors of speeds slower than ANSI Speed Group E *shall not* be used for intraoral radiography. Faster receptors *should* be evaluated and adopted if found acceptable" (NCRP, 2004). This means that offices do not have to switch to digital but rather could switch to E- or F-speed film but *must* switch to at least E-speed film in order to be in compliance with this report. This is but one example of practicing ALARA. In the United States, federal and nationally recognized agencies such as the Food and Drug Administration (FDA)

and the NCRP issue guidelines and best practice recommendations; however, laws are enforced on the state level, which results in a confusing patchwork of various regulations, and dentists sometimes confuse what must be done with what should be done, especially because a colleague in a neighboring state must follow different laws. For example, although it is recommended by the NCRP but not legally required in many states, the state of Maryland now legally requires dentist to practice ALARA (Maryland, 2013), although the neighboring state of Virginia does not specifically require this in their radiation protection regulations(Commonwealth of Virginia, 2008). Therefore, in the state of Maryland, in order to satisfy legal requirements, dentists will soon be replacing D-speed film with either F-speed film or digital systems. Internationally, groups such as the International Commission on Radiological Protection (ICRP), the United Nations Scientific Committee on the Effects of Atomic Radiation (UNSCEAR), and the Safety and Efficacy in Dental Exposure to CT (SEDENTEXCT) have provided well-researched recommendations on the use of imaging in dentistry and guidance on the information of the effects of ionizing radiation on the human body (ICRP, 1991; Valentin, 2007; Ludlow *et al.*, 2008; UNSCEAR, 2001; Horner, 2009).

When a clinician goes through the process of examining a patient and formulating a diagnostic question, he or she is justifying the radiographic examination. This principle of *justification* is one of the primary principles of radiation safety. With digital radiography, our radiation doses are very low: so low, in fact, that if we have a diagnostic question that can only be answered with the information obtained from a dental radiograph, the risk from the radiograph is low enough that the "risk to benefit analysis" is always in favor of exposing the radiograph. There will always be enough of a benefit to the patient to outweigh the very small risk of the radiographic examination, as long as there is significant diagnostic information to be gained from the X-rays.

The principle of *limitation* means that the X-ray machine operator is doing everything possible to limit the actual size of the X-ray beam: that is, collimation of the X-ray beam. For intraoral radiography, rectangular collimation is recommended for routine use by the NCRP and there are various methods available to achieve collimation of the beam. Rectangular collimation reduces the radiation dose to the patient by approximately 60%. In panoramic imaging, the X-ray beam is collimated to a slit-shape. Moreover, in cone-beam CT, the X-ray beam has a cone shape.

In late 2012, the FDA and ADA issued the latest recommendations for selection criteria of the dental patient. These guidelines give the dentist several common scenarios that are seen in practice and offer suggestions on which radiographs may be appropriate. This article provides an excellent review of the topic and is best summarized by a sentence found in its conclusion: "Radiographs should be taken only when there is an expectation that the diagnostic yield will affect patient care" (ADA & FDA, 2012).

How does digital radiography assist with managing radiation safety? As mentioned earlier, digital receptors require less radiation dose than film receptors. In the 2012 NCRP Report #172, section 6.4.1.3, it is recommended that US dentists adopt a diagnostic reference level (DRL) for intraoral radiographs of 1.2 mGy. This dose is the median dose for E- and F-speed film systems, and it is higher than the dose for digital systems. This means that in order to predictably achieve this ambitious goal, US dentists who are still using D-speed film will need to either switch to F-speed film or transition to a digital system (NCRP, 2012).

Radiation dosimetry

The dental profession owns more X-ray machines than any other profession; and, we expose a lot of radiographs. Our doses are very small, but today our patients expect us to be able to educate them and answer their questions about the safety of the radiographs that we are recommending and it is part of our professional responsibility to our patients. Let's review some vocabulary first. The International System uses the *Gray* (Gy) or milliGray (mGy), and microGray (μGy) to describe the amount of radiation dose that is absorbed by the patient's skin (skin entrance dose) or by their internal organs. This dose is measured by devices such as ionization chambers or optically stimulated dosimeters (OSLs). There

are different types of tissues in our body and they all have a different response or sensitivity to radiation; for instance, the child's thyroid gland seems to be the most sensitive tissue that is in the path of our X-ray beams while the mature mandibular nerve may be the least sensitive tissue type in the maxillofacial region (Hall and Giaccia, 2012). Of course, we only deal with diagnostic radiation, but there are other types of radiation such as gamma rays, alpha particles, and beta particles; in order to provide a way to measure the effect on the body's various tissues when exposed by radiation from the various sources, a term known as *equivalent dose* is used. This term is expressed in *Sieverts* (S) or milliSieverts (mSv), and microSieverts (μSv). Finally, another term known as *effective dose* is used to compare the risk of radiographic examinations. This is the most important term for dental professionals to be familiar with as this is the term that accounts for the type of radiation used (diagnostic in our case) and the type of tissues exposed by the X-ray beam in the examination, whether it is a bitewing, a panoramic, a cone beam CT or a chest X-ray, and so on. Using this term is like comparing apples with apples. By using this term, we can compare the risk of a panoramic radiograph with the risk of an abdominal CT or a head CT and so on.

When patients ask us about how safe a particular radiographic examination may be, they are really asking whether that X-ray is going to cause a fatal cancer. Moreover, when medical physicists estimate the risk of X-rays in describing effective dose as measured in Sieverts and microSieverts for dentistry, they are talking about the risk of developing a fatal cancer. The risk is usually given as the rate of excess cancers per million. In order to accurately judge this number, the clinician needs to know the background rate of cancer (and fatal cancer) in the population. According to the American Cancer Society, the average person, male or female, in the population of the United States has a 40% chance of developing cancer during his or her lifetime; furthermore, the rate of fatality of that group is 50%; therefore, the overall fatal cancer rate in the United States is 20%, or 200,000 per million people (Siegel *et al.*, 2014). Now, when you read in the radiation dosimetry table (Table 1.2) that if a million people had a panoramic exposure and the excess cancer rate in those one million people was 0.9 per million, you will know that the total cancer rate changed from 200,000 per million to 200,000.9 per million. On a percentage basis, that is very small indeed – a 0.00045% risk of developing cancer. Of course, these are population-based numbers and are the best estimates groups like the NCRP can come up with, and you should also know that a very generous safety factor is built in. At the very low doses of ionizing radiation seen in most dental radiographic examinations experts such as medical physicists and molecular biologists do not know the exact mechanisms of how the human cell responds to radiation. So, to be safe and err on the side of caution, which is the prudent course of action, we all assume that some cellular and some genetic damage is possible due to a dose–response model known as the *linear no-threshold* model of radiation interaction, which is based on the assumption that in the low dose range of radiation exposures, any radiation dose will increase the risk of excess cancer and/or heritable disease in a simple proportionate manner (Hall and Giaccia, 2012).

There is one more column in Table 1.2 that needs some explanation – background equivalency. We live in a veritable sea of ionizing radiation, and the average person in the United States receives approximately 8 μSv of effective dose of ionizing radiation per day (NCRP, 2009). Take a look at the first examination – panoramic exposure; it has an effective dose of approximately 16 μSv; if you divide 16 μSv by 8 μSv per day, the result is 2 days of background equivalency. Using this method, you now know that the amount of effective dose in the average panoramic examination equals the same amount of radiation that the average person receives over the course of 2 days. This same exercise has been completed for the examinations listed in the table; and, for examinations not listed, you can calculate the background equivalency by following the aforementioned simple calculations. The intended use of effective dose is to compare population risks; however, this use as described earlier is a quick and easy patient education tool that most of our patients can quickly understand.

Uses of 2D systems in daily practice

The use of standard intraoral and extraoral imaging for clinical dentistry have been available for many years and include caries and periodontal diagnosis, endodontic diagnosis, detection, and evaluation of oral and maxillofacial pathology and evaluation of craniofacial developmental disorders.

Caries diagnosis

The truth is that diagnosing early carious lesions with bitewing radiographs is much more difficult than it appears to be than at first impression. Most researchers have found that a predictably accurate caries diagnosis rate of 60% would be very acceptable in most studies. In a 2002 study, Mileman and van den Hout compared the ability of Dutch dental students and practicing general dentists to diagnose dentinal caries on radiographs. The students performed almost as well as the experienced dentists (Mileman and Van Den Hout, 2002; Bader et al., 2001; Bader et al., 2002; Dove, 2001). We will explore caries diagnosis and how modern methods of caries diagnosis are changing the paradigm from the past ways of diagnosing caries (Price, 2013).

Caries detection is a basic task that all dentists are taught in dental school. In principle, it is very simple – detect mineral loss in teeth visually, radiographically, or by some other adjunctive method. There can be many issues that affect this task, including training, experience, and subjectivity of the observer; operating conditions and reliability of the diagnostic equipment; these factors and others can all act in concert and often, the end result is that this "simple" task becomes complex. It is important to realize that the diagnosis of a carious lesion is only one aspect of the entire management phase for dental caries. In fact, there are many aspects of managing the caries process besides diagnosis. The lesion needs to be assessed as to whether the caries is limited to enamel or if it has progressed to dentin. A determination of whether the lesion progressed to a cavity needs to be made because a cavitated lesion will continue to trap plaque and will need to be restored. The activity level of the lesion

Table 1.2   Risks from various dental radiographic examinations.

Effective Doses from Dental and Maxillofacial X-Ray Techniques and Probability of Excess Fatal Cancer Risk Per Million Examinations			
Technique	Dose Microsieverts	CA Risk Per Million Examinations	Background Equivalency
Panoramic–indirect digital	16	0.9	2 days
Skull/Cephalometrics–indirect digital	5	0.3	17 hours
FMX (PSP or F-speed film-rectangular collimation)	35	2	4.3 days
FMX (PSP or F-speed film-round collimation)	171	9	21 days
FMX (D-speed film-round collimation)	388	21	47 days
Single PA or Bitewing (PSP or F-speed film-rect. collimation)	1.25	0.1	3.6 hours
Single PA or Bitewing (PSP or F-speed film-round collimation)	9.5	0.5	1 day
Single PA or Bitewing (D-speed film-round collimation)	22	1.2	2.6 days
4 Bitewings (PSP or F-speed film-rectangular collimation)	5	0.3	17 hours
4 Bitewings (PSP or F-speed film-round collimation)	38	2	4 days
4 Bitewings (D-speed film-rectangular collimation)	88	5.5	11 days
Conventional Tomogram (8 cm × 8 cm field of view)	10	0.5	1 day
Cone Beam CT examination (Carestream 9300 10 × 10 cm Full Jaw)	79	5	10 days
Cone Beam CT examination (Carestream 9300 5 × 5 cm, post mand)	46	3	6 days
Cone Beam CT examination (Sirona Galileos)	70	4	8 days
Maxillo-mandibular MDCT	2100	153	256 days

Permission granted by Dr. John Ludlow.

needs to be determined; a single evaluation will only tell the clinician the condition of the tooth at that single point in time; not whether the demineralization is increasing or, perhaps whether it is decreasing; larger lesions will not require a detailed evaluation of activity, but smaller lesions will need this level of examination and follow-up. Finally, the therapeutic or operative management options for the lesion need to be considered based on these previous findings.

One thing to keep in mind is that most of the past research on caries detection has focused on occlusal and smooth surface caries. There are two reasons for this – first of all, from a population standpoint, more new carious lesions are occlusal

lesions today than in the past (NIH, 2001; Zandoná et al., 2012; Marthaler, 2004; Pitts, 2009) and, secondly, many studies rely on screening examinations without intraoral radiographic capability (Bader et al., 2001; Zero, 1999). Let look at the traditional classification system that US dentists have used in the past and a system that is being taught in many schools today.

Caries classifications

The standard American Dental Association (ADA) caries classification system designated dental caries as initial, moderate, and severe

Table 1.3   ADA caries classification system.

ADA Caries Classification System
No caries – Sound tooth surface with no lesion
Initial enamel caries – Visible non cavitated or cavitated lesion limited to enamel
Moderate dentin caries – Enamel breakdown or loss of root cementum with non-cavitated dentin
Severe dentin caries – Extensive cavitation of enamel and dentin

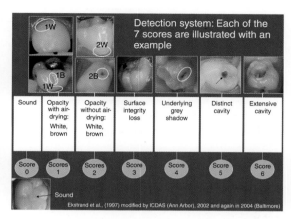

Figure 1.1 ICDAS caries classification. (Printed with permission of professor Kim Ekstrand.)

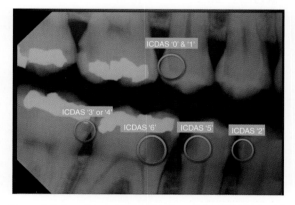

Figure 1.2 A radiographic application of the ICDAS classification for interproximal caries compiled by the author.

(Table 1.3); this was commonly modified with the term "incipient" to mean demineralized enamel lesions that were reversible (Zero, 1999; Fisher and Glick, 2012). There have been many attempts over the years to develop one universal caries classification system that clinical dentists as well as research dentists can use not only in the United States, but also internationally. As the result of the International Consensus Workshop on Caries Clinical Trials (ICW-CCT) held in 2002, the work on the International Caries Detection and Assessment System (ICDAS) was begun in earnest, and today it has emerged as the leading international system for caries diagnosis (Ismail et al., 2007; ICDAS, 2014). The ICDAS for caries diagnosis offers a six-stage, visual-based system for detection and assessment of coronal caries. It has been thoroughly tested and has been found to be both clinically reliable and predictable. Perhaps its' greatest strengths are that it is evidence based, combining features from several previously existing systems and does not rely on surface cavitation before caries can be diagnosed (Figures 1.1 and 1.2). Many previous systems relied on conflicting levels of disease activity before a diagnosis of caries; but, with the ICDAS, leading cariologists have been able to standardize definitions and levels of the disease process. The ICDAS appears to be the new and evolving standard for caries diagnosis internationally and in the United States.

Ethics of caries diagnosis

One of the five principles of the American Dental Association's Code of Ethics is nonmaleficence, which states that dentists should "do no harm" to his or her patients (ADA, 2012). By enhancing their caries detection skills, dental practitioners can detect areas of demineralization and caries at the earliest possible stages; these teeth can then be managed with fluorides and other conservative therapies (Bravo et al., 1997; Marinho et al., 2003; Petersson et al., 2005). This scenario for managing teeth with early caries will hopefully make some inroads into the decades old practice of restoring small demineralized areas because they are going to need fillings anyway and you might as well fill them now instead of waiting until they get bigger (Baelum et al., 2006). Continuing to stress the preventive approach to managing early caries begins with early diagnosis, and what better way to "do no harm" to our patients than to avoid placing restorations in these teeth with early demineralized enamel lesions and remineralize them instead?

Computer-aided diagnosis of radiographs

The use of computer-aided diagnosis (CAD) of disease is well established in medical radiology, having been utilized since the 1980s at the University of Chicago and other medical centers for assistance with the diagnosis of lung nodules, breast cancer, osteoporosis, and other complex radiographic tasks (Doi, 2007). A major distinction has been made in the medical community between automated computer diagnosis and computer-aided diagnosis. The main difference is that in automated computer diagnosis, the computer does the evaluation of the diagnostic material, that is, radiographs, and reaches the final diagnosis with no human input, while in computer-aided diagnosis, both a medical practitioner and a computer evaluate the radiograph and reach a diagnosis separately. Computer-aided diagnosis is the logic behind the Logicon Caries Detector (LCD) software marketed by Carestream Dental LLC, Atlanta, GA (Gakenheimer, 2002).

The Logicon system has been commercially available since 1998 and has seen numerous updates since that time. The Logicon software contains within its database teeth with matching clinical images, radiographs, and histologically known patterns of caries; as a tooth is radiographed and an interproximal region of interest is selected for evaluation, this database is accessed for comparison purposes. The software will then, in graphic format, give the dentist a tooth density chart and the odds ratio that the area in question is a sound tooth or simply decalcified or frankly carious and requires a restoration. In addition, the dentist can adjust the level of false positives, or specificity, that he or she is willing to accept (Gakenheimer, 2002; Tracy et al., 2011; Gakenheimer et al., 2005). The author used the Logicon system as part of his Trophy intraoral digital radiology installation in a solo general practice from 2003 to 2005 and found the Logicon system to be very helpful, particularly in view of its intended use as a computer-aided diagnosis device, which is also known as computerized "second opinion."

In a 2011 study, Tracy et al. describe the use of Logicon whereby 12 blinded dentists reviewed 17 radiographs from an experienced practitioner who meticulously documented the results that he obtained from the use of Logicon. Over a period of 3 years, he followed and treated a group of patients in his practice and photographed the teeth that required operative intervention for documentation purposes. In addition, he documented those teeth that did not have evidence of caries or had evidence of caries only in enamel that did not require operative treatment. The study included a total of 28 restored surfaces and 48 nonrestored surfaces in the 17 radiographs. His radiographic and clinical results were then compared to the radiographic diagnoses of the 12 blinded dentists on these 17 radiographs. The true positive, or actual diagnosis of caries when caries is present, is where the Logicon system proved to be of benefit. With routine bitewing radiographs and unadjusted images, the dentists diagnosed 30% of the caries; with sharpened images, only 39% of the caries. When using Logicon, the caries diagnosis increased to 69%, a significant increase in the ability to diagnose carious lesions. The other side of the diagnostic coin is specificity, or ability to accurately diagnose a sound tooth; both routine bitewing and Logicon images were equally accurate, diagnosing at a 97% and a 94% rate (Tracy et al., 2011). These results offer evidence that by using the Logicon system, dentists are able to confidently double the numbers of carious teeth that they are diagnosing without affecting their ability to accurately diagnose a tooth as being free from decay. The Logicon system appears to be a very worthwhile technological advancement in caries detection.

Non radiographic methods of caries diagnosis

Quantitative light-induced fluorescence

It has been shown that tooth enamel has a natural fluorescence. By using a CCD-based intraoral camera with specially developed software for image capture and storage (QLFPatient, Inspektor Research Systems BV, Amsterdam, The Netherlands), quantitative light-induced fluorescence (QLF) technology measures (quantifies) the refractive differences between healthy enamel and demineralized, porous enamel with areas of caries and demineralization showing less fluorescence. With the use of a fluorescent dye which can be applied to dentin, the QLF system can also be used to detect dentinal lesions in addition to enamel lesions. A major advantage of the QLF system is that these changes in tooth mineralization levels can be tracked over time using the documented measurements of fluorescence and the images from the camera. In addition, the QLF system has shown to have reliably accurate results between examiners over time as well as all around good ability to detect carious lesions when they are present and not mistakenly diagnose caries when they are not present (Angmar-Månsson and Ten Bosch, 2001; Pretty and Maupome, 2004; Amaechi and Higham, 2002; Pretty, 2006).

Laser fluorescence

The DIAGNOdent uses the property of laser fluorescence for caries detection. Laser fluorescence detection techniques rely on the differential refraction of light as it passes through sound tooth structure versus carious tooth structure. As described by Lussi et al. in 2004, a 650 nm light beam, which is in the red spectrum of visible light, is introduced onto the region of interest on the tooth via a tip containing a laser diode. As part of the same tip, there is an optical fiber that collects reflected light and transmits it to a photo diode with a filter to remove the higher frequency light wavelengths, leaving only the lower frequency fluorescent light that was emitted by the reaction with the suspected carious lesion. This light is then measured or quantified, hence the name "quantified laser fluorescence." One potential drawback with the DIAGNOdent is the increased incidence of false-positive readings in the presence of stained fissures, plaque and calculus, prophy paste, existing pit and fissure sealants, and existing restorative materials. A review of caries detection technologies published in the *Journal of Dentistry* in 2006 by Pretty that compared the DIAGNOdent technology with other caries detection technologies such as ECM, FOTI, and QLF showed that the DIAGNOdent technology had an extremely high specificity or ability to detect caries (Lussi et al., 2004; Tranaeus et al., 2005; Côrtes et al., 2003; Lussi et al., 1999; Pretty, 2006).

Electrical conductance

The basic concept behind electrical conductance technology is that there is a differential conductivity between sound and demineralized tooth enamel due to changes in porosity; saliva soaks into the pores of the demineralized enamel and increases the electrical conductivity of the tooth.

There has been a long-standing interest in using electrical conductance for caries detection; original work on this concept was published as early as 1956 by Mumford. One of the first modern devices was the electronic caries monitor (ECM), which was a fixed-frequency device used in the 1990s. The clinical success of the ECM was mixed as evidenced by the lack of reliable diagnostic predictability (Amaechi, 2009; Mumford, 1956; Tranaeus et al., 2005).

Alternating current impedance spectroscopy

The CarieScan device uses multiple electrical frequencies (alternating current impedance spectroscopy) to detect and diagnose occlusal and smooth surface caries. By using compressed air to keep the tooth saliva free, one specific area on a tooth can be isolated from the remaining areas and one small region of interest can be examined. If an entire surface needs to be evaluated, an electrolyte solution is introduced and the tip of the probe is placed over the larger area to allow for examination of the entire surface. The diagnostic reliability of this device is more accurate and reliable than the ECM, and, according to the literature, stains and discolorations do not interfere with the proper use of the device. It appears to have good potential as a caries detection technology (Tranaeus et al., 2005; Amaechi, 2009; Pitts et al., 2007; Pitts, 2010).

Frequency-domain laser-induced infrared photothermal radiometry and modulated luminescence (PTR/LUM)

This technology has recently been approved by the FDA and is known as the Canary system (Quantum Dental Technologies, Inc., Toronto, CA). It relies on the absorption of infrared laser light by the tooth with measurement of the subsequent temperature change, which is in the 1 °C range. This optical to thermal energy conversion is able to transmit highly accurate information regarding tooth densities at greater depths than visual only techniques. Early laboratory testing shows better sensitivity for caries detection for this technology than for radiography, visual, or DIAGNOdent technology; laboratory testing of an early OCT commercial model meant for the dental office has been accomplished; and clinical trials were successfully completed before the FDA approval (FDA, 2012; Amaechi, 2009; Jeon *et al.*, 2007; Jeon *et al.*, 2010; Sivagurunathan *et al.*, 2010; Matvienko *et al.*, 2011; Abrams *et al.*, 2011; Kim *et al.*, 2012).

Cone beam computed tomography

Dental cone beam computed tomography (CBCT) is arguably the most exciting advancement in oral radiology since panoramic radiology in the 1950s and 1960s and perhaps since Roentgen's discovery of X-rays in 1895 (Mozzo *et al.*, 1998). The concept of using a cone-shaped X-ray beam to generate three-dimensional (3D) images has been successfully used in vascular imaging since the 1980s (Bushberg *et al.*, 2012) and, after many iterations, is now used in dentistry. Many textbooks offer in-depth explanations of the technical features of cone beam CT (White and Pharoah, 2014; Miles, 2012; Sarment, 2014; Brown, 2013; Zoller and Neugebauer, 2008), so, we will offer a summary using a full maxillofacial field of view CBCT as an example. While the X-ray source is rotating around the patient, most manufacturers today design the electrical circuit to pulse the source on and off approximately 15 times per second; the best analogy to use is that the computer is receiving a low-dose X-ray movie at a quality of about 15 frames per second. At the end of the image acquisition phase for most systems, the reconstruction computer then has about 200 basis or projection images. These images are then processed using any one of several algorithms. The original, classic algorithm is the *back projection reconstruction* algorithm that was a key element of the work of Sir Godfrey Hounsfield and Allan McCormack who shared the Nobel Peace Prize in Medicine in 1979 (Bushberg *et al.*, 2012). Today, many other algorithms such as the Feldkamp algorithm, the cone beam algorithm, and the iterative algorithm are used in various forms as well as metal artifact reduction algorithms. In addition, manufacturers have their own proprietary algorithms that are applied to the CBCT volumes as well. The end result of the processing is not only 3D volumes, but also *multi-planar reconstructed* (MPR) images that can be evaluated in the three following standard planes of axial, coronal, and sagittal images (Figure 1.3). In addition, it is a generally accepted standard procedure to reconstruct a panoramic curve within the dental arches that is similar to a 2D panoramic image except for the lack of superimposed structures (Figure 1.4). In addition, any structure can be evaluated from any desired 360 degree angle. The strength of CBCT is the ability to view any mineralized anatomic structure within the field of view, from any angle. These images have zero magnification, and unless there are patient motion artifacts or patients have a plethora of dental restorations, these anatomic structure can be visualized without distortions.

Limitations of CBCT

The most significant limitation of CBCT is the increased radiation dose to the patient when compared to panoramic imaging. It is the duty of the ordering clinician to remain knowledgeable regarding the radiation doses of the CBCT examinations he or she orders for his or her patients. Earlier in this chapter, we referred to the risk to benefit analysis; this concept should be applied to CBCT decision making as well when the clinician is considering ordering a CBCT for the patient. The dentist should consider the following questions: (i) What is the diagnostic question? (ii) Is it likely that the information gained from the CBCT yield

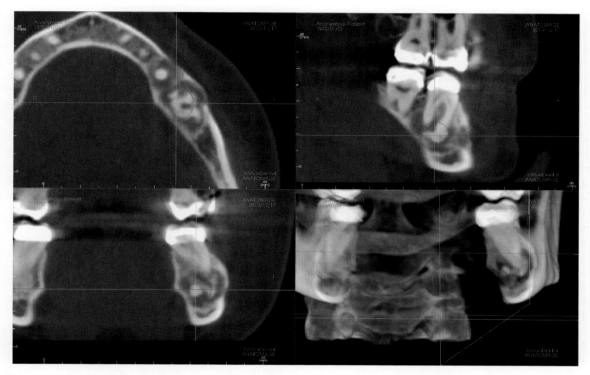

Figure 1.3 A typical MPR image of the posterior left mandible; note the expansion and mixed density lesion inferior to the apex of #19. The software is InVivo Dental by Anatomage, and the patient was scanned on a Carestream 9300 CBCT machine.

information will improve the treatment outcome? (iii) What is the risk to the patient? and (iv) Is the risk worth the improved outcome? Fortunately, in almost every instance, the risk to the patient is so small that the diagnostic information obtained from the CBCT will be worth the risk of the CBCT. On the other hand, if there is not a definite diagnostic question, then the risk outweighs the benefit (there is no defined benefit to the patient if there is no diagnostic question); therefore, do not take the CBCT. One other weakness of the technique is that due to scatter radiation, only high density objects such as bone and teeth are clearly and reliably seen in CBCT images while details in soft tissue objects such as lymph nodes and blood vessels are not seen. The outline of the airway can be seen due to the dramatic difference in density between air and soft tissue; however, the details of the soft tissues that form the borders of the airway cannot be discerned.

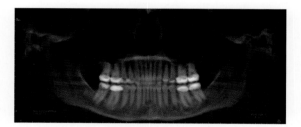

Figure 1.4 A reconstructed panoramic image from a Carestream 9300 CBCT machine; the patient is the same patient as in Figure 1.3 and the software is InVivo Dental by Anatomage.

In multi-detector CT (MDCT) used in medical imaging, both the primary X-ray beam and the remnant X-ray beam are collimated so that the X-ray beam that reaches the detector has a signal-to-noise ratio (SNR) of approximately 80%, while in CBCT, the SNR is only about 15–20%. This feature of the imaging physics of CBCT results in images with excellent details of high density objects and no details of the low density objects. This does appear to be a weakness, but let us examine this further. The most common diagnostic tasks that CBCT is used for are dental implant planning, localization of impacted teeth, pathosis of hard tissues in the maxillofacial region, endodontic diagnoses, evaluation of growth and development, and airway assessments. These tasks do not require the evaluation of soft tissue details; as a matter of fact, if soft tissue details were evident on CBCT scans, the amount of training and expertise required to interpret these scans would increase significantly. Advanced imaging modalities such as MDCT, magnetic resonance imaging (MRI), and ultrasound are available to assist with examinations of the soft tissues of the maxillofacial region when indicated. Therefore, this "weakness" of CBCT is actually a positive for us in dentistry as CBCT only images the hard tissues of the maxillofacial region and these are the tissues that are of primary interest to the dental professional.

Other limitations of CBCT include image artifacts such as *motion artifacts, beam hardening,* and *metal scatter*. Motion artifacts are the most common image artifact and can be managed in the following ways: use short scan times of 15 seconds or less; secure the chin and head during image acquisition; use a scanning appliance, a bite tab or even cotton rolls for the patient to occlude against during acquisition; instruct the patient to keep the eyes closed to prevent "tracking" of the rotating gantry; and use a seated patient technique when possible to eliminate patient movement.

The diagnostic X-ray beam used in dental CBCT (and in all other oral radiographic examinations) is polychromatic, which means that there is a range of energies in the primary X-ray beam. The term kVp means peak kilovoltage, so that if an 80 kVp setting is selected for a CBCT exposure, the most energetic X-ray photons will have an energy of 80 kVp and the average beam energy will be approximately 30 to 40 kVp. When the primary beam strikes a dense object such as titanium implant, a gold crown, an amalgam, or an endodontic post, these dense restorations selectively attenuate practically all of the lower energy X-ray photons and the only X-ray photons that might reach the detector are a few of highest energy photons, the 80 kVp photons in our example. In addition, this restoration is not centered within the patient, so as the X-ray source and receptor are rotating around the patient, this dental restoration is also rotating which causes this selective attenuation to constantly move in relation to the source and receptor. Beam hardening is due to the sudden attenuation of the lower energy X-ray photons and describes the increased average energy change from 30 to 40 kVp to close to 80 kVp. It is also manifested by the dark line seen around dense restorations, again, due to the border between the sudden difference in density between the very dense restoration and the not so dense tooth structure. Metal scatter is the bright colored, star-shaped pattern of X-ray images that are associated with these dense dental restorations (Bushberg *et al.*, 2012).

Common uses of CBCT in dentistry

As discussed earlier, dental CBCT provides for 3D imaging of the maxillofacial region. As such, there is great potential to affect how the dental professional can visualize the patient; after all, our patients are 3D objects. We will explore several of the areas of dentistry where CBCT is proving to be extremely useful.

Dental implant planning

The most common use of CBCT has been for dental implant planning. It appears that approximately two-thirds of the CBCT scans ordered are for dental implant planning purposes. Several professional organizations have recommended using CBCT for implant planning, including the American Association of Oral & Maxillofacial Radiologists (AAOMR), the International Congress of Oral Implantologists (ICOI), and the International Team for Implantology (ITI) among others (Tyndall *et al.*, 2012; Benavides *et al.*, 2012; Dawson *et al.*, 2009).

The most valuable information obtained from the CBCT scan is highly accurate information on alveolar ridge width and height in addition to the density of the bone. The earliest implant planning software used medical CT scans, which of course used CT numbers, also known as *Hounsfield numbers*, to precisely measure bone density. As these medical CT scanners have been replaced with CBCT scanners, many manufacturers have continued to use Hounsfield numbers as a matter of tradition, but be careful with this "tradition." A more accurate way to use these numbers in CBCT is to consider them as a relative gray density scale and not a precise number as in medical CT. Owing to the scatter issue discussed earlier, there is an approximate ± 100 range of error in the "Hounsfield" number seen in the common implant planning software packages (Mah *et al.*, 2010; Reeves *et al.*, 2012).

One other feature of evaluating the alveolar ridge is the principle of orthogonality; this means that the point of view of the viewer should be at a ninety degree angle to the buccal surface of the alveolus. How does one ensure this feature? Most software programs have a method to locate the panoramic curve; it is this position of the panoramic curve that determines the angulation of the buccal views as well as the orientation of the coronal slices through the alveolar ridges. The recommended way to draw the maxillary or mandibular arch panoramic curve is to place the panoramic curve points every 5 mm or so in a curvilinear manner in the center of the ridge. This will ensure that the "tick" marks on the axial slice will enter the buccal cortical plate at the desired 90 degree angle. You may ask why this is important. When measuring the ridge width in a potential implant site, the most accurate ridge width is the one taken at the ninety degree angle, straight across the ridge and not a measurement taken at an oblique angle across the ridge. Geometry will tell us that an error of 10–15 degrees can yield an error of 0.5–1.0 mm in some ridges, which may be clinically significant (Misch, 2008)

Using CBCT, clinicians can precisely identify anatomic features such as the maxillary sinus, nasal fossae, nasopalatine canal, mandibular canal, mental canal, incisive canal, submandibular fossae, localized defects, and undercuts and make preoperative decisions regarding bone grafting and/or implant placement. Implant planning software allows for the virtual placement of physically accurate models of implants, so not only can the alveolar ridge be measured, but the 3D stereolithographic implant model can also be placed into an accurately modeled alveolus to assist with determining the appropriate emergence profile and position of the implant. Surgical guides can be fabricated to duplicate these virtual implant surgeries (Sarment *et al.*, 2003; Ganz, 2005; Rothman, 1998; Tardieu and Rosenfeld, 2009; Guerrero *et al.*, 2006). These topics will be covered in much greater detail in Chapter 7. The use of CBCT for dental implant treatment planning has been at the forefront of CBCT research and development since the early days of CBCT and will continue to be a leader in the clinical application of CBCT.

Endodontics

In 2010, the American Association of Endodontists (AAE) was the first specialty group besides oral radiologists to issue a recommendation on the use of CBCT (AAE and AAOMR, 2011). Perhaps one of the reasons is that endodontists are often faced with the complex anatomy and surrounding structures of teeth and the maxillofacial region that make interpretation of 2D X-ray "shadows" difficult. The advent of CBCT has made it possible to visualize the anatomical relationship of structures in 3D. Significantly increased use of CBCT is evidenced by a recent Web-based survey of active AAE members in the United States and Canada, which found that 34.2% of 3,844 respondents indicated that they were utilizing CBCT. The most frequent use of CBCT among the respondents was for the diagnosis of pathosis, preparation for endodontic treatment or endodontic surgery, and for assistance in the diagnosis of trauma related injuries (AAE and AAOMR, 2011).

Many CBCT machines exist in the market that can be categorized by various criteria but the most common is the "field of view". CBCT can have craniofacial (large), maxillofacial (medium), and limited volume. Smaller scan volumes generally produce higher resolution images and deliver a smaller exposure dose, and as endodontics relies on detecting disruptions in the periodontal ligament space measuring approximately 100 μm, optimal resolution selection is necessary. For most endodontic applications, limited volume CBCT is preferred over medium or large volume CBCT for the following reasons: (i) the high spatial resolution increases the accuracy of endodontic-specific tasks such as the detection of features such as accessory canals, root fractures, apical deltas, calcifications, and fractured instruments and evaluation of the canal shaping and filling; (ii) the small field of view decreases the exposed surface for the patient, resulting in a decrease in radiation exposure; and (iii) the small volume limits the time and expertise required to interpret the anatomical content and allows the clinician or radiologist to focus on the area of interest (AAE & AAOMR, 2011).

- As seen in Table 1.2, CBCT scans have a significantly lower exposure than medical CT, but even limited volumes have a higher exposure than either conventional film or digital radiographs and their use must be justified based on the patient's history and clinical examination. In their 2010 document, the AAE recommended an initial radiographic examination with a periapical image and then described how CBCT use should be limited to the assessment and treatment of complex endodontic conditions, such as:
- Identification of potential accessory canals in teeth with suspected complex morphology based on conventional imaging;
- Identification of root canal system anomalies and determination of root curvature;
- Diagnosis of dental periapical pathosis in patients who present with contradictory or nonspecific clinical signs and symptoms, who have poorly localized symptoms associated with an untreated or previously endodontically treated tooth with no evidence of pathosis identified by conventional imaging, and in cases where anatomic superimposition of roots or areas of the maxillofacial skeleton is required to perform task-specific procedures;
- Diagnosis of non endodontic origin pathosis in order to determine the extent of the lesion and its effect on surrounding structures;
- Intra- or postoperative assessment of endodontic treatment complications, such as overextended root canal obturation material, separated endodontic instruments, calcified canal identification, and localization of perforations;
- Diagnosis and management of dentoalveolar trauma, especially root fractures, luxation and/or displacement of teeth, and alveolar fractures;

- Localization and differentiation of external from internal root resorption or invasive cervical resorption from other conditions, and the determination of appropriate treatment and prognosis;
- Presurgical case planning to determine the exact location of root apex/apices and to evaluate the proximity of adjacent anatomical structures.

In summary, as in the other areas of dentistry, use the risk to reward analysis procedure and let the potential information obtained from the radiographic examination guide you in deciding whether there is a good probability that the information obtained from the CBCT will affect the treatment outcome. If the information seems likely to be beneficial, then order the scan; however, if there does not appear to be any significant additional information to be gained from the scan, perhaps the risk to the patient is not worth the additional burden of the ionizing radiation.

Growth and development

The area of growth and development encompasses not only the growth and maturation of the dentoalveolar arches but also the airway. Orthodontists use CBCT imaging for many tasks including, but not limited to, evaluation for asymmetric growth patterns and localization of impacted or missing teeth, in particular maxillary canines and congenitally absent maxillary incisors, cases of external root resorption (Figures 1.5 and 1.6), and abnormal airway growth. A working group consisting of orthodontists as well as oral radiologists convened by the AAOMR published a position statement in 2013 that reviewed the general indications for the use of CBCT technology for orthodontics. The conclusions of this group were to: use image selection criteria when considering CBCT, assess the radiation dose risk, minimize patient radiation exposure, and to maintain professional competency in performing and interpreting CBCT examinations. These are very similar to the standard principles of radiation safety that were reviewed earlier in this section (AAOMR, 2013).

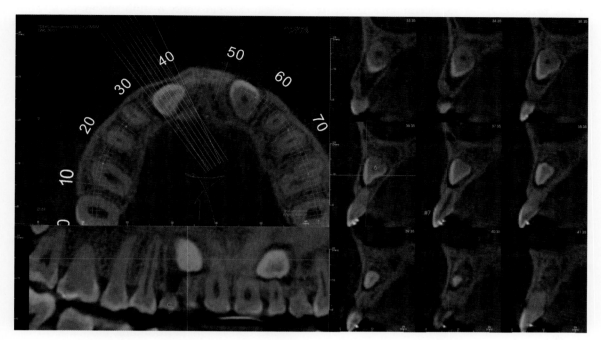

Figure 1.5 A multiplanar view of an impacted maxillary right canine (taken with Sirona Galileos).

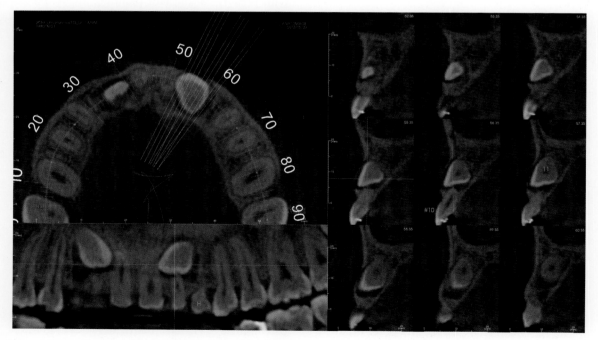

Figure 1.6 A multiplanar view of an impacted maxillary left canine (same patient as Figure 1.5 and taken with Sirona Galileos).

The primary issue in deciding whether to use conventional panoramic and cephalometric imaging for the growth and development patient versus CBCT imaging is the potential difference in the amount of radiation doses involved in the two protocols. Children and adolescents are ten to fifteen times more sensitive to ionizing radiation than adults and, therefore, obviously represent the group of patients that demand our greatest attention in the realm of radiation safety. Furthermore, most orthodontic patients are adolescents, so even small savings in radiation doses in this age group are magnified when viewed over the growing child's lifetime potential to develop cancer as a result of an exposure to ionizing radiation (Hall and Giaccia, 2012).

The difference in these aforementioned imaging protocols is best illustrated in the recently published AAOMR position paper on orthodontic imaging published in *The Oral Surgery, Oral Medicine, Oral Pathology, Oral Radiology Journal* in 2013. As Table 1.4 illustrates, an adolescent receiving a conventional regimen of a pretreatment panoramic and lateral cephalometric, a mid-treatment panoramic, and a posttreatment panoramic and lateral cephalometric would receive approximately 47 µSv of effective dose of radiation. On the opposite extreme, a patient who received a large field of view CBCT with a dose of 83 µSv radiation at each of these three time intervals would receive a total dose of approximately 249 µSv. This is a fivefold difference in radiation dose (AAOMR, 2013). Of course, this is a hypothetical situation, but it is entirely possible that there are unsuspecting practitioners who have exposed their patients to this regimen. There are CBCT manufacturers who are developing low-dose protocols especially for use in the mid- and posttreatment time periods when the image quality is not of paramount importance, which allows for lower dose to the patient. As time passes, clinical studies will need to be accomplished to evaluate the optimal strategies for when and how to incorporate CBCT imaging into the orthodontic practice (Ludlow, 2011; Ludlow and Walker, 2013).

The AAOMR, ADA, AAO, and other organizations have joined forces with a movement known as "Image Gently." "Image Gently" was begun as an educational entity within the radiology profession to train medical radiology technologists and radiologists of the need to optimize radiation doses for the pediatric patient. It has now spread to the dental community and is making a difference in decreasing the radiation dose for our most radiation-sensitive segment of the population (Image Gently, 2014; Sidhu *et al.*, 2009).

More complete details on digitally managing and creating the virtual orthodontic patient will be illustrated in Chapter 10.

Oral & maxillofacial surgery

There are several oral surgical diagnostic questions in which CBCT technology is proving to be very helpful. Localizing third molar position in relation to the mandibular canal is a common task (Figure 1.7). In addition, localizing other impacted teeth such as maxillary canines and determining the presence or absence of external resorption of the surrounding incisor teeth is a commonly accomplished task (Figures 1.5 and 1.6). Evaluation of the dental implant patient with presurgical implant planning; evaluation of patients with soft and hard tissue pathosis such as odontogenic cysts and tumors (Larheim and Westesson, 2006; Koenig, 2012); and evaluation of maxillofacial trauma as well as diagnosis of the orthognathic surgery patient are all diagnostic dilemmas in which CBCT is proving to be very helpful. In particular, these last three examples can often benefit from 3D modeling in which virtual surgery can be performed within the software, then various models and stents can be generated either with direct 3D or stereolithographic printing methods, and then the live patient surgery can be performed with the assistance of the stents.

Several software programs for orthognathic surgery treatment simulation, guided surgery, and outcome assessment have been developed. 3D surface reconstructions of the jaws are used for preoperative surgical planning and simulation in patients with trauma and skeletal malformation coupled with dedicated software tools, simulation of virtual repositioning of the jaws, virtual osteotomies, virtual distraction osteogenesis, and other surgical interventions can now be successfully performed on a trial basis to test

Table 1.4   Examples of the relative amounts of radiation associated with the specific imaging protocols used in orthodontics.

Protocol	Modality	Stage of Treatment			Dose (µSv)	
		Initial Diagnostic	Mid-Treatment	Post-treatment	Sub-total	Total
Conventional imaging	Panoramic*	+	+	+	36	47.2
	Lateral ceph[†]	+	–	+	11.2	
Conventional + small FOV CBCT	Panoramic	+	+	+	36	107.2
	Lateral ceph	+	–	+	11.2	
	Small FOV CBCT[‡]	+	–	–	60	
Large FOV CBCT + conventional imaging	Panoramic	–	+	+	24	112.6
	Lateral ceph	–	–	+	5.6	
	Large FOV CBCT[§]	+	–	–	83	
Large FOV CBCT	Large FOV CBCT	+	+	+	249	249

(AAOMR, 2013)

CBCT, cone beam computed tomography; FOV, field of view; Sub-total, product of the times when the modality is used at each stage over a course of treatment by the average effective dose per modality exposure; Total, sum of sub-totals for a particular orthodontic imaging protocol.

*Average panoramic dose of 12 µSv per exposure.
[†]Average lateral cephalometric dose of 5.6 µSv per exposure.
[‡]Small FOV i-CAT Next Generation Maxilla 6 cm FOV height, high resolution at 60 µSv dose per exposure.
[§]Large FOV i-CAT Next Generation 16 × 13 cm at 83 µSv per exposure.

the outcome before irreversible procedures are accomplished on the patient. Multiple imaging techniques include not only the regular CBCT volume but also a 3D soft tissue image along with optical images of the impressions; all of these images can then be merged into one virtual patient to create an almost perfect duplicate of the patient. Subsequently, a preview of the planned osseous surgery can be made with the software, which will give the operator an assessment of the hard and soft tissue outcomes. The patient will be able to see how they will look after the surgery with high accuracy. Pre- and postoperative images can also be registered and merged with high accuracy to assess the amount and position of alterations in the bony structures of the maxillofacial complex following orthognathic surgery (Cevidanes *et al.*, 2005; Cevidanes *et al.*, 2006; Cevidanes *et al.*, 2007; Hernández-Alfaro and Guijarro-Martínez, 2013; Swennen *et al.*, 2009a; Swennen *et al.*, 2009b; Plooij *et al.*, 2009). Further exploration of oral and maxillofacial surgery techniques will be reviewed in Chapter 11.

Future imaging technology

Polarization-sensitive optical coherent tomography (OCT)

OCT uses near infrared light to image teeth with confocal microscopy and low coherence interferometry resulting in very high resolution images at approximately 10–20 µm. The accuracy of OCT is so detailed that early mineral changes in teeth can be detected *in vivo* after exposure to low pH acidic solutions in as little as 24 hours by using differences in reflectivity of the near infrared light. In addition, tooth staining and the presence of dental plaque and calculus do not appear to affect the accuracy of OCT (Amaechi, 2009).

Advancements in the logicon computer-aided diagnosis software

The Logicon software continues to be refined. According to Dr. David Gakenheimer, the principal developer of the Logicon system, the next

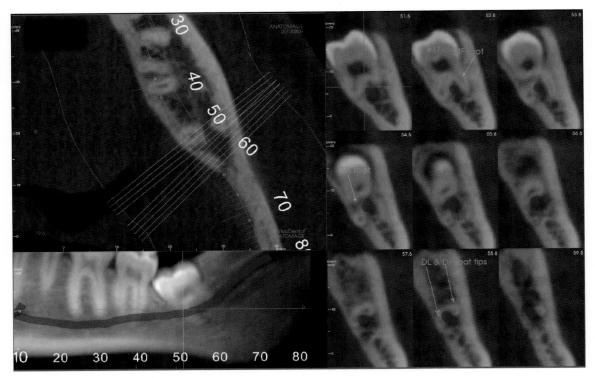

Figure 1.7 The mandibular canal passes through the furcation of an impacted third molar in a distal-to-mesial direction and bifurcates the mesial and distal roots (the CBCT volume is exposed by a Carestream 9300, and the software is InVivo Dental by Anatomage).

generation of Logicon will have a new routine called PreScan that will automatically analyze all of the proximal surfaces in a bitewing radiograph in 10–15 seconds. This feature is presently under review at the FDA. The dentist will continue to first perform a visual evaluation of the radiograph as always, then run manual Logicon calculations on suspicious surfaces as per the normal routine, and finally, the PreScan routine will be run to verify the dentist's initial assessments (Gakenheimer, 2014).

Other potential refinements include analyzing more than one bitewing at a time; for example, all four BW's taken in an FMS, or any four different BW's taken at different patient visits of the same quadrant over time to track how the carious lesion is changing. In addition, other updates may include modifying Logicon for the ability to evaluate primary teeth and to evaluate teeth for recurrent caries.

MRI for dental implant planning

The potential use of MRI in the area of dental implant planning has very good potential. Of course, the primary interest is due to the fact that MRI uses magnetic resonance energy detection and so far there is little, if any, known safety issues for the average person as compared to the potential hazards of exposure to ionizing radiation. There have been several published pilot studies on the use of MRI and it appears that the reported margin of error is within a reasonable level. This may one day be an accepted modality (Gray *et al.*, 1998; Gray *et al.*, 2003; Aguiar *et al.*, 2008).

MRI for caries detection

Moreover, the use of MRI technology for caries detection has a great deal of appeal as there is no ionizing radiation involved with the use of MRI. There are several drawbacks, however, that need to be addressed before the use of MRI is ready for clinical use: improvement of the signal to noise ratio due to small size of the average carious lesion and relatively low powered magnetic fields induced during diagnostic imaging; relatively high per image cost as compared to routine intraoral radiography; acquisition times of 15 minutes and longer for MRI; potential for artifacts from surrounding metal restorations; and, finally, potential magnetic interference from ferromagnetic metals such as nickel and cobalt. In addition, further clinical exploration is required before we see this technique routinely used (Lancaster *et al.*, 2013; Tymofiyeva *et al.*, 2009; Bracher *et al.*, 2011; Weiger *et al.*, 2012).

Dynamic MRI

Functional MRI for dental use appears to be of interest for evaluating the tissues of the temporomandibular joint apparatus while the patient is experiencing occlusal loading forces. By using MRI, this imaging modality adds the ability to see the soft tissues of the joint, including the articular disk and ligaments. Now, by adding the dynamic component of the force along with the fourth dimension of time, the clinician can also, for the first time, visualize the effects on these tissues of occlusal forces. This is information that has never been available before and will require a significant amount of study and affirmation before the results can be fully appreciated and utilized clinically (Tasali *et al.*, 2012; Hopfgartner *et al.*, 2013).

Low dose CBCT

Low dose CBCT protocols can potentially bring the radiation dose of CBCT into the realm of panoramic imaging. If this were to happen, 3D imaging would truly become the standard of care for almost every dental procedure. X-ray detector efficiency can be improved, and processing algorithms are being improved. Most dentists in the United States are accustomed to "nice looking" images whereas the medical community is moving to images that are diagnostic although they may not be as pleasing to the eye as they once

were (Schueler *et al.*, 2012; Schueler *et al.*, 2013; ACR & AAPM, 2013; Rustemeyer *et al.*, 2004). In dentistry, we will be forced to accommodate to images that while they may not be as pretty as the images that we have used in the past, they will be just as diagnostic. For example, if we are planning for dental implants, we really need to see the outlines of cortical borders, which we can do at 250–300 µm resolution. Thus, we do not need an image taken at 75 or 100 µm resolution, which would require a much higher radiation dose.

Summary

Advanced technology is used routinely today as we move through our daily lives. In the United States, the number of mobile subscriptions per 100 people has doubled during the last 10 years to over 98 subscriptions per 100 people, and 69% of US cellphones are smartphones, for a total of 230 million smartphones in use in the United States. These 230 million people using smartphones routinely use technology such as digital photography with the built in camera on their phone, as well as the texting, emailing, and internet surfing features (ICT, 2013). These same people, our dental patients, expect the technology that their dentist uses to at least be comparable to the technology found on today's typical smartphone (Douglass and Sheets, 2000).

This chapter has examined the use of radiology in digital dentistry and has reviewed the areas of primary importance to the dentist who is considering how to incorporate digital radiographic techniques into the modern dental practice. The remaining chapters will examine how the different specialties are utilizing digital technology to its full advantage in examining and managing today's modern dental patient.

References

Image Gently [Online]. 2014 The Alliance for Radiation Safety in Pediatric Imaging. Available: http://www.pedrad.org/associations/5364/ig/ [Accessed April 29, 2014].

AAE & AAOMR (2011) Use of cone beam computed tomography in endodontics: Joint Position Statement of the American Association of Endodontists and the

American Academy of Oral & Maxillofacial Radiology. *Oral Surgery, Oral Medicine, Oral Pathology, Oral Radiology, and Endodontics*, **111**, 234–237.

AAOMR (2013) Clinical recommendations regarding use of cone beam computed tomography in orthodontic treatment. Position statement by the American Academy of Oral and Maxillofacial Radiology. *Oral Surgery, Oral Medicine, Oral Pathology, Oral Radiology*, **116**, 238–257.

Abrams, S., Sivagurunathan, K., Jeon, R., Silvertown, J., Hellen, A., Mandelis, A., Hellen, W., Elman, G., Amaechi, B. & Finer, Y. (2011) Multi-Center Study Evaluating Safety and Effectiveness of the Canary System. *The Preliminary Program for IADR/AADR/ CADR 89th General Session and Exhibition (March 16-19th, 2011)*. San Diego, CA.

ACR & AAPM (2013) ACR-AAPM Practice Guideline for Diagnostic Reference Levels and Achievable Doses in Medical X-ray Imaging. American College of Radiology, Reston, VA.

ADA (2012) Principles of Ethics and Code of Professional Conduct. American Dental Association, Chicago, IL.

ADA & FDA (2012) Dental Radiographic Examinations: Recommendations for Patient Selection and Limiting Radiation Exposure. ADA & FDA, Chicago, IL.

Aguiar, M., Marques, A., Carvalho, A., & Cavalcanti, M. (2008) Accuracy of magnetic resonance imaging compared with computed tomography for implant planning. *Clinical Oral Implants Research*, **19**, 362.

Amaechi, B.T. (2009) Emerging technologies for diagnosis of dental caries: The road so far. *Journal of Applied Physics*, **105**, 102047.

Amaechi, B.T. & Higham, S.M. (2002) Quantitative light-induced fluorescence: a potential tool for general dental assessment. *Journal of Biomedical Optics*, **7**, 7–13.

Angmar-Månsson, B. & Ten Bosch, J. (2001) Quantitative light-induced fluorescence (QLF): a method for assessment of incipient caries lesions. *Dentomaxillofacial Radiology*, **30**, 298–307.

Bader, J.D., Shugars, D.A., & Bonito, A.J. (2001) Systematic reviews of selected dental caries diagnostic and management methods. *Journal of Dental Education*, **65**, 960–968.

Bader, J.D., Shugars, D.A., & Bonito, A.J. (2002) A systematic review of the performance of methods for identifying carious lesions. *Journal of Public Health Dentistry*, **62**, 201–213.

Baelum, V., Heidmann, J., & Nyvad, B. (2006) Dental caries paradigms in diagnosis and diagnostic research. *European Journal of Oral Sciences*, **114**, 263–277.

Benavides, E., Rios, H.F., Ganz, S.D., *et al.* (2012) Use of cone beam computed tomography in implant dentistry: the International Congress of Oral Implantologists Consensus Report. *Implant Dentistry*, **21**, 78–86.

Berkhout, W.E., Verheij, J.G., Syriopoulos, K., Li, G., Sanderink, G.C., & Van Der Stelt, P.F. (2007) Detection of proximal caries with high-resolution and standard resolution digital radiographic systems. *Dento Maxillo Facial Radiology*, **36**, 204–210.

Bracher, A.K., Hofmann, C., Bornstedt, A., *et al.* (2011) Feasibility of ultra-short echo time (UTE) magnetic resonance imaging for identification of carious lesions. *Magnetic Resonance in Medicine*, **66**, 538–545.

Bravo, M., Baca, P., Llodra, J.C., & Osorio, E. (1997) A 24-month study comparing sealant and fluoride varnish in caries reduction on different permanent first molar surfaces. *Journal of Public Health Dentistry*, **57**, 184–186.

Jr Brown, C.F. (2013) Galileos Cone-Beam & CEREC Integration. iBookstore: Apple.

Bushberg, J.T., Seibert, J.A., Leidholdt, J., Edwin, M., & Boone, J.M. (2012) The Essential Physics of Medical Imaging 3rd edn. Lippincott Williams & Wilkins, a Wolters Kluwer business, Philadelphia, PA.

Bushong, S. (2008) Radiologic Science for Technologists: Physics, Biology, and Protection. Mosby Elsevier, St. Louis, MO.

Cevidanes, L.H., Bailey, L.J., Tucker, G.R., Jr,, *et al.* (2005) Superimposition of 3D cone-beam CT models of orthognathic surgery patients. *Dento Maxillo Facial Radiology*, **34**, 369–375.

Cevidanes, L.H., Bailey, L.J., Tucker, S.F., *et al.* (2007) Three-dimensional cone-beam computed tomography for assessment of mandibular changes after orthognathic surgery. *American Journal of Orthodontics and Dentofacial Orthopedics*, **131**, 44–50.

Cevidanes, L.H., Styner, M.A., & Proffit, W.R. (2006) Image analysis and superimposition of 3-dimensional cone-beam computed tomography models. *American Journal of Orthodontics and Dentofacial Orthopedics*, **129**, 611–618.

Côrtes, D., Ellwood, R., & Ekstrand, K. (2003) An in vitro comparison of a combined FOTI/visual examination of occlusal caries with other caries diagnostic methods and the effect of stain on their diagnostic performance. *Caries Research*, **37**, 8–16.

Dawson, A., Chen, S., Buser, D., Cordaro, L., Martin, W., & Belser, U. (2009) The SAC Classification in Implant Dentistry. Quintessence Publishing Co Limited, Berlin.

Doi, K. (2007) Computer-aided diagnosis in medical imaging: historical review, current status and future potential. *Computerized Medical Imaging and Graphics: the Official Journal of the Computerized Medical Imaging Society*, **31**, 198.

Douglass, C.W. & Sheets, C.G. (2000) Patients' expectations for oral health care in the 21st century. *The Journal of the American Dental Association*, **131**, 3S–7S.

Dove, S.B. (2001) Radiographic diagnosis of dental caries. *Journal of Dental Education*, **65**, 985–990.

Farman, A.G., Levato, C.M., Gane, D., & Scarfe, W.C. (2008) In practice: how going digital will affect the dental office. *The Journal of the American Dental Association*, **139**(Suppl), 14S–19S.

FDA. (2012) The Canary System Gains 510(k) Clearance From FDA [Online]. Quantum Dental Technologies, Inc. Available: http://www.thecanarysystem.com/documents/2012-10-29TheCanarySystemGains510kClearancefromFDA.pdf [Accessed May 5, 2013].

Fisher, J. & Glick, M. (2012) A new model for caries classification and management: The FDI World Dental Federation Caries Matrix. *The Journal of the American Dental Association*, **143**, 546–551.

Gakenheimer, D., Farman, T., Farman, A., *et al.* (2005) Advancements in Automated Dental Caries Detection using DICOM Image Files (International Congress Series), pp. 1250–1255. Elsevier.

Gakenheimer, D.C. (2002) The efficacy of a computerized caries detector in intraoral digital radiography. *The Journal of the American Dental Association*, **133**, 883–890.

Gakenheimer, D.C. 2014 *RE: Update on Logicon*. Private communication to Price, J.B. [Accessed April 29, 2014]

Ganz, S. (2005) Presurgical planning with CT-derived fabrication of surgical guides. *Journal of Oral and Maxillofacial Surgery*, **63**, 59–71.

Gray, C., Redpath, T., & Smith, F. (1998) Low-field magnetic resonance imaging for implant dentistry. *Dentomaxillofacial Radiology*, **27**, 225.

Gray, C., Redpath, T., Smith, F., & Staff, R. (2003) Advanced imaging: magnetic resonance imaging in implant dentistry: a review. *Clinical Oral Implants Research*, **14**, 18–27.

Guerrero, M., Jacobs, R., Loubele, M., Schutyser, F., Suetens, P., & Van Steenberghe, D. (2006) State-of-the-art on cone beam CT imaging for preoperative planning of implant placement. *Clinical Oral Investigations*, **10**, 1–7.

Hall, E.J. & Giaccia, A.J. (2012) Radiobiology for the Radiologist. Lippincott Williams & Wilkins, a Wolters Kluwer business, Philadelphia.

Hernández-Alfaro, F. & Guijarro-Martínez, R. (2013) New protocol for three-dimensional surgical planning and CAD/CAM splint generation in orthognathic surgery: an in vitro and in vivo study. *International Journal of Oral and Maxillofacial Surgery*, **42**, 1547–1556.

Hildebolt, C.F., Couture, R.A., & Whiting, B.R. (2000) Dental photostimulable phosphor radiography. *Dental Clinics of North America*, **44**, 273–297.

Hopfgartner, A.J., Tymofiyeva, O., Ehses, P., *et al.* (2013) Dynamic MRI of the TMJ under physical load. *Dento Maxillo Facial Radiology*, **42**, 20120436.

Horner, K. (2009) Radiation Protection: Cone Beam CT For Dental And Maxillofacial Radiology Provisional Guidelines 2009. SedentextCT.

Huda, W., Rill, L.N., Benn, D.K., & Pettigrew, J.C. (1997) Comparison of a photostimulable phosphor system with film for dental radiology. *Oral Surgery, Oral Medicine, Oral Pathology, Oral Radiology, and Endodontics*, **83**, 725–731.

ICDAS. (2014) Leeds, UK: International Caries Detection and Assessment System. Available: http://www.icdas.org/home [Accessed May 2, 2014].

ICRP (1991) ICRP publication 60: 1990 recommendations of the International Commission on Radiological Protection. *Annals of the ICRP*, **21**, 1–201.

ICT (2013) The World in 2013: ICT Facts and Figures (ed B. Sanou). International Telecommunication Union. Geneva, Switzerland.

Ismail, A.I., Sohn, W., Tellez, M., *et al.* (2007) The international caries detection and assessment system (ICDAS): an integrated system for measuring dental caries. *Community Dentistry and Oral Epidemiology*, **35**, 170–178.

Jeon, R., Sivagurunathan, K., Garcia, J., Matvienko, A., Mandelis, A., & Abrams, S. (2010) Dental diagnostic clinical instrument. *Journal of Physics: Conference Series*, **214**, 012023.

Jeon, R.J., Matvienko, A., Mandelis, A., Abrams, S.H., Amaechi, B.T., & Kulkarni, G. (2007) Detection of interproximal demineralized lesions on human teeth in vitro using frequency-domain infrared photothermal radiometry and modulated luminescence. *Journal of biomedical optics*, **12**, 034028.

Kim, J., Mandelis, A., Matvienko, A., Abrams, S., & Amaechi, B. (2012) Detection of dental secondary caries using frequency-domain infrared photothermal radiometry (ptr) and modulated luminescence (LUM). *International Journal of Thermophysics*, **33**, 1778–1786.

Koenig, L. (2012) Diagnostic Imaging: Oral and Maxillofacial. Amirsys, Manitoba, Canada.

Lancaster, P., Carmichael, F., Britton, J., Craddock, H., Brettle, D., & Clerehugh, V. (2013) Surfing the spectrum - what is on the horizon? *British Dental Journal*, **215**, 401–409.

Langland, O.E., Sippy, F.H., & Langlais, R.P. (1984) Textbook of Dental Radiology. Charles C.Thomas, Springfield, IL.

Larheim, T.A. & Westesson, P.-L. (2006) Maxillofacial Imaging. Springer, Berlin, Germany.

Li, G., Sanderink, G., Berkhout, W., Syriopoulos, K., & Van Der Stelt, P. (2007) Detection of proximal caries in vitro using standard and task-specific enhanced images from a storage phosphor plate system. *Caries Research*, **41**, 231–234.

Ludlow, J. (2011) A manufacturer's role in reducing the dose of cone beam computed tomography examinations: effect of beam filtration. *Dentomaxillofacial Radiology*, **40**, 115.

Ludlow, J.B., Davies-Ludlow, L.E., & White, S.C. (2008) Patient risk related to common dental radiographic examinations: the impact of 2007 International Commission on Radiological Protection recommendations regarding dose calculation. *The Journal of the American Dental Association*, **139**, 1237–1243.

Ludlow, J.B. & Walker, C. (2013) Assessment of phantom dosimetry and image quality of i-CAT FLX cone-beam computed tomography. *American Journal of Orthodontics and Dentofacial Orthopedics*, **144**, 802–817.

Lussi, A., Hibst, R., & Paulus, R. (2004) DIAGNOdent: an optical method for caries detection. *Journal of Dental Research*, **83**, Spec No C: C80–C83.

Lussi, A., Imwinkelried, S., Pitts, N., Longbottom, C., & Reich, E. (1999) Performance and reproducibility of a laser fluorescence system for detection of occlusal caries in vitro. *Caries Research*, **33**, 261–266.

Mah, P., Reeves, T.E., & Mcdavid, W.D. (2010) Deriving Hounsfield units using grey levels in cone beam computed tomography. *Dentomaxillofacial Radiology*, **39**, 323–335.

Marinho, V., Higgins, J., Logan, S., & Sheiham, A. (2003) Fluoride mouthrinses for preventing dental caries in children and adolescents. *Cochrane Database of Systematic Reviews*, 1–3.

Marthaler, T. (2004) Changes in dental caries 1953–2003. *Caries Research*, **38**, 173–181.

Maryland, State of (2013) Regulatory Guidelines for Dental Radiation Machines. Issued by the Radiological Health Program, Air and Radiation Management Administration, Maryland Department of the Environment (ed.) *Code of Maryland Regulations 26.12.01.01*. 1800 Washington Boulevard, Baltimore, MD 21230: State of Maryland.

Matvienko, A., Amaechi, B., Ramalingam, K., *et al.* (2011) PTR-LUM-based detection of demineralization and remineralization of human teeth. *The Preliminary Program for IADR/AADR/CADR 89th General Session and Exhibition (March 16–19th, 2011)*. San Diego, CA.

McCoy, J.D. (1919) Dental and Oral Radiography: A Textbook For Students and Practitioners of Dentistry. C.V. Mosby Company, St. Louis, MO.

Mileman, P. & Van Den Hout, W. (2002) Comparing the accuracy of Dutch dentists and dental students in the radiographic diagnosis of dentinal caries. *Dentomaxillofacial Radiology*, **31**, 7–14.

Miles, D.A. (2012) Atlas of Cone Beam Imaging for Dental Applications. Quintessence Publishing.

Misch, C.E. (2008) Contemporary Implant Dentistry. St. Louis, MO, Mosby Elsevier.

Mouyen, F., Benz, C., Sonnabend, E., & Lodter, J.P. (1989) Presentation and physical evaluation of RadioVisio Graphy. *Oral Surgery, Oral Medicine, Oral Pathology*, **68**, 238–242.

Moyal, A.E. (2007) Nationwide Evaluation of X-ray Trends (NEXT): Tabulation and Graphical Summary of the 1999 Dental Radiography Survey 2nd edn. Conference of Radiation Control Program Directors, Inc., Frankfort, KY.

Mozzo, P., Procacci, C., Tacconi, A., Martini, P.T., & Andreis, I.A. (1998) A new volumetric CT machine for dental imaging based on the cone-beam technique: preliminary results. *European Radiology*, **8**, 1558–1564.

Mumford, J. (1956) Relationship between the electrical resistance of human teeth and the presence and extent of dental caries. *British Dental Journal*, **100**, 10.

NCRP. (2004) NCRP Report #145: Radiation Protection in Dentistry.National Council on Radiation Protection and Measurements,Bethesda, MD.

NCRP (2009) NCRP Report #160: Ionizing Radiation Exposure of the Population of the United States. National Council on Radiation Protection and Measurements,Bethesda, MD.

NCRP (2012) NCRP Report #172: Reference Levels and Achievable Doses in Medical and Dental Imaging: Recommendations for the United States. National Council on Radiation Protection and Measurements, Bethesda, MD.

NIH (2001) Diagnosis and management of dental caries throughout life. *2001 NIH Consensus Development Conference on Diagnosis and Management of Dental Caries Throughout Life*.National Institutes of Health, Washington DC.

Petersson, L., Lith, A., & Birkhed, D. (2005) Effect of school-based fluoride varnish programmes on approximal caries in adolescents from different caries risk areas. *Caries Research*, **39**, 273–279.

Pitts, N.B. (2009) Detection, Assessment, Diagnosis and Monitoring of Caries. Karger, Basle, Switzerland.

Pitts, N., Losb, P., Biesakb, P., *et al.* (2007) Ac-Impedance Spectroscopy technique for monitoring dental caries in human teeth. *Caries Research*, **41**, 321–322.

Pitts, N.B. (2010) How electrical caries detection and monitoring with cariescan can help deliver modern caries management. *Oral Health*, **100**, 34.

Plooij, J., Swennen, G., Rangel, F., *et al.* (2009) Evaluation of reproducibility and reliability of 3D soft tissue analysis using 3D stereophotogrammetry. *International Journal of Oral & Maxillofacial Surgery*, **38**, 267–273.

Pretty, I.A. (2006) Caries detection and diagnosis: novel technologies. *Journal of Dentistry*, **34**, 727–739.

Pretty, I.A. & Maupome, G. (2004) A closer look at diagnosis in clinical dental practice: part 5. Emerging technologies for caries detection and diagnosis. *Journal of Canadian Dental Association*, **70**(9), 540a–540i.

Price, J.B. (2013) A Review of Dental Caries Detection Technologies. Available: http://www.ineedce.com/coursereview.aspx?url=2424%2FPDF%2F1306cei_price_web.pdf&scid=15056 [Accessed July 9, 2013].

Reeves, T., Mah, P., & Mcdavid, W. (2012) Deriving Hounsfield units using grey levels in cone beam CT: a clinical application. *Dentomaxillofacial Radiology*, **41**, 500–508.

Rogers, E.M. (2003) Diffusion of Innovations. Free Press, New York, NY.

Rothman, S.L.G. (1998) Dental Applications of Computerized Tomography. Quintessence Publishing Co.Inc, Chicago.

Russ, J.C. (2007) The Image Processing Handbook. CRC Press Taylor & Francis Group, Boca Raton, FL.

Rustemeyer, P., Streubühr, U., & Suttmoeller, J. (2004) Low-dose dental computed tomography: significant dose reduction without loss of image quality. *Acta Radiologica*, **45**, 847–853.

Sarment, D.P. (2014) Cone Beam Computed Tomography: Oral and Maxillofacial Diagnosis and Applications. Ames, IA, John Wiley & Sons Inc.

Sarment, D.P., Sukovic, P., & Clinthorne, N. (2003) Accuracy of implant placement with a stereolithographic surgical guide. *The International Journal of Oral & Maxillofacial Implants*, **18**, 571–577.

Schueler, B., Abbara, S., Bettmann, M., Hevezi, J., Madsen, M., Morin, R., Strauss, M. & Zhu, X. (2012) ACR Appropriateness Criteria Radiation Dose Assessment Introduction [Online]. American College of Radiology. Available: http://www.acr.org/%7E/media/A27A29133302408BB86888EAFD460A1F.pdf [Accessed September 9, 2012].

Schueler, B., Cody, D., Abbara, S., *et al.* (2013) ACR Appropriateness Criteria: Radiation Dose Assessment Introduction. American College of Radiology.

Sidhu, M., Goske, M., Coley, B., *et al.* (2009) Image gently, step lightly: increasing radiation dose awareness in pediatric interventions through an international social marketing campaign. *Journal of Vascular and Interventional Radiology*, **20**, 1115–1119.

Siegel, R., Ma, J., Zou, Z., & Jemal, A. (2014) Cancer statistics, 2014. *CA: A Cancer Journal for Clinicians*, **64**, 9–29.

Sivagurunathan, K., Abrams, S., Jeon, R., *et al.* (2010) Using PTR-LUM ("The Canary System") for in vivo detection of dental caries: clinical trial results. *Caries Research*, **44**, 171–247.

Swennen, G., Mollemans, W., De Clercq, C., *et al.* (2009a) A cone-beam computed tomography triple scan procedure to obtain a three-dimensional augmented virtual skull model appropriate for orthognathic surgery planning. *Journal of Craniofacial Surgery*, **20**, 297.

Swennen, G., Mommaerts, M.Y., Abeloos, J., *et al.* (2009b) A cone-beam CT based technique to augment the 3D virtual skull model with a detailed dental surface.

International Journal of Oral & Maxillofacial Surgery, **38**, 48–57.

Tardieu, P.B. & Rosenfeld, A.L. (eds) (2009) The Art of Computer-Guided Implantology. Quintessence Publishing Co, Inc, Chicago, IL.

Tasali, N., Cubuk, R., Aricak, M., *et al.* (2012) Temporomandibular joint (TMJ) pain revisited with dynamic contrast-enhanced magnetic resonance imaging (DCE-MRI). *European Journal of Radiology*, **81**, 603–608.

Tracy, K.D., Dykstra, B.A., Gakenheimer, D.C., *et al.* (2011) Utility and effectiveness of computer-aided diagnosis of dental caries. *General Dentistry*, **59**, 136.

Tranaeus, S., Shi, X.Q., & Angmar-Månsson, B. (2005) Caries risk assessment: methods available to clinicians for caries detection. *Community Dentistry and Oral Epidemiology*, **33**, 265–273.

Tymofiyeva, O., Boldt, J., Rottner, K., Schmid, F., Richter, E.J., & Jakob, P.M. (2009) High-resolution 3D magnetic resonance imaging and quantification of carious lesions and dental pulp in vivo. *Magnetic Resonance Materials in Physics, Biology and Medicine*, **22**, 365–374.

Tyndall, D.A., Price, J.B., Tetradis, S., Ganz, S.D., Hildebolt, C., & Scarfe, W.C. (2012) Position statement of the American Academy of Oral and Maxillofacial Radiology on selection criteria for the use of radiology in dental implantology with emphasis on cone beam computed tomography. *Oral Surgery, Oral Medicine, Oral Pathology and Oral Radiology*, **113**, 817–826.

UNSCEAR. (2001) Hereditary effects of radiation: UNSCEAR 2001 report to the General Assembly, with scientific annex, The Committee.

Valentin, J. (2007) ICRP Publication 103: The 2007 Recommendations of the International Commission on Radiological Protection. *Annals of the ICRP*, **37**, 1–332.

Commonwealth of Virginia (2008) Commonwealth of Virginia Radiation Protection Regulatory Guide. Commonwealth of Virginia, Richmond,VA.

Weiger, M., Pruessmann, K.P., Bracher, A.K., *et al.* (2012) High-resolution ZTE imaging of human teeth. *NMR in Biomedicine*, **25**, 1144–1151.

Wenzel, A. (2006) A review of dentists' use of digital radiography and caries diagnosis with digital systems. *Dentomaxillofacial Radiology*, **35**, 307–314.

Wenzel, A., Haiter-Neto, F., & Gotfredsen, E. (2007) Influence of spatial resolution and bit depth on detection of small caries lesions with digital receptors. *Oral Surgery, Oral Medicine, Oral Pathology, Oral Radiology, and Endodontics*, **103**, 418–422.

Wenzel, A. & Møystad, A. (2010) Work flow with digital intraoral radiography: a systematic review. *Acta Odontologica Scandinavica*, **68**, 106–114.

White, S.C. & Pharoah, M.J. (2014) Oral Radiology: Principles and Interpretation. St. Louis, MO, Elsevier Mosby.

Zandoná, A.F., Santiago, E., Eckert, G., *et al.* (2012) The natural history of dental caries lesions a 4-year observational study. *Journal of Dental Research*, **91**, 841–846.

Zero, D.T. (1999) Dental caries process. *Dental Clinics of North America*, **43**, 635.

Zoller, J.E. & Neugebauer, J. (2008) Cone-beam Volumetric Imaging in Dental, Oral and Maxillofacial Medicine: Fundamentals, Diagnostics and Treatment Planning. Quintessence Publishing Co. Ltd., London, UK.

2 Digital Impressions

Gary D. Hack, Ira T. Bloom, and Sebastian B. M. Patzelt

Introduction

Television sets initially consisted of an array of vacuum tubes. They resembled a collection of various sized light bulbs that when lit up made the television turn on and operate. The chassis that contained these early television sets were enormous by today's standards, in order to accommodate the large internal electronic devices. Likewise, the first computers of the 1940s and 1950s were also very large, unstable, only allowed a single user to perform a single job, contained 19,000 vacuum tubes, and had the computational power of today's pocket calculator (Berkeley, 1949). Necessity being the "mother of invention," transistors came into being in the late 1940s and early 1950s. In 1958, the microchip was developed. This allowed the ability to place circuits and miniaturized transistors onto a small piece of silicon. The microchip was born, and the rest is history.

All of us whether we like it or not have been thrust into a digital age. We have moved from the rotary telephone to the cell phone, from television sets that were 18 inches deep to TVs that are now less than an inch thick. Moreover, GPS systems have replaced paper maps, and communicating by the written hand has morphed into email. Computer power has exploded to the extent that the computing capability of our current cell phones is greater than that of all of the computing power used on the first space flights to the moon by NASA (Kaku, 2011). Today's students have been raised in this digital world.

Digital technology has profoundly impacted the dental profession. Significant progress has already been made in computerized digital technologies, such as digital cast scanners, intraoral digital impression-capture devices, cone beam computed tomography, three-dimensional (3D) printers, laser sintering units, and milling machines (Beuer *et al.*, 2008). It can be expected that in the not-too-distant future, the art of making conventional impressions will become nonessential. Just as students today have grown up knowing the Internet, the new generation of dentists entering dental schools will learn to practice dentistry using intraoral scanners to make their dental impressions instead of using custom trays and conventional impression materials.

Consider the fact that dental X-ray film has been replaced by digital radiography and cone beam technology. Photographic film, for patient documentation, has evolved into the digital memory

Clinical Applications of Digital Dental Technology, First Edition. Edited by Radi Masri and Carl F. Driscoll.
© 2015 John Wiley & Sons, Inc. Published 2015 by John Wiley & Sons, Inc.

card. The manually written appointment book has been transformed into practice management software, and dental advertising has changed from paper to Web-based. Digital impressions or optical scans are moving in the direction of overtaking the use of conventional dental impressions. While approximately 16% of general dentists in the United States have adopted this technology, it is predicted that in the near future, the majority of impressions sent by dentists to dental laboratories will be digital (Christensen and Child, 2011) and probably in the next 5–10 years, it will approach 100%. Whether realized or not, dentists are now receiving digital dentistry from their dental laboratories. Major transitions are now taking place in dental laboratories as a result of these new digital technologies. Laboratories are scanning dies, stone casts, and conventional impressions and designing restorations digitally on computers. Dental laboratories are eliminating wax and wax spatulas. It is estimated that approximately 50% of US dental laboratories are now utilizing these digital technologies. The technology is such that now almost anything that you might expect a dental laboratory to produce can be done digitally and therefore more consistently, quicker, and at a reduced cost (Touchstone et al., 2010; Van Noort, 2012). It is not only interesting to know where dentistry is going, but it is important to understand from where it has come from. Digital imaging for making dental impressions is not new.

This chapter will focus primarily on data acquisition with some reference to processing and manufacturing.

Historical overview

In the early 1970s, Dr. Francois Duret, conceptualized how digital technology being used in industry might be adapted to dentistry for digital impression making. He conceived of the idea of an application of laser imaging to make optical impressions of teeth and milling out a restoration, representing the original process for capturing data used in what ultimately became the computer-assisted design/computer-assisted manufacturing (CAD/CAM) of dental restorations, with digital data being transferred to a production-milling unit to fabricate various dental restorations. Interestingly, however, his enthusiasm was not shared by others at the time who dismissed his ideas as nonsense.

Dr. Duret's concept was further developed in 1980 when Professor Werner Mörmann of Zurich, Switzerland, in collaboration with Dr. Marco Brandestini began experiments in the machining of dental restorations. By December of 1980, Professor Mörmann obtained the first patient for dental scanning. Two years later, in 1982, the first handheld intraoral 3D scanner was developed. By 1983, the first optical impression of an inlay was successfully made at the bench, and in 1985 the first functional 3D camera for intraoral imaging was commercially introduced – the CEREC 1 (Sirona, Bensheim, Germany). This acquisition unit was called the RedCam (infrared light emitting diodes as the light source; Mörmann et al., 1987), which was replaced in 2009 with the BlueCam (blue light emitting diodes). Today, the Omnicam, a powder-free, real-time, full color, high-definition video scanning system, is the latest advancement in the CEREC family.

Dental CAD/CAM's evolution over the past 30 years has centered on the chairside market, beginning with CEREC® (Sirona). This is in part because the appeal of the CAD/CAM concept is that it offers dental professionals and their patients the convenience of same-day dentistry.

While the concept of scanning teeth has not yet exceeded conventional impression making, it is anticipated that digital scanning of teeth will continue to grow until it does eventually become the predominant method (Miyazaki et al., 2009). The development of CAD/CAM is based around three elements: data acquisition, data processing and design, and manufacturing. One can now not only acquire digital impressions, but design and mill fixed dental restorations for teeth and implants chairside utilizing in-office milling units. A further development in CAD/CAM technology is the transition from closed file format to open access file systems, which opens up access to a much wider range of manufacturing technology such that the most appropriate manufacturing processes and associated materials can be selected (van Noort, 2012).

Conventional impression versus digital impression making

The significant question is, why utilize digital impressions in the first place? The answer to this question is the same as the answer to the question of why use cell phones, computers, digital photography, or GPS. These technologies make our lives easier, better, and more efficient. Likewise, digital impressions, help to make dentistry easier, better, and more efficient and lead to an increase in patients' satisfaction (Seelbach *et al.*, 2013; Lee and Gallucci, 2013; Yuzbasioglu *et al.*, 2014).

When looking into a conventional impression, one sees a negative image of the tooth preparations. It is difficult, if not sometimes impossible, to critically evaluate the quality of a preparation simply by looking at the negative of the preparation. When using conventional impression materials, one can only accurately evaluate the quality of the impression itself. Are the margins adequately captured? Are there voids or tears and pulls in the impression material? If a triple tray was used for instance, did it flex or distort, or if using a full arch tray, did the tray adhesive perform adequately or did the impression material pull slightly away from the tray? It is difficult for the clinician to evaluate the preparation until the impression is poured in stone and a positive cast of the preparation is produced.

Digital impression making has improved this process and the ability to evaluate the preparation in real-rime. Having the capability of acquiring a scan of a prepared tooth and visualizing it on a computer monitor eliminates the issues associated with conventional impressions. The dentist is now able to see a magnified high-resolution image of exactly what is present in the oral cavity and not just a negative representation. This improved visualization enables the dentist to see and evaluate, in exquisite detail, the quality of the preparations, while the patient is still in the chair. Factors such as preparation taper, quality of margins, undercuts, inter-occlusal clearance, and path of draw can be color-coded displayed and directly corrected if necessary, and a new digital impression can be made within seconds. In essence, the dentist is receiving immediate feedback on their work avoiding additional appointments,

new impressions and the patient is spared the inconvenience of additional anesthesia, cord packing, and re-provisionalization. Moreover, it is interesting to note that of the approximately 40 million conventional impressions taken each year, more than 50% of these do not capture the entire preparation margin, thus impacting the quality of the final restoration (Christensen, 2005).

All of the currently available conventional impression materials exhibit some degree of dimensional change that builds distortion and inaccuracy into the final restoration. Digital impressions can reduce the possibility of dimensional change (shrinkage) that is evident with all conventional impression materials. Voids, tears, and pulls that are routinely experienced with conventional materials are no longer an issue with digital scans. Research has demonstrated that the accuracy of digital impressions is clinically comparable with conventional impressions (Leu *et al.*, 2008; Holmes *et al.*, 1989; Ender and Mehl, 2011, 2013, 2015; Patzelt *et al.*, 2014a).

In addition to the sole scans, in some cases, it might be required to obtain a physical dental cast. For this, some companies provide stereolithographic (3D printed) or milled casts based on the data from the digital impression. Casts from digital impressions are not poured in a stone die material as are those fabricated from conventional impressions (Hack *et al.*, 2011) eliminating the risk of additional inaccuracies due to the expansion of the stone and the possible movement or shifting of the individual dies when sectioned from the cast. In contrast, casts fabricated from digital impressions are produced using a polyurethane material, printed in layers in order to build the dental cast or by milling a solid block of material. The produced CAD/CAM-based casts show a clinically acceptable accuracy (~50 μm) comparable to stone casts (Nizam, 2006; Hack *et al.*, 2011; Ender and Mehl, 2011; Patzelt *et al.*, 2014a; Leu *et al.*, 2008; Holmes *et al.*, 1989). This falls well within the range of clinically acceptable marginal discrepancies for cast and ceramic restorations (McClean and von Fraunhofer, 1971).

The automated fabrication of physical casts, die trimming, and virtual articulation of the dental casts all add to the inherent accuracy and predictability of CAD/CAM systems.

Economics of computer-aided impression making

Digital impressions also improve the efficiency and profitability of the dental practice and may be up to 20 minutes faster than conventional impression making (Patzelt *et al.*, 2014b). Remakes of digital impressions take only seconds, and they are inexpensive compared to the time needed and the cost of materials required in remaking a conventional impression. Moreover, conventional impressions need to be disinfected prior to sending them to the dental laboratory. There is obviously no need to disinfect a digital impression; however, the wand needs a proper disinfection or sterilization. Digital impressions are less costly and easier to store, as they do not take up any physical space. Finally, there is little or no gagging with digital impressions, as there is no runny impression material that is placed in the patient's mouth. The ability to fabricate crowns, bridges, inlays, onlays, and veneers and deliver them in one appointment, makes digital impressions a great marketing tool for the dental practice.

Although, these facts suggest a superiority of digital impression making, there is still room for improvement. It is still necessary to pack cord for capturing subgingival preparation margins as there is currently no digital impression system that is capable of capturing an image through tissue, saliva, and blood. Moreover, the purchase costs appear relatively high but will be paid off when applying a proper workflow. Further and similar to conventional impressions, a critical evaluation of the individual clinical situation before the actual impression making is essential and one has to consider that not all clinical scenarios are suitable for digital impressions at this time (completely edentulous jaws).

Digital acquisition units

Two major categories of digital acquisition systems can be distinguished. One category allows for the acquisition of digital data only – a sole impression system. The second category of digital acquisition systems allows the dentists to not only acquire digital impressions, but also affords the ability to digitally design restorations, and subsequently mill the restorations chairside in the dental office – CAD/CAM impression systems.

Sole impression systems

These systems do not have the ability to design or mill the restorations chairside. The acquired digital information must be sent to a qualified dental laboratory via the Internet for processing and fabrication of the restoration. The patient's prepared tooth will therefore need to be provisionalized, and the patient will need to return in order to receive the final restoration. Acquisition units in this category are for example the iTero system (Align Technology Inc., San Jose, California), the True Definition Scanner (3M, St. Paul, Minnesota), or the TRIOS scanner (3shape, Copenhagen, Denmark).

CAD/CAM *impression systems*

These systems allow for "one day or one appointment" dentistry. The patient receives the final restoration in one appointment. This category currently consists of the PlanScan (Planmeca Oy, Helsinki, Finland), the CEREC 3D BlueCam and OmniCam (Sirona, Bensheim, Germany), as well as the Carestream CS 3500 (Carestream Dental, Atlanta, Georgia) (Figure 2.1a–e; Table 2.1).

The pros and cons should be investigated and evaluated by the individual dental practitioner in order to choose a system that best fits their specific needs and style of practice. A summary of some commercially available systems and their specifications are described in the following sections:

iTero

The iTero digital impression scanner utilizes parallel confocal imaging technology to capture a color 3D digital impression of the tooth surfaces, contours, and surrounding gingival tissues. The system captures up to 3.5 million

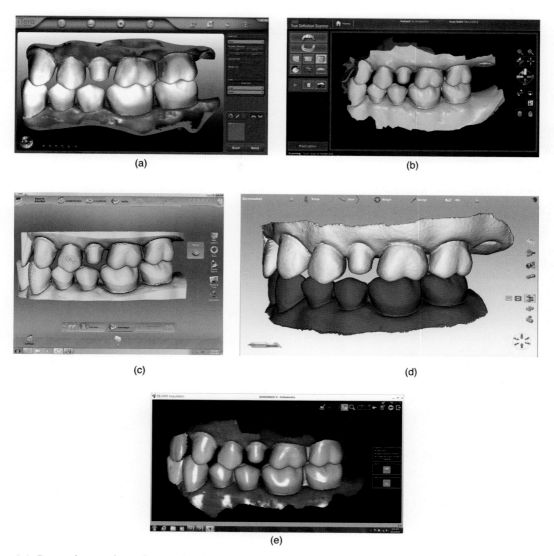

Figure 2.1 Captured screenshots of a partial arch digital impression done with the iTero (a), the 3M True Definition Scanner (b) the CEREC AC with Bluecam (c), the PlanScan (d), and the CareStream CS 3500 (e).

data points per each arch scan. The scanner has the ability to capture preparations for crowns, bridges, inlays, and onlays.

During scanning, a series of visual and verbal prompts are given that are customized for the patient being treated and guide the clinician through the scanning process. For each preparation, a facial, lingual, mesio-proximal, and disto-proximal view is recorded in approximately

15–20 seconds, after which the adjacent teeth are scanned from the facial and lingual aspects.

The iTero system is only used for digital impression making and does not come with a dedicated milling machine, although its open platform can integrate with design software and third-party milling units. If required, it is possible to obtain milled iTero CAD/CAM resin (polyurethane) casts.

Table 2.1   Comparison chart of some of the digital impression systems (company reports, time sensitive estimates).

		3M true definition	Cerec bluecam	Cerec omnicam	Align itero	Plan scan	3Shape trios
Technology		**Continuous video data Capture**	**Visible Blue Light**	**Continuous 3D Color Capture**	**Red laser with parallel confocal imaging**	**Blue Laser**	**Confocal Microscopy**
Indications	**Single unit crowns**	Yes	Yes	Yes	Yes	Yes	Yes
	Long-span restorations	Laboratory fabricated	Milled Emax 3 to 4 units	Milled Emax 3 to 4 units	Laboratory fabricated	Milled Emax 3 to 4 units	Laboratory fabricated
Usability	**Weight**	~200 g	~280 g	~313 g	~1.5 kg	~337 g	~1 kg
	Wand Tip (~)	14.4 mm × 16.2 mm	22 mm × 17 mm	16 mm × 16 mm	25 mm × 25 mm	30 mm × 23 mm with standoff	–
	Powder	Light	Yes	No	No	No	No
	User interface	Touch screen	Menus, ball, foot	Menus, ball, foot	Menus, mouse, foot	Icons, mouse, foot	–
	Novel features	–	–	Color streaming	Speech synthesizer	Impression scanning	Shade measurement
Connections	**Open file format**	Yes	No	No	Yes	Yes	Yes
	Chairside CAD/CAM	Yes	Yes	Yes	Yes	Yes	Yes
	Laboratory network	Yes	Yes	Yes	Yes	Yes	Yes
	Cloud storage	Yes	No	No	Yes	No	No
	Open cast	Yes	Yes	Yes	Yes	Yes	Yes
	Cast production	SLA	Milled/SLA	Milled/SLA	Milled	Quad cast only	No cast solution
	Implant impression	Yes	Yes	Yes	Yes	No	Yes
	CBCT integration	No	Galileos only	Galileos only	Yes	Yes	No

3M true definition scanner

The 3M True Definition Scanner (Figure 2.2) is a digital scanning system only; however, similar to the iTero scanner, it is an open platform system offering the ability to connect to a certified design software and chairside milling machine. Unlike the confocal imaging of the iTero system, the 3M system uses a blue LED light and an active wavefront sampling video imaging system to capture the data and create a virtual cast. By moving the camera over the tooth surfaces, the video feed develops a virtual cast. The clinical technique used with the 3M system requires proper isolation of the desired area to be captured as well as a light dusting of the teeth with a specific titanium

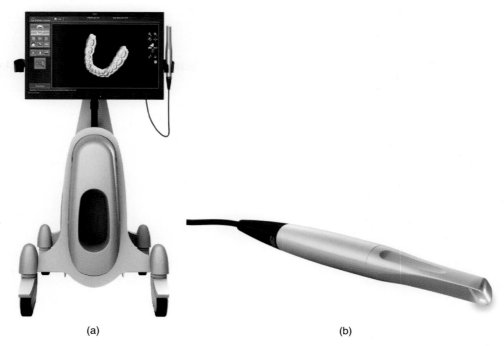

(a)   (b)

Figure 2.2 3M True Definition intraoral scanning system (a) and its wand (b). (Reproduced with permission of 3M.)

oxide powder. This digital impression technique has been shown to be very accurate (Guth *et al.*, 2012; Patzelt *et al.*, 2014a; Patzelt *et al.*, 2014b). After scanning of the teeth and the creation of the virtual cast, the acquired data ($\approx$ 70–80 MB) is sent to 3M for processing and available for download in minutes. If required, a physical dental cast using stereolithography can be obtained from the manufacturer (typically after 48–72 hours).

CEREC systems

This CAD/CAM technology has the longest track record of any of the currently available systems. The CEREC system has been in existence in one form or another for close to three decades (Mörmann *et al.*, 1987). The CEREC AC digital impression system with BlueCam, brought to the market in 2009, has a number of improved technologies, over the older RedCam system, including an image-capturing system that automatically determines the focus of the subject and instantly saves the image, eliminating the need for the clinician to click a button or pedal to acquire the image, as was the case with the RedCam. Included in the auto-capture with the BlueCam is an anti-shake function with a broad depth of field. The BlueCam requires a proper antireflective powdering to opaque the teeth (da Costa *et al.*, 2010). Sirona's latest digital impression system is the CEREC AC with Omni-Cam unit (Figure 2.3), released in the summer of 2012. In contrast to the BlueCam, where imaging is done via the stitching of individual images together creating a monochromatic yellow stone-like digital cast, the OmniCam captures without powdering via digital streaming a full color digital cast. Similar to the BlueCam, one can also design and mill the final restoration using the Sirona chairside milling units. In addition, the data can be sent via the CEREC Connect Internet Protal to a laboratory for fabrication of a cast or prosthesis ($\approx$ file size 16–25 MB).

In the laboratory, casts for the CEREC systems, can be fabricated using steriolithography. Once the restoration is designed, it can be milled in a variety

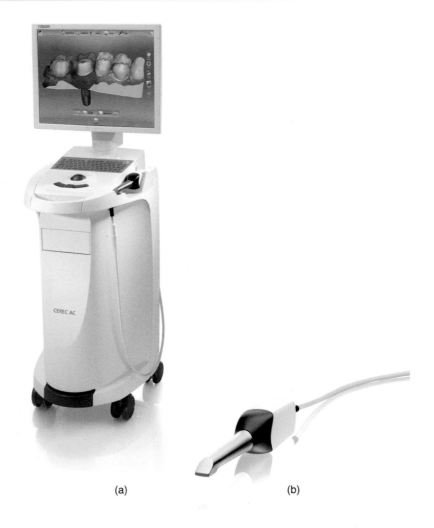

(a)   (b)

Figure 2.3 CEREC OmniCam intraoral scanning system (a) and its wand (b). (Reproduced with permission of Sirona Dental GmbH.)

of materials, including resin-based provisional materials, lithium disilicate, feldspathic porcelain, and leucite-reinforced porcelain. Zirconia-based single-unit and multiunit fixed partial dentures can also be fabricated if the office is equipped with the appropriate ovens to sinter the zirconia. The CEREC software is robust enough to design and mill single-unit inlays, onlays, veneers, crowns, and fixed partial dentures, both provisional and permanent and also implant abutments.

PlanScan

The Planmeca PlanScan (driven by E4D Technologies) system is designed to be used in a similar manner to Sirona's CEREC systems, as it can be used as a digital impression system as well as chairside design and milling system (Figure 2.4). The PlanScan system uses blue laser light with real-time video-streaming technology to capture the dental data, and it is powder-free. It accurately captures both hard and soft tissues of various

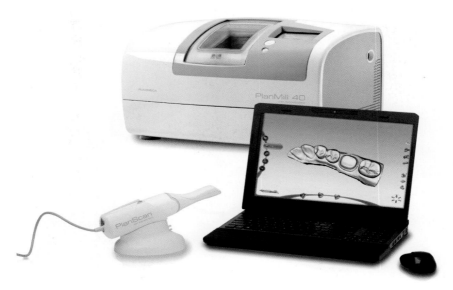

Figure 2.4 PlanScan intraoral scanning system with PlanMill milling machine and laptop. (Reproduced with permission of Planmeca – USA.)

translucencies, dental restorations, models, and conventional impressions. Removable scanner tips with built-in heated mirrors allow for no down time between patients, as well as high-level disinfection. The scanner tips can now be auto-claved as well as being available in different sizes. The Planmeca PlanCAD Design Center includes scanning software, design software, a mouse, and a laptop. The digital casts can be used to design inlays, onlays, crowns, bridges, and veneers. If needed, the scans can be sent to the laboratory for processing, designing, and manufacturing of the restorations or the restorations can be milled chairside using the PlanMill 40 milling machine.

CS3500 intraoral digital impression scanner

The CS 3500 intraoral scanner (Figure 2.5) is one of the latest available powder-free intraoral scanners that enables dental professionals to scan patients' teeth to create color 3D images. Similar to the CEREC BlueCam, it is a click-and-point system. Thus, it requires the user to keep the wand still during capturing. Additionally, adequate overlapping of the single images (≥50% of the previous image) is essential. The scanner can

be used to design a single crown, bridge, inlay, onlay, and veneer through the CS Restore software and milled with the optional carestream milling machine (CS 3000) or the data can be sent to a laboratory for design and milling. Moreover, the colored 3D image are supposed to help drawing margin lines easily and identifying the differences between natural tooth structure and existing restorations. A light guidance system allows the user to focus on the acquisition of the image in the patient's mouth, and not on the monitor.

Digital impression technique

Although the practitioner should follow the specific protocol suggested by the manufacturer of the various imaging systems, the basic principles for acquiring an accurate digital impression are the same as they are for conventional impressions. Thus, if one cannot visualize the structure to be captured one cannot capture the actual structure. With systems that require powder, dryness is more critical than with systems that do not require powder. However, hemostasis is essential with all systems, as neither the digital camera nor conventional material can tolerate bleeding.

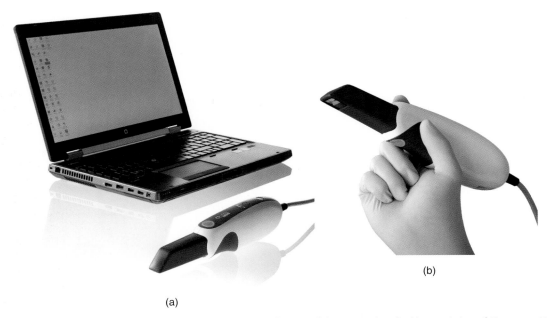

(a)

(b)

Figure 2.5 Carestream CS 3500 intraoral scanning system (a) and its wand (b). (Reproduced with permission of Carestream.)

Interestingly, it has been reported that there is work in progress in developing methods (e.g., optical coherence tomography) that allow intraoral data acquisition without the necessity of tissue displacement, as the technique apparently can distinguish between tooth structure and soft tissue (Kachalia and Geissberger, 2010; Fasbinder and Poticny, 2010).

Visualization of the margins is as critical with all imaging systems as it is with conventional impressions. Retraction cord or a soft tissue diode laser may be utilized for hemostasis and for retracting gingival tissues. As conventional impressions require the use of an impression tray, a rubber dam for retracting surrounding soft tissues (cheeks, tongue, etc.) and developing a dry field is not possible. Cotton rolls, dry angles, a saliva evacuation system, and an excellent dental assistant are essential. With digital impressions, however, a rubber dam or other device such as the Optradam or Optragate (Ivoclar Vivadent, Liechtenstein), and the Isolite (Isolite Systems, Santa Barbara, California) can facilitate the procedure.

As with conventional impression techniques, when using digital imaging, we do not capture an image (impression) of just a single tooth. We are typically capturing a minimum of one tooth on either side of the prepared tooth, a full quadrant or in some cases even a whole arch. All of the available systems allow an opposing arch scan and a buccal bite scan to be able to articulate the obtained data as close as possible to the actual patient's intraoral jaw relation. Some of the available systems even offer the ability to simulate movements of the digital scans in a virtual articulator.

Applications and limitations of computer-aided impression making

Digital impression technology can be applied to most areas in dentistry where we now use conventional impression material. Our primary focus for its use is with fixed restorations, such as crowns, inlays, onlays, veneers, and fixed partial dentures. The dentist can utilize digital impressions to fabricate and mill restorations in one appointment chairside. If multiple appointments are necessary to complete treatment, the dentist may also use digital impressions to design and mill provisional restorations in minutes. In addition, the dentist can send digital impressions via the Internet to his laboratory for design and fabrication of physical casts and/or prostheses.

Current digital imaging systems are so efficient that we have the ability to successfully and accurately image into the dental pulp chamber. This enables us to apply digital imaging to an interesting technique for restoring endodontically treated teeth. The method is referred to as the "Endo Crown" whereby a ceramic crown and core are milled as one unit (Biacchi *et al.*, 2013; Lander and Dietschi, 2008)

Contraindications to making digital impressions are few. The major contraindication is the inability to access the area with the digital camera. Either the camera head is too large or the patient does not have the ability to open wide enough to accommodate the camera head. Sizes and weight of camera heads vary with different systems, but the trend in development is toward a smaller camera size. Another contraindication for digital impressions is lack of patient cooperation. Stillness on the part of the patient is needed to capture adequate images.

Future innovations

Dentistry and dental imaging have come a long way. More and more companies are developing dental imaging systems, and more will be developing them as the digital platforms become more open. The cameras are steadily improving, and the technologies of imaging are changing from single image point-and-click to real-time video streaming. With the elimination of the need for powdering during imaging, the systems are also becoming increasingly user-friendly. 3M, the world's largest manufacturer of conventional impression material, has invested millions of dollars into digital imaging to eventually replace conventional impression making. As the dental profession is typically 10–20 years behind industry in the acceptance of new technological innovation (Rogers, 2003), this transition will take some time. The trend, however, is happening now. It is predicted and statistics show that by the year 2015 a majority of dental impressions

sent to dental laboratories will be digital. This does not include dentists that are using digital impressions for in-office design and milling. The latest statistics from Sirona indicate that every 7 seconds somewhere in the world, a CEREC restoration is being placed.

Future innovations in the area of digital impressions can only be limited by the imagination. Research is now being done with the use of SONAR technology in capturing images. Radiation-free Optical Coherence Tomography (OCT) has been used in optometry for a while, but now, applications in dentistry are evolving (Hsieh *et al.*, 2013). OCT produces real time images as deep as 3 mm into the tissue structure. This would make imaging systems even more user-friendly by eliminating the interference of blood and soft tissue in making impressions. Will camera imaging even remain necessary in the future? Cone beam technology has already been linked with digital imaging for the treatment planning of implant placement and the design and milling of implant abutments and restorations. Perhaps in the future, we will be able to design and mill restorations directly from 3D cone beam imaging.

In the past 30 years since CEREC was introduced as a fringe technology, more and more systems tried to make it to the dental market each year. Other technologies are either just being released or are on the verge of joining the ever growing CAD/CAM market. CAD/CAM dentistry, whether it is something you choose to incorporate as just an imaging system, or as an imaging and milling system, is now a mainstream dental procedure (Mörmann, 2006).

Summary

For today's dental students, digital is all that they know. Previous generations sometimes find it difficult, if not impossible, to adapt to new technology, but to the younger generation it is second nature and in fact demanded. Digital technology has affected and is affecting the profession of dentistry in the same way. Whether we as individuals like it or not, digital impression making is here to stay. Patients like digital dentistry, as it minimizes the discomfort associated with traditional impressions. Moreover, it minimizes chair and office time, making the office significantly more efficient, reduces remakes, reduces seating time of restorations, and lowers or eliminates laboratory bills. Moving to digital dentistry leads to improvements in the quality of oral care, offers a better patient experience, and improves the productivity and economics of the dental practice (Davidowitz and Kotick, 2011).

Studies have shown that digital impressions are at least as accurate as conventional impressions. Retakes are quick, easy, and inexpensive. Digital impressions are easier to store, because they do not take up space. There is no need for disinfectants. Pulls, bubbles, tears, and shrinkage are mostly eliminated.

Predicting the future is difficult, but trends and developments can guide one to the correct answer. Technology is advancing exponentially, and there are many exciting new technologies on the horizon. The reducing cost of processing power will ensure that these developments will continue as exemplified by the recent introduction of a new range of digital intraoral scanners.

References

Berkeley, E.C. (1949) Giant Brains or Machines that Think. John Wiley & Sons, Inc., New York.

Beuer, F., Schweiger, J., & Edelhoff, D. (2008) Digital dentistry: an overview of recent developments for CAD/CAM generated restorations. *British Dental Journal*, **204**(9), 505–511.

Biacchi, G.R., Mello, B., & Basting, R.T. (2013) The endocrown: an alternative approach for restoring extensively damaged molars. *Journal of Esthetic and Restorative Dentistry*, **25**(6), 383–390.

Christensen, G.J., (2005) The state of fixed prosthodontics impressions: room for improvement. *Journal of the American Dental Association*. **136**, 343–346.

Christensen, G.J. & Child, P.L. Jr. (2011) Fixed prosthodontics: time to change the status quo. *Dent Today*. **30**(9) 66, 68, 70–73.

da Costa, J.B., Pelogia, F., Hagedorn, B., & Ferracane, J.L. (2010) Evolution of different methods of optical impression making on the marginal gap of onlays with CEREC 3D. *Operative Dentistry*, **35**(3), 324–329.

Davidowitz, G. & Kotick, P.G. (2011) The use of CAD/CAM in Dentistry. *Dental Clinics of North America*, **55**(3), 559–570.

Ender, A. & Mehl, A. (2011) Full arch scans: conventional versus digital impressions – an in-vitro study. *International Journal of Computerized Dentistry*, **14**(1), 11–21.

Ender, A. & Mehl, A. (2013) Accuracy of complete-arch dental impressions: A new method of measuring trueness and precision. *The Journal of Prosthetic Dentistry*, **109**(2), 121–128.

Ender, A. & Mehl, A. (2015) In-vitro evaluation of the accuracy of conventional and digital methods of obtaining full-arch dental impressions. *Quintessence International*, **46**(1), 9–17. DOI: 10.3290/j.qi.a32244.

Fasbinder, D.J. & Poticny, D.J. (2010) Accuracy of occlusal contacts for crowns with chairside CAD/CAM techniques. *International Journal of Computerized Dentistry*, **13**(4), 303–316.

Guth, J.F., Keul, C., Stimmelmayr, M., Beuer, F., & Edelhoff, D. (2012) Accuracy of digital casts obtained by direct and indirect data capturing. *Clinical Oral Investigations*, **17**(4), 1201–1208.

Hack, G.D., Barns, D., & Depaola, L. (2011) In vitro evaluation of the ITero digital impression system. *ADA Professional Product Review*, **6**(2), 6–10.

Holmes, J.R., Bayne, S.C., Holland, G.A., & Sulik, W.D. (1989) Considerations in measurement of marginal fit. *Journal of Prosthetic Dentistry*, **62**(4), 405–408.

Hsieh, Y.S., Ho, Y.C., Lee, S.Y., *et al.* (2013) Dental optical coherence tomography. *Sensors (Basel, Switzerland)*, **13**(7), 8928–8949.

Kachalia, P.R. & Geissberger, M.J. (2010) Dentistry a la carte: in-office CAD/CAM technology. *Journal of the California Dental Association*, **38**(5), 323–330.

Kaku, M. (2011) Physics of the Future: How Science will Shape Human Destiny and our Daily Lives by the Year 2100 1st edn. Doubleday, New York.

Lander, E. & Dietschi, D. (2008) Endocrowns: a clinical report. *Quintessence International*, **39**(2), 99–106.

Lee, S.J. & Gallucci, G.O. (2013) Digital vs. conventional implant impressions: efficiency outcomes. *Clinical Oral Implants Research*, **24**(1), 111–115.

Leu, M.C., Parthiban, D., & Walker, M.P. (2008) Digital design and fabrication in dentistry. In: Bio-Materials and Prototyping Applications in Medicine (eds P. Bártolo & B. Bidanda), pp. 124–155. Springer, USA.

McClean, J.W. & von Fraunhofer, J.A. (1971) The estimation of cement film thickness by an in vivo technique. *British Dental Journal*, **131**(3), 107–111.

Mörmann, W.H. (2006) The evolution of the CERECC system. *Journal of the American Dental Association*, **137**, 7S–13S.

Mörmann, W.H., Brandestini, M., & Lutz, F. (1987) The Cerec system: computer-assisted preparation of direct inlays in one setting. *Quintessence International*, **38**(3), 457–470.

Miyazaki, T., Hotta, Y., Kunii, J., Kuriyama, S., & Tamaki, Y. (2009) A review of dental CAD/CAM: Current status and future perspectives from 20 years of experience. *Dental Materials Journal*, **28**(1), 44–56.

Nizam, A., Gopal, R.N., & Naing, L., *et al.* (2006) Dimensional accuracy of the shull casts produced by rapid prototyping technology using steriolithography apparatus. *Archives of Orofacial Sciences*, **1**, 60–66.

Patzelt, S.B., Emmanouilidi, A., Stampf, S., Strub, J.R., & Att, W. (2014a) Accuracy of full-arch scans using intraoral scanners. *The journal Clinical Oral Investigations*, **18**(6), 1687–1694.

Patzelt, S.B., Lamprinos, C., Stampf, S., & Att, W. (2014b) The time efficiency of intraoral scanners: An in vitro comparative study. *The Journal of the American Dental Association*, **145**(6), 542–551.

Rogers, E.M. (2003) Diffusion of Innovations 5th edn. Simon & Shuster Inc., New York.

Seelbach, P., Brueckel, C., & Wöstmann, B. (2013) Accuracy of digital and conventional impression techniques and workflow. *The journal Clinical Oral Investigations*, **17**(7), 1759–1764.

Touchstone, A., Nieting, T., & Ulmer, N. (2010) Digital transition: the collaboration between dentists and laboratory technicians on CAD/CAM restorations. *The Journal of the American Dental Association*, **141**(2), 15S–19S.

Van Noort, R. (2012) The future of dental devices is digital. *Dental Materials*, **28**(1), 3–12.

Yuzbasioglu, E., Kurt, H., Turunc, R., & Bilir, H. (2014) Comparison of digital and conventional impression techniques: evaluation of patients' perception, treatment comfort, effectiveness, and clinical outcomes. *BMC Oral Health*, **14**, 10.

3

Direct Digital Manufacturing

Gerald T. Grant

Introduction

Advances in medical imaging, light and laser scanning technologies, development of dental and medical design software, as well as adaptation of computer manufacturing techniques have all contributed to the digital revolution. Over the past two decades, medical images have merged with digital fabrication processes to become an essential process in the fabrication of medical models and have been used extensively in creating cranial implants for the US military (Gronet *et al.*, 2003). Indeed, these days, medical modeling of cranial defects is routine for US military medical facilities for cranioplasty and craniofacial reconstructions (Taft *et al.*, 2011) (Figure 3.1).

Several digital impression systems are available in the market (see Chapter 2). They offer excellent scanning accuracy and user-friendly software and allow for a seamless integration of CAD/CAM techniques in the dental office and laboratory. CAD/CAM techniques have the potential to streamline the conventional dental laboratory process, by minimizing or eliminating traditional impressions and lost wax casting techniques; thus, reducing the time to deliver a dental restoration. Faced with a shortage of skilled dental laboratory technicians, alternative methods that provide dental prostheses in a timely manner are becoming more attractive. The Bureau of Labor Statistics (United States Department of Labor, 2013) reports that they expect little or no change in the job outlook of dental laboratory technicians for the next 10 years citing a less than 1% growth with a median annual wage of about $35,000. As CAD/CAM and other direct digital manufacturing (DDM) techniques become more advanced, the traditional skills of the dental laboratory technician will necessarily be redefined to include more digital knowledge. As CAD/CAM skills replace traditional craftsman skill sets in dental laboratory, increased productivity should offset the shortage of laboratory technicians.

The use of DDM techniques in dentistry and medicine is based on the "Scan, Plan, and Manufacture" principle of digital workflow paradigm (Figure 3.2). Each part of this workflow paradigm is based on distinct technologies: scanning technology to capture the anatomy, software applications to digitally compose the design, and DDM technology to render the design into a durable restoration or prosthesis. The

Clinical Applications of Digital Dental Technology, First Edition. Edited by Radi Masri and Carl F. Driscoll.
© 2015 John Wiley & Sons, Inc. Published 2015 by John Wiley & Sons, Inc.

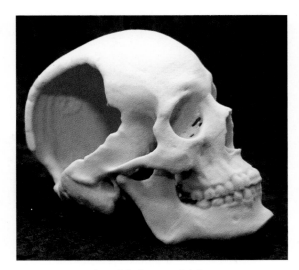

Figure 3.1 Printed model of a cranial defect.

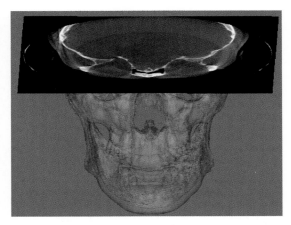

Figure 3.3 Medical images such as a CT scan are a stack of axial slices that can be stacked to build a 3D image.

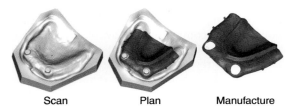

Scan   Plan   Manufacture

Figure 3.2 Diagram to describe how a cast is planned, a metal denture base is designed, and the metal denture base is manufactured using a direct digital workflow.

development of all of these technologies continues to improve, characterized by the number of new hardware and "advancements" or upgrades of each step of the process.

Scanning devices

Intraoral scanning devices discussed in Chapter 2 preclude the need for impressions and casts, which streamlines the dental restoration to a purely digital process. However, many of the digital scanning technologies still depend on traditional impression and casts to generate a digital copy of the oral anatomy. Whether intraoral scanning is used or a scan of the impression or cast is used, the captured digital files of the oral anatomy possess sufficient

detail resolution to fabricate a well fitting restoration by a variety of DDM approaches. Scanning technologies are based on a variety of optical or laser surface capture approaches, which present no exposure risk to the patient, unlike conventional medical imaging techniques that currently cannot match this level of detail resolution.

Conventional medical imaging from CT, MRI, and ultrasound has transitioned from stacks of film to a standardized digital format (Figure 3.3). Digital imaging and communications in medicine (DICOM) is the current standard for digital storage and retrieval of medical images, DICOM files are compatible with a variety of medical image viewers from different vendors.

Software has been developed that allows DICOM images to be converted into a three-dimensional (3D) surface model, providing access to the use of CAD manipulation for virtual surgical manipulation, design of surgical guides, custom fixation devices, medical devices, and their digital manufacturing as a device or model. Although these images generally lack the details necessary for direct restoration planning, they do offer a picture of the internal anatomy at sufficient resolution for treatment planning and development of treatment aids, such as oral surgery guides. When translated into a standard 3D digital format, anatomy from medical images and oral scanning techniques may be merged in CAD/CAM applications.

Digital manufacturing

Prostheses designed using a CAD application are fabricated by a DDM device. These devices generally fall into one of two categories, Subtracting Manufacturing Technology (SMT) or Additive Manufacturing Technology (AMT). SMT is the more common technology; based on conventional Computer Numerical Control (CNC) milling (Figure 3.4). SMT technologies are generally limited by geometric complexity and are not suitable to produce all shapes; however, AMT can fabricate the far more complex organic forms (Figure 3.5). Although SMT-based CNC milling systems have been the predominant DDM technology in dentistry, the advancement of AMT will provide the flexibility in design, fabrication, and economy

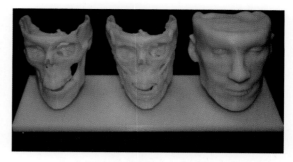

Figure 3.5 Example of the irregular organic shapes that are best fabricated using additive manufacturing techniques.

of cost to support digital manufacturing in the future.

SMT approaches generally process the model into tool paths to direct a cutting tool and spindle. AMT generally slices the 3D model into regular planes with instructions for material deposition, polymerization, or fusing in each plane. AMT is more sensitive to the integrity of these 3D model files as opposed to the SMT process.

File format in the digital workflow

To date, most dental CAD/CAM systems have been generally "closed" systems; the image file, CAD application, the CAD output file, and tool paths (instructions of movement to the cutter of a milling system) are compatible only in that system; therefore, there has been no ability to select different imaging systems, design software, and digital manufacturing as a preference. As newer technologies and a better understanding of CAD/CAM technologies by the dental profession begin to prevail, there will be a demand for flexibility between scanners, design software, and manufacturing devices, forcing more open options (interoperability) to be available.

System interoperability is dependent on the use of a common file format form the "Scan" step forward in the workflow. This has been achieved in medical imagery with the near universal adoption of the DICOM file format, developed by the National Electrical Manufacturers Association (NEMA) for storage of all medical images. MRI, CT, ultrasound, and other medical imaging systems all use this file format to describe their

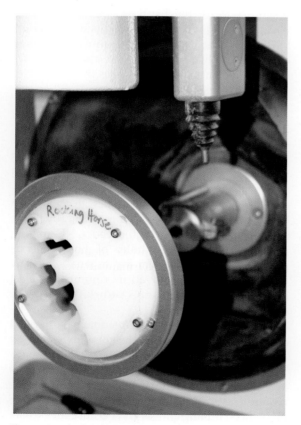

Figure 3.4 A 5-axis computer numerical control (CNC) milling machines.

images. DICOM enables the integration of scanners, servers, workstations, printers, and network hardware from multiple manufacturers into a picture archiving and communication system. The different devices come with DICOM conformance statements that clearly state which DICOM classes they support. DICOM has been widely adopted by hospitals and the Department of Defense Medical Care systems. However, the standard is not widely accepted in dentistry, demonstrated by the proprietary image formats common in some cone beam CT scanners, intraoral scanners, and dental CAD/CAM systems.

Interoperability during planning and manufacturing stages depends on the use of a common 3D file format between the imaging output, the CAD application, and the DDM device. A number of suitable digital file formats exist: .ply, .obj, .vrml, .amf to list but a few; however, the most common digital file format is the .stl (surface tessellation format) file format. The STL file format enables the approximation of the shape of a part or the entire assembly using triangular surface facets (Figure 3.6).

Generally, the smaller the facet, the higher the quality of the surface produced. When linked together into a closed surface, these triangular facets compose a 3D approximation of an object such as the patient's anatomy or a prosthesis design. This 3D surface is processed into machine code to direct the DDM fabrication, usually using

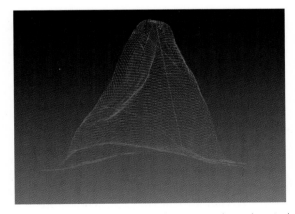

Figure 3.6 An example of the mesh structure of a tooth typical of an .stl file used in direct digital manufacturing.

vendor specific software applications provided with the DDM device.

The .stl file format is limited to surface geometry, which is a suitable definition for most currently available DDM devices. However, the future direction of AMT-based DDM will allow for esthetic and mechanical material properties to be varied in the fabrication process. New 3D file formats, such as .amf (additive manufacturing format), are under development which will allow for the 3D definition of shape, esthetic properties and mechanical properties in 3D. Future workflow will necessarily be based on a common 3D file format that supports these additional pieces of information.

Additive versus subtractive manufacturing technologies

As discussed earlier, DDM technologies can manufacture parts by two basic approaches: (i) SMT in which material is selectively removed from a bulk billet by mechanical cutting, chemical processes, electrical discharge, or directed energy and (ii) AMT in which materials are selectively fused or deposited, typically in layers.

Subtractive manufacturing technology

SMT has been the dominant method for dental fabrication since the advent of dental CAD/CAM systems. A wide range of dental restorative materials, from composites, to ceramics, to metals can be processed by these systems. Typically these systems are based on high-speed CNC milling technology, whereby a billet of homogeneous material is shaped by removal of small chips by one or more cutters moved in a number of axis, and/or rotated, with respect to the work piece (Figure 3.7).

The number of degrees of freedom of cutter and material movement limits the complex geometry and features of the manufactured part. Typically, SMT milling devices have three to five degrees of freedom; four or more degrees of freedom are required to mill overhang features. They utilize high-speed milling cutters and because they rotate much faster than conventional milling machines, the cutting forces remain small. Thus cooling is not

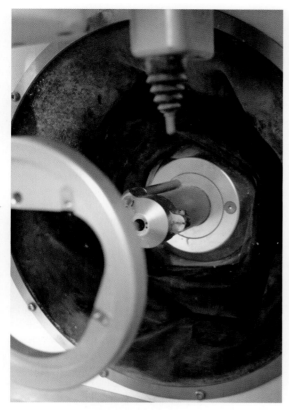

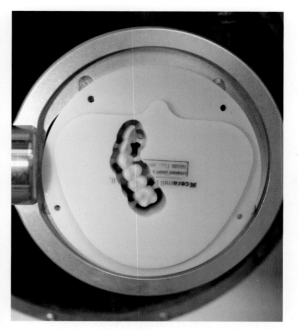

Figure 3.8 Milling requires that the design needs structures to maintain the part with the bulk of the material.

Figure 3.7 A 5-axis milling is achieved not only by moving the milling burs in the *x*, *y*, and *z* axes, but also by moving the material different axis of rotation as well.

needed since the removal of the chips buffers the heat and vibrations can be minimized (Gunnink, 1998). Minimum feature size and surface finish quality are governed by the cutter tool size and rotational speed.

A 3D geometry from a CAD file is used to create tool paths to direct the SMT device. Posts, or sprues, must be added to the manufactured shape to hold the work piece during the fabrication process. Next, a digital file is generated, which specifies the tool selection: spindle movement paths, work piece movement, and spindle speeds (Figure 3.8). Generally vendor specific software provided with the SMT device prepares this file. These software packages often limit the user to specific material billets, in specific shapes ("blocks" or "pucks"). Depending on the material employed, some post-processing manipulation

of the material is necessary, such as sintering of a green ceramic restoration, or application of esthetic treatments, such as stain and glazing, or stacking conventional porcelains to a coping.

The advantages of SMT include:

- SMT is well suited for fabrication when the surface finish and shape is important;
- Ease of use – the process of removing material is not complicated, therefore chances of failure are low;
- Capable of handling incorrect STL files– systems are not sensitive to small inconsistencies in solid geometry and can even handle single surfaces with minimal thickness;
- Choice of materials – any material can be manufactured;
- Definable accuracy – the distance between the tool paths can be chosen, generally from 0.01 mm to 10 mm or larger. However, building speed is slower the greater the resolution;
- Cost – light CNC milling machines can be less than one thousand US dollars;

The disadvantages of SMT include:

- Not suited for cross-sectional fabrication – cannot produce structures within structures or enclosed hollow structures;
- Limited Axis of rotation – there is some limitation of the accuracy and achievability of an organic shape due to the number of axis the mill allows. The basic CNC machine uses 3 controlled axes: x, y, and z. Advanced machines may be equipped with a fourth axis (rotation table), or with 5 axes where the tool can be rotated to approach the geometry from different directions;
- Cutter Wear – due to the nature of the technology, cutters can become dull and inefficient if hard materials are desired. In dental fabrication, non-sintered materials are often used to increase cutter life.

Additive manufacturing technology

AMT techniques have been commercially available for nearly 30 years at the time when the process known as Stereolithography (SLA) was patented (see below). This process formed three-dimensional geometries, of arbitrary complexity, by exposing thin layers of a photopolymer with a concentrated beam of ultraviolet light. Since then, this process of "printing" thin layers has progressed to different technologies with an array of materials. AMT has had many different names: Rapid Prototyping, Layered Manufacturing Technology (LMT), eManufacturing, freeform fabrication, and generally as 3D Printing. However, the American Society for Testing and Materials (ASTM International) adopted a standard term for this class of manufacturing process: Additive Manufacturing (AM). AM is described under the ASTM F2792-12a – Standard for terminology of Additive Manufacturing as per Table 3.1.

The majority of commercially available AM processes build a part in sequential layers, stacked vertically (z axis). Material is deposited in a plane transverse to the vertical ($x–y$ plane) and layers are sequentially deposited. Depending on the process, additional support structures are often necessary to fix the part during the layering process and support overhangs against the force of gravity.

Secondary processes, performed after the AMT device had completed layering, are often necessary to complete the fabrication process. These processes include: support structure removal, excess material removal, green part curing, or reinforcement material infusion. Tertiary surface finishing and esthetic treatment processes are also generally necessary.

Unlike the SMT, long associated with traditional manufacturing, AMT offers not only the flexibility to produce more organic shapes but also a more conservative process with greater access to the point of consumption with a greater labor cost savings) (Cozmei and Caloian, 2012); however, some devices can produce inhomogeneous materials, by digitally mixing droplets of different photopolymers (Stratasys). These parts can be composed of a mixture of two base polymers, for instance, opaque teeth within a clear mandible. The full potential for manufacturing is still in its development and is somewhat limited to specialty items such as medical models, dental prostheses, customized fittings, and difficult metal devices in conjunction with CNC processes.

Unlike SMT, there are widely different fabrications methods used in AMT; however, we can generalize the advantages and disadvantages.

The advantages of AMT devices include:

- Design Freedom – it is virtually unlimited as to what can be designed for AMT to include hollow and functioning devices/rapid prototypes;
- Produce complex geometry – a complex des ign can be produced in one fabrication cycle, unlike in SMT where different parts would need to be fabricated and assembled;
- Ease of use – the complexity of the system is in the design of the .stl file for fabrication. Items can be scaled and easily oriented on fabrication platforms, once the platform is virtually "loaded," it is pretty much a "click OK" and fabrication commences.

The disadvantages of AMT include:

- Cost – the initial cost of most of commercially available AMT devices can be well over $100,000 US. However, some of the smaller

Table 3.1   AM processes and materials.

Type	Process/technology	Material
Vat photopolymerization	SLA (stereolithography)	UV curable resins
		Waxes
		Ceramics
Material jetting	MJM (multi-jet modeling)	UV curable resins
		Waxes
Binder jetting	3DP (3D printing)	Composites
		Polymers, ceramics
		Metals
Material extrusion	FDM (fused deposition modeling)	Thermoplastics
		Waxes
Powder bed fusion	SLS (selective laser sintering)	Thermoplastics
		Metals
	SLM (selective laser melting)	Metals
	EBM (electron beam melting)	Metals
Sheet lamination	LOM (laminated objet modeling)	Paper
		Metals
		Thermoplastics
Directed energy deposition	LMD/LENS (laser metal deposition/laser engineered net shaping	Metals

producing machines can fall in the range of 15,000–60,000 US dollars.

- Finish – Generally the products produced need some post-processing and polishing, especially with the metal AMT. There is a need to provide some post-polishing by either CNC or manual methods, although the resolution of the machines and the powder sizes continue to be improved and will eventually rival the surfaces seen from milling.
- Materials – the range of materials is specific to the AMT being used. Unlike CNC that can generally be used on any material that can withstand the milling forces, the method of production has limitations in the materials can use.
- Product design – although there is a lot of design freedom, AMT is very sensitive to inconsistency in the STL file to include open triangles and a need for "watertight" designs. In addition, the software to manipulate the files can be expensive.

Materials extrusion technologies

Material extrusion is the ASTM classification of any AM process whereby a liquefied material is extruded through a nozzle and selectively deposited onto a platform layer by layer. Material extrusion devices are known by the trademark name fused deposition modeling (FDM™) printers or by the generic term fused filament fabrication (FFF) printers (Figure 3.9).

The material is most often a solid filament that is progressed through a heated nozzle, similar to a glue gun, where the material melts then solidifies after being deposited. This process is applicable to any liquid material, which will solidify rapidly

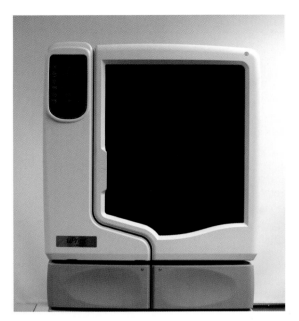

Figure 3.9 The Uprint Deposition modeling machine from Stratasys.

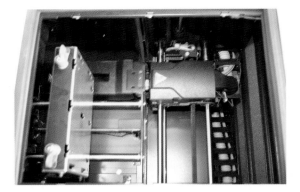

Figure 3.10 Nozzle and platform arrangement of the typical fused deposition modeling device.

after deposition from a nozzle. The typical layer thickness for thermoplastics used in material extrusion is on the order of 0.25 mm (0.010 in); however, layers as fine as 0.04 mm (0.0016 in.) can be deposited with certain materials. The materials available are thermoplastics, waxes, and some eutectic metals. In dentistry, wax filaments are available that can be used to fabricate a wax pattern to design and fabricate removal and fixed denture frameworks and there are complete systems that are commonly used for fabricating wax jewelry patterns for casting.

Aside from extruding filaments in FFF fabrication, there are systems which employ a reservoir of liquid materials that are extruded through a nozzle as deposited in a similar fashion. The Envisiontec 3D-Bioplotter™ uses this approach, a wide range of materials are available such as ceramic pastes for creating porous bone scaffolds, bioresorbable polymers and a host of materials as carriers for cells that are used in organ printing (van Noort, 2012). The 3D-Bioplotter™ has a resolution of a few micrometers that make it ideal for fabricating microstructural patterns to enhance cell profusion through a porous structure (Zein et al., 2002). Using a micro syringe, structures that are fine enough to provide

guidance for blood vessels growing into the scaffolds can be fabricated (Muller et al., 2010).

Material extrusion devices are relatively simple in comparison to other AM approaches. One or more extrusion nozzles are moved relative to the workpiece by servo motors. The nozzles are first moved transverse to the vertical to deposit a layer of material, then stepped vertically to the height of the next layer and the process is repeated, building upon the last layer. Material is selectively deposited at desired locations in the plane of the layer by modulating flow from the nozzle; multiple materials in a layer are possible if multiple extrusion heads are employed. Since material is being deposited as a liquid, support of overhanging structure is generally necessary. Overhang support is achieved with removable structures or an auxiliary support material, which is typically removed by dissolution after fabrication. Most of the FFF devices marketed for home use some variation of the described approach to fabricate parts in thermoplastics using a single nozzle (Figure 3.10).

Powder bed fusion

Powder bed fusion systems use powders as their source of material that are fused or sintered into a solid shape. The materials most commonly used in this type of manufacturing are metals, thermoplastic materials, and ceramics. This process shows the most promise in the fabrication of custom medical devices and dental fixed and removable prosthesis due to the flexibility of AMT to use freeform shapes and use of similar materials.

Selective laser melt

Selective laser melt (SLM), also known by the trademark name DMLS, is a laser powder fusion process. In this AMT process, powdered metal is welded into a solid form by a high-power laser, layer by layer. All welding related problems as shrinkage, distortion, cracks; residual stress and surface hardening are to be expected. To control this complex set of parameters, the process runs under a shielding gas. Fine grained powders are applied and sophisticated scan strategies are used to govern the exposure by the laser beam. Furthermore, heat treatment of the completed parts is generally necessary to relieve residual stresses in the finished part. In general, the residual stress profile consists of two zones of large tensile stresses at the top and bottom of the part and a large zone of intermediate compressive stress in between. The most important parameters determining the magnitude and shape of the residual stress profiles are the material properties, the sample and substrate height, the laser scanning strategy, and the heating conditions (Mercelis and Kruth, 2006). The surrounding unfused powder generally supports layers of fused material; however, owing to the internal stresses in the part under fabrication, fixing supports are necessary to prevent the part from warping.

To achieve fine detail resolution and a minimum of stair stepping artifacts on the vertical surfaces, a small layer thickness and a small laser beam diameter are necessary. Fiber lasers used in SLM are generally greater than 100 W, with beam diameters in the range of 0.2–0.4 μm with a layer thickness in the range of 30 μm. Commercially available metal powders with grain size in the range of 20–50 μm can be used in this process (Gebhards *et al.*, 2010). The SLM process has been successfully applied to a wide range of metals, including: stainless steel alloys, nickel alloys, Cr-Co, aluminum, and titanium. Optimized SLM parameters lead to part densities up to 99.98% for titanium. Strength and stiffness, corrosion behavior, and process accuracy fulfill requirements for medical or dental parts. Surface roughness analyses show some limitations of the SLM process. However, dental frameworks can be produced efficiently and with high precision (Vandenbrouchke and Kruth, 2007).

Electron beam melting

Electron beam melting (EBM) is a rapid manufacturing process in which fully dense parts with properties equal to those of wrought materials are built layer by layer. A bed of conductive powdered metal is heated to near the melting temperature. Next, an electron beam is raster scanned over the top layer of the powder to selectively fuse particles into the desired cross-sectional shape; the process is repeated for subsequent layers until the part is complete. Since the process takes place under vacuum, EBM is suited to manufacture parts in reactive materials with a high affinity for oxygen, such as titanium. Since the EBM process operates at an elevated temperature, typically between 700 and 1000 °C, finished parts are virtually free from residual stress; thus, heat treatment after the build is not necessary. The melt rate is up to 80 cm^3/hour with a minimum layer thickness of 0.05 mm (0.0020 in.) and a tolerance capability: ±0.2 mm; this results in a faster build rate than SLM, but at the sacrifice of the fine detail resolution of SLM. After melting and solidifying one layer of metal powder, the process is repeated for subsequent layers until the part is complete. The additive process opens the door to new design configurations and weight-reduction alternatives (Hiemenz, 2009). This solid free form fabrication method produces fully dense metal parts directly from metal powder with characteristics of the target material. The EBM machine reads data from a 3D CAD model and lays down successive layers of powdered material. These layers are "melted" together utilizing a computer controlled electron beam generated from a filament to build the parts. Usually minimum supports are required and the parts are recovered from a block of unsintered metal. The process takes place under vacuum, which makes it suited to manufacture parts in reactive materials with a high affinity for oxygen such as titanium (Figure 3.11).

The material is a pure alloy in powder form of the final material to be fabricated with no fillers;

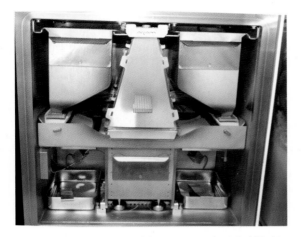

Figure 3.11 Internal setup of the EBM, powder is held in bins on both sides of the heat shield, powder is racked across the platform and the beam is exposed to the powder fusing the powder in an oxygen free chamber.

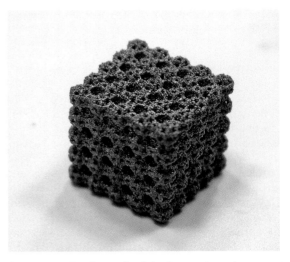

Figure 3.12 3D cube made of titanium, a shape that cannot be fabricated using a milling processes.

therefore, it does not require additional thermal treatment to obtain the full mechanical properties of the parts. That aspect allows classification of EBM with SLM where competing technologies like selective laser sintering SLS and DMLS require thermal treatment after fabrication. Compared to SLM and DMLS, EBM has a generally superior build rate because of its higher energy density and scanning method (Figure 3.12).

Selective heat sintering

Selective heat sintering (SHS) AMT was launched in 2011. It is similar to SLS, but instead of using a laser, SHS uses a thermal print head, which is mechanically scanned over the surface of the powder bed. The powder bed is held at an elevated temperature so the thermal print head only has to elevate the temperature slightly above the powder's melting temperature to selectively bond it. Like other AMT, a 3D model is designed and sliced into layers (minimum of 1 mm), the printer spreads plastic powder in a thin layer across the build chamber, selectively fuses materials in the layer to form a cross section of layer across the build chamber, selectively fuses materials to form a cross section of the part on the top layer, and the process continues until the 3D geometry is

complete. SHS does not require support structures since each cross section is surrounded by unfused powder, which provides a foundation for the next layer. Finished parts must be removed from the powder bed and excess unfused powder must be removed from the part.

The SHS process is limited to a white thermoplastic material; presently there are no metals available for this technique. Unused powder is 100% recyclable and there is no need for additional support materials.

Selective laser sintering

SLS is an additive manufacturing layer technology that involves the use of a high power laser to fuse small particles of plastic, metal (direct metal laser sintering), ceramic, or glass powders into a mass that has a desired 3D shape. The laser selectively fuses powdered material by scanning cross sections generated from a 3D digital description of the part on the surface of a powder bed. After each cross section is scanned, the powder bed is lowered by one layer thickness, a new layer of material is applied on top, and the process is repeated until the part is completed. Much like the EBM process, the powder is elevated to a temperature near the melting point of the material to minimize energy necessary to fuse the material particles. Because finished part density depends on peak laser power, rather than laser duration, an SLS machine typically uses a pulsed laser. As opposed to SLM and EBM technologies, metal powders are not fully melted, but sintered into a mass with greater porosity and inferior mechanical properties to wrought material. The SLS machine preheats the bulk powder material in the powder bed somewhat below its melting point, to make it easier for the laser to raise the temperature of the selected regions the rest of the way to the melting point.

Similar to EBM, SLS does not require support structures due to the fact that the part being constructed is surrounded by unsintered powder at all times, this allows for the construction of previously impossible geometries. However, residual stresses are found to be very large in SLS parts. In general, the residual stress profile consists of two zones of large tensile stresses at the top and bottom of the part and a large zone of intermediate compressive stress in between. The most important parameters determining the magnitude and shape of the residual stress profiles are the material properties, the sample and substrate height, the laser scanning strategy and the heating conditions (Mercelis and Kruth, 2006).

Optimized SLS parameters lead to part densities up to 99.98% for titanium. Strength and stiffness, corrosion behavior, and process accuracy fulfill requirements for medical or dental parts. Surface roughness analyses show some limitations of the SLM process. However, dental frameworks can be produced efficiently and with high precision (Vandenbrouchke and Kruth, 2007).

Binder jetting

Plaster-based 3D printing

Plaster-based 3D printing (PP) is another method that consists of an inkjet 3D printing system. The printer creates the cast one layer at a time by spreading a layer of powder (plaster or resins) and printing with a liquid binder in the cross section of the part using an inkjet-like process. This is repeated until every layer has been printed. This

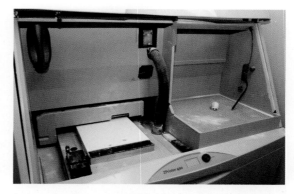

Figure 3.13 The printing and cleaning chamber of a binder-jet 3D printer.

technology allows the printing of full color prototypes, overhangs, and elastomer parts. Supports for fabrication are not needed as the process uses the powder bed for support. The relative strength of the fabricated product is poor; however, the strength of bonded powder prints can be enhanced with wax, sealed with cyanoacrylate, or infiltrated with a resin (Figure 3.13).

Sheet lamination

Laminated object manufacturing (LOM)

Layers of adhesive-coated paper, plastic, or metal laminates are successively glued together and cut to shape with a knife or laser cutter. The original process worked in the following manner: a sheet is adhered to a substrate with a heated roller, a laser traces desired dimensions of prototype and cross hatches non-part area to facilitate waste removal. The platform with completed layer moves down and out of the way, a fresh sheet of material is rolled into position, the platform moves up into position to receive next layer and the process is repeated.

Recently, the process was modified by MCORE; they developed an adhesive dispensing system that deposits thousands of tiny glue dots on each layer. Fewer dots are applied to the "throw-away" areas, allowing for easy removal of the waste area. Unlike the original process in which the adhesive was universal, which made cleanup a bit laborious (Figure 3.14).

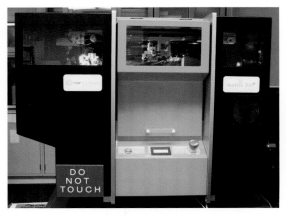

Figure 3.14 The Mcore Iris color sheet lamination printer uses plain and colored paper.

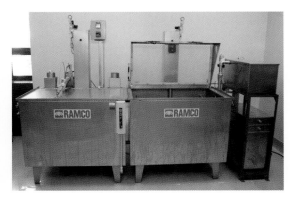

Figure 3.15 Parts washers are needed to clean the SLA pieces from the residual photopolymers.

LOM is low cost due to the readily available raw material, paper models have wood-like characteristics, therefore can be sanded and sealed, and the dimensional accuracy is reported to be slightly less than that of SLA and SLS.

Vat photopolymerization

Stereolithography

The term "Stereolithography" (SLA) was coined in 1986 by Charles Hull, who patented it as a method and apparatus for making solid objects by successively "printing" thin layers of an ultraviolet curable material one on top of the other with a concentrated beam of ultraviolet light (laser) focused onto the surface of a vat filled with liquid photopolymer (Figure 3.15). For each layer, the laser beam traces a cross section of the part pattern on the surface of the liquid resin. Exposure to the ultraviolet laser light cures and solidifies the pattern traced on the resin and joins it to the layer below, a complex process, which requires automation. After the pattern has been traced, the SLA's elevator platform descends by a distance equal to the thickness of a single layer, typically 0.05–0.15 mm (0.002–0.006 in.). Then, a resin-filled blade sweeps across the cross section of the part, re-coating it with fresh material. On this new liquid surface, the subsequent layer pattern is traced, joining the previous layer. This process

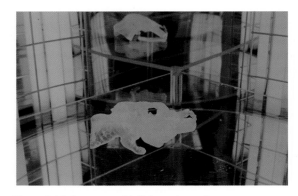

Figure 3.16 Post-cure with light curing unit.

forms a complete 3D part. After being built, parts are immersed parts washer with solvent in order to be cleaned of excess resin and are subsequently cured in an ultraviolet oven (Figure 3.16).

SLA requires the use of supporting structures, which serve to attach the part to the elevator platform, prevent deflection due to gravity and hold the cross sections in place so that they resist lateral pressure from the re-coater blade. Supports are generated automatically during the preparation of 3D CAD models for use on the SLA machine, although they may be manipulated manually. Supports must be removed from the finished product manually, unlike in other, less costly, rapid prototyping technologies (Figure 3.17).

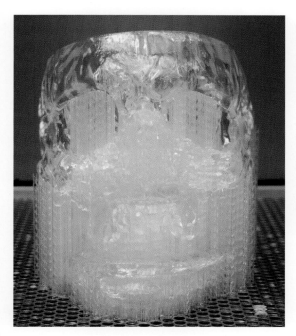

Figure 3.17 Model of a skull with supports.

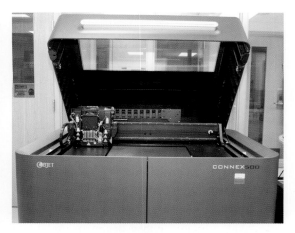

Figure 3.18 A Connex 500 Polyjet printer.

Digital light processing

Much like SLA, digital light processing exposes a liquid polymer to light from a digital light processing (DLP) projector, which hardens the polymer layer by layer until the object is built and the remaining liquid polymer is drained off. This has recently been the focus of many of the home use options.

Materials jetting

Polyjet 3D printing

PolyJet 3D printing is similar to inkjet document printing. But instead of jetting drops of ink onto paper, PolyJet 3D printers jet layers of liquid photopolymer onto a build tray and cures them with UV light. The layers build up one at a time to create a 3D cast or prototype (Figure 3.18). Fully cured casts can be handled and used immediately, without additional post-curing. Along with the selected cast materials, the 3D printer also jets a gel-like support material specially designed to uphold overhangs and complicated geometries. It is easily removed by hand and with water.

PolyJet 3D printing technology has many advantages for rapid prototyping, including superior quality and speed, high precision, and a very wide variety of materials. Based on PolyJet technology, Objet Conned 3D Printers from Stratus are presently the only additive manufacturing systems that can combine different 3D printing materials within the same 3D printed cast, in the same print job (Figure 3.19).

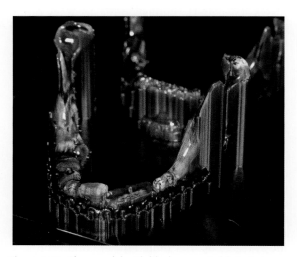

Figure 3.19 Clear model with black supports fabricated on a polyjet printer.

Applications of digital manufacturing in medicine and dentistry

Over the past couple of decades, digital manufacturing has become more available and accepted for use in dental and medical treatment of patients. Additive manufacturing companies such a Materialise (Leuven, Belgium) developed software (Mimics) specifically aimed at the medical industry, converting DICOM files into the required 3D file structures resulting in the development of medical anatomical model design, virtual surgical treatment planning, and digital manufacturing of models, guides, and medical devices. In the early 2000, the US military began to use digital manufacturing to address reconstruction needs of wounded warriors using both FDM and SLA, specifically in the fabrication of cranial implants. Digital methods cut the fabrication time to about a fourth of the time of manual fabrication as well as reduced operating times in half (Taft *et al.*, 2011).

In addition to the military experience, the use of digital models have become more widely accepted in treatment planning for oral and maxillofacial surgery; vascular models provide better visualization of vascular defects; for neurosurgery, spine, hip, and pelvis models allow for measurement and preoperative bending of reconstruction plates in orthopedics; and cardiac models of vessels and valves have provided support for cardiologists (Esses *et al.*, 2011). Studies on the accuracy of the models from DICOM scanned data and digital fabrication of models support fabrication of custom cutting guides, positioning guides, and reconstruction plates (Roser *et al.*, 2010; Taft *et al.*, 2011) (Figure 3.20).

Future of DDM

Although milling systems have been the predominant method of dental CAD/CAM, additive manufacturing techniques for dentistry may provide the technology to produce direct dental frameworks for fixed and removable prosthetics as well as custom fixation devices for craniofacial reconstructions in a more efficient and economic manner. As more custom materials are developed, there may also be a shift from the more

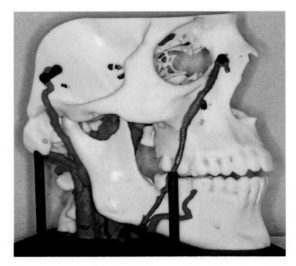

Figure 3.20 Vascular models from a CT with contrast fabricated on a binder jetting printer allows for color to be applied to the vessels.

conventional metals and porcelains for other biocompatible, tough polymers, ceramics, and eutectic metals as dental restorative materials

DDM will define how dentistry is practiced in the future, and advances in the digital processes of scanning, virtual design, and digital manufacturing of dental prostheses will have an impact on the conventional methods of tooth preparation, impression, and custom dental prostheses fabrication, decreasing the time, access to care, and the eventual cost of delivery of a dental restoration. Digital dental laboratories will see a shift in the traditional "craftsman" skills to a more computer savvy technician, with the potential to be more productive and provide more consistent quality with more advanced materials. Although we cannot abandon the conventional principles in how we have practiced medicine and dentistry in the past, dental and medical professionals are now challenged to embrace technology for their patients.

References

Cozmei, C. & Caloian, F. (2012) Additive manufacturing flickering at the beginning of existence. *Procedia Economics and Finance*, **3**, 457–462.

Esses, S.J., Berman, P., & Bloom, A.I., *et al.* (2011) Clinical applications of physical 3D models derived from MDCT data and created by rapid prototyping. *AJR. American Journal of Roentgenology*, **196**, W683–W688.

Gebhards, A., Schmidt, F.M., & Hotter, J.S., *et al.* (2010) Additive Manufacturing by selective laser melting the realizer desktop machine and its application for the dental industry. *Physics Procedia*, **5**, 543–549.

Gronet, P.M., Waskewicz, G.A., & Richardson, C. (2003) Preformed acrylic cranial implants using fused deposition modeling: a clinical report. *The Journal of Prosthetic Dentistry*, **90**, 429–433.

Gunnink, J.W. (1998) Multi-axis high speed milling, how to speed up prototyping and tooling processes by using STL technology, *TCT'98 Proceedings*, 43–65.

Hiemenz, J. (2009) Electrom beam melting. *Advanced Materials and Processes*, **165**, 45–46.

Mercelis, P. & Kruth, J. (2006) Residual stresses in selective laser sintering and selective laser melting. *Rapid Prototyping Journal*, **12**, 254–265.

Muller, D., Chim, H., & Bader, A., *et al.* (2010) Vascular guidance: microstructural scaffold patterning for inductive neovascularization. *Stem Cells International*, **2011**, 547247.

Roser, S.M., Ramachandra, S., & Blair, H., *et al.* (2010) The accuracy of virtual surgical planning in free fibula mandibular reconstruction: comparison of planned and final results. *Journal of Oral and Maxillofacial Surgery*, **68**, 2824–2832.

Taft, R.M., Kondor, S., & Grant, G.T. (2011) Accuracy of rapid prototype models for head and neck reconstruction. *The Journal of Prosthetic Dentistry*, **106**, 399–408.

United States Department of Labor (2013) Dental Laboratory Technicians. In: Occupational Outlook Handbook, p. 429. United States Department of Labor.

van Noort, R. (2012) The future of dental devices is digital. *Dental Materials*, **28**, 3–12.

Vandenbrouchke, B. & Kruth, J.P. (2007) Selective laser melting of biocompatible metals for rapid manufacturing of medical parts. *Rapid Prototyping Journal*, **13**, 196–2013.

Zein, I., Hutmacher, D.W., & Tan, K.C., *et al.* (2002) Fused deposition modeling of novel scaffold architectures for tissue engineering applications. *Biomaterials*, **23**, 1169–1185.

4 Digital Application in Operative Dentistry

Dennis J. Fasbinder and Gisele F. Neiva

Introduction

The most common application of CAD/CAM dentistry is the fabrication of permanent restorations for teeth and implants. As discussed in earlier chapters, there are three sequences included in the CAD/CAM workflow. The first sequence is to record the geometry of the patient's intraoral condition to a computer system using an intraoral camera. This is referred to as a digital impression. A software program is used in the second sequence to create a volume proposal of the restoration. Once the design has been completed, a machining device is used to produce the designed restoration in the third sequence (Beuer *et al.*, 2008).

Computerized systems for use in the dental office can be divided arbitrarily into two general categories. Digital impression systems focus on the first step of the CAD/CAM process to accurately record the patient's intraoral condition (see Chapter 2). The digital file is transmitted to the dental laboratory for fabrication of the desired restoration.

Chairside CAD/CAM systems are the other category. These systems also rely on a digital impression and include the ability to design and mill the restoration employing all three steps of the CAD/CAM process in the dental office, usually during a single dental appointment. This affords a significant improvement in efficiency and convenience for the patient as there is no need for a provisional restoration or a second appointment to deliver the final restoration.

Conventional impression materials and techniques have been essential for the fabrication of an indirect restoration. Digital impression systems focus on a similar outcome, a replica of the patient's dentition to utilize during case fabrication. However, they avoid a number of factors that negatively influence restoration outcomes, such as volumetric changes in the manipulation of impression materials and stone models, distortion of impressions or casts, abrasion or fracture of the casts, and problems created during shipment of cases. Digital impressions are not susceptible to changes in accuracy once they are recorded and electronic transmission of the files to dental laboratories is completed efficiently with no loss of accuracy (see Chapter 2 for more details on digital impressions).

Clinical Applications of Digital Dental Technology, First Edition. Edited by Radi Masri and Carl F. Driscoll.
© 2015 John Wiley & Sons, Inc. Published 2015 by John Wiley & Sons, Inc.

Case selection

Treatment planning cases to be treated with digital systems is generally not different than planning cases to be treated with conventional impression materials and techniques. The type of restoration that is indicated for the clinical situation is the primary consideration rather than the impression process used to fabricate the restoration. For example, subgingival margin placement should be considered relative to the ability to isolate the margin for adhesive cementation if an adhesive ceramic restoration is planned regardless of whether a conventional or digital impression is planned. Intraoral access for the camera may be a concern for patients with a restricted vertical opening. However, if a dental handpiece can be used to prepare the tooth, generally there is sufficient intraoral access for use of the intraoral scanner. Conventional impressions for patients with a severe gag reflex may be problematic due to the stimulation of the gag reflex through physical contact with the impression material and/or tray. Digital impressions can be less stimulating to the gag reflex as no actual contact with the soft or hard tissues is required while recording the dentition.

Tooth preparation for computerized restorations

Computerized dentistry systems rely on digitally recording the tooth preparation for fabrication of the desired restoration. The digital impression does not dictate the type of restoration any more than a conventional impression dictates a specific restoration. It is just the means to replicate the patient's intraoral condition from which to make the planned restoration.

Tooth preparation guidelines for specific types of restorations are generally based on the features of the restorative material to be used for the case. For example, the occlusal reduction required for a metal crown is more conservative in thickness than for an all-ceramic crown as ceramics require a greater thickness for strength of the crown compared to a metallic crown. However, there are several tooth preparation guidelines that will enhance the ease of recording and accuracy of a digital impression.

Intraoral digital scanners are line of sight cameras. They will record what is directly visible to the camera. Maximum data is recorded when the camera lens is parallel to the tooth surface and the field of view is angled perpendicular to the surface of the tooth as this affords maximum surface of the tooth to be visible to the camera. As the camera lens is moved to be more perpendicular to the surface of the tooth and the field of view is angled to be more parallel to the tooth surface, less tooth surface data is made available to the direct line of sight of the camera. This feature of intraoral digital scanners can influence the ease of recording tooth preparations. Margin designs for all ceramic restorations require a bulk of material at the margin to ensure strength of the ceramic. This is usually accomplished with a shoulder, sloped shoulder, or heavy chamfer margin design. These margin designs are readily visible to the intraoral digital scanner as the margins are approximately parallel to the occlusal surface of the preparation allowing maximum recording of the tooth data from an occlusal direction. Margin designs for metallic restorations require adequate bulk of metal at the margins to facilitate good fitting margins and prevent distortion. This is usually accomplished with a chamfer or beveled margin design. These margin designs approach a more perpendicular angle with the occlusal surface of the preparation and the intraoral digital scanner must be rotated at a greater angle to the facial or lingual direction to increase the available tooth surface for recording these designs. The proximal surface of the adjacent tooth as well as soft tissue contours may be limiting factors as to how far the intraoral digital scanner may be rotated laterally and still have visible access to the thinner margin design.

In the case of an inlay or onlay preparation, the location of the proximal box wall margins relative to an adjacent tooth is generally determined based on the need to be able to finish the margins for the restoration after it has been cemented. The clearance of the proximal wall margin from the adjacent tooth is often times evaluated by the ability to clear the proximal contact with the tip of the explorer. For digital impressions, the proximal box wall margin must be visibly open from the adjacent tooth so the intraoral digital scanner can distinguish the margin from the adjacent tooth surface. This is particularly a factor when adjacent teeth have root approximation with the prepared tooth. A similar concern may also occur if the proximal contour of the adjacent tooth has drifted excessively toward the prepared tooth due to a longstanding missing proximal surface of the prepared tooth.

It is not uncommon to encounter significant undercuts in the tooth preparation due to previous large restorations or caries. These generally must be blocked out to a great extent prior to making a conventional impression so as not to distort the impression when removing it from the mouth. This is not a factor for digital impressions. The intraoral digital scanner will accurately record the undercuts to the extent that the digital scanner is rotated to visualize the entire undercut. However, it does not adversely affect the accuracy of the digital impression and is easily managed in the digital design and processing steps.

Clinical guidelines for digital impressions

It is axiomatic that the accuracy of the final restoration can only be as good as the accuracy of the replica of the tooth preparation. The margin fit and internal adaptation of the final restoration are directly related to the accuracy of the recorded tooth preparation. This is true for both digital and conventional impressions. There are several basic concepts that are essential for making an accurate impression and these concepts must be equally applied for both digital and conventional impressions. The cavity preparation must be well isolated from moisture contamination, soft tissues retracted for visualization of preparation margins, and all areas of the dentition and soft tissues affecting the final restoration are accurately recorded.

No matter how easy and efficient it would be to digitally record tooth preparations through saliva, blood, and soft tissues, this is not possible today. Digital recordings or scans are as sensitive to moisture contamination and soft tissue retraction as are traditional impression materials. Moisture, such as saliva or blood, obscures the preparation surface and prevents accurate recording of the

tooth and soft tissues. Similarly, inadequate retraction of soft tissues may obscure the marginal areas. Digital cameras can only record what is visible and isolated. Careful control of the intraoral scanning environment ensures an accurate digital file essential to a well fitting restoration.

Conventional impressions require that soft tissues be retracted laterally sufficient to allow for a bulk of impression material at the margin to avoid tearing of the impression upon removal from the mouth. Soft tissues must also be retracted at least 1 mm cervically past the margin to ensure accurate reproduction and visualization of the margin in the impression material. Digital impressions have an advantage in that the soft tissues only need to be retracted sufficiently laterally to visualize the margins. This dimension may be as little as 150 μm for the digital scanner to record the margin of the tooth separate from the soft tissues. For this reason, diode lasers are particularly popular adjunctive instruments for digital impressions as they can create lateral retraction while preventing bleeding and a moisture free margin environment (Figure 4.1).

A critical element of digital impressions is the difference between "calculated" data and "real" or "actual" data. It should be obvious that to have an accurate digital impression actual data of the intraoral condition is required and not extrapolated or calculated data. This is also true of conventional impressions. Local areas of folds, tears, voids, or bubbles in a conventional impression in a noncritical area relative to the

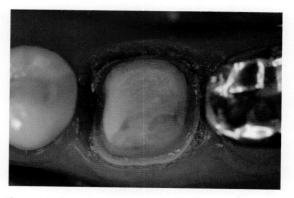

Figure 4.1 Crown preparation with diode laser retraction of the gingiva.

planned restoration are replicated in the stone cast and may be considered "calculated" data as they do not accurately replicate the intraoral condition. This calculated data is acceptable in a conventional impression as long as it does not affect the accuracy of the final restoration. If it does, a new impression must be made as there is no technique to accurately modify the existing impression or stone cast. The evaluation of "calculated" data as critical or noncritical to the accuracy of the final restoration is similar for digital impressions as well. Rather than evaluating the impression, the actual recorded virtual cast can be magnified and rotated on the computer monitor to search for missing or distorted scan data. A particular advantage of a digital impression is the ability to additionally scan missing data and have it added to the existing virtual cast rather than remake the entire digital impression. This results in a much more efficient process than having to remake a conventional impression.

Digital impression workflow

The clinical workflow for making a digital impression varies between the available systems primarily in the function of the camera and navigation of the software program. Once the tooth preparation has been completed and the margins of the preparation visualized and the area isolated from moisture, the preparation is lightly coated with a titanium dioxide powder to enhance the speed and accuracy of scanning process (Box 4.1). The scanning does not have to be completed in a single pass but instead can be recorded in overlapping sections and the software program will combine the scan sections into a single virtual cast. A common practice is to scan the preparation and adjacent teeth first, evaluate the accuracy of the scan, and then scan any missing data as well as the remaining teeth desired to be included in the final cast. The opposing cast is scanned separate from the preparation cast.

The ability to record the contact relationships of the patient's opposing dentition is critical to reproducing accurate occlusal contacts on the planned restoration. The most common technique for digital impressions is to first separately record the maxillary and mandibular virtual casts. The

patient is guided into maximum intercuspation and a digital scan is made of the facial surfaces of the opposing teeth in this static position. The software program uses the buccal scan to match the facial surfaces of the maxillary and mandibular virtual casts and reproduce the patient's vertical dimension of occlusion. No current digital impression system has the capability of reproducing the lateral or protrusive functional movements of the dentition, although several software programs are expected to make this feature available in the near future. One study has reported the accuracy of the buccal scan to reproduce the vertical dimension of occlusion using a digital impression system based on active wavefront sampling (Poticny and Fasbinder, 2011). There was no significant difference in the occlusal vertical dimension between the master mounting and the buccal scan mounting of the virtual casts generated from digital impressions.

Once the virtual casts have been recorded, several evaluation screens can be accessed for the case. One option is to visualize the preparation at a higher magnification on the monitor. This affords the opportunity to critically determine if the preparation margins have been accurately recorded prior to transmitting the case to the dental laboratory. A second option is to quantitatively evaluate the occlusal clearance of the tooth preparation from the opposing cast. This can ensure adequate thickness for the proposed restoration exists, preventing the problem of trying to fabricate the restoration and making modifications at the delivery appointment (Figure 4.2).

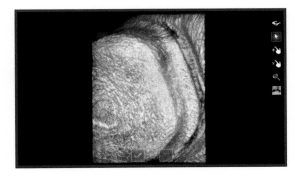

Figure 4.2 High-magnification image of a crown preparation margin with the True Definition digital impression system software.

Box 4.1 Workflow chart #1: Digital Impression Workflow (True Definition/3M ESPE).

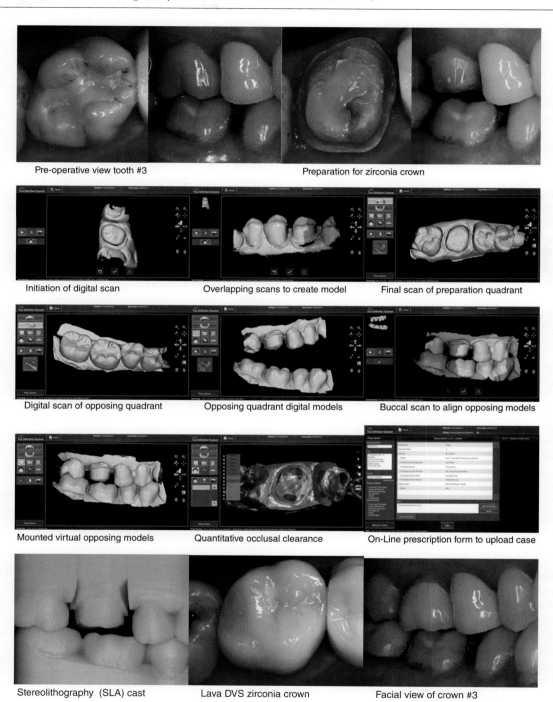

Pre-operative view tooth #3   Preparation for zirconia crown

Initiation of digital scan   Overlapping scans to create model   Final scan of preparation quadrant

Digital scan of opposing quadrant   Opposing quadrant digital models   Buccal scan to align opposing models

Mounted virtual opposing models   Quantitative occlusal clearance   On-Line prescription form to upload case

Stereolithography (SLA) cast   Lava DVS zirconia crown   Facial view of crown #3

Digital impressions of the intraoral condition are stored in a data file commonly referred to as a stereolithography file (.stl file). At the completion of the scan process, a laboratory prescription is completed on the system software and the data file is electronically transmitted by the internet to the dental laboratory for processing. The dental laboratory downloads the data file to its software system and is faced with several options of how to utilize the data file. One option is to forward the data file to a processing center and have resin or polyurethane casts fabricated for the case. The articulated casts are returned to the dental laboratory and the restoration can be fabricated on the casts with any conventional laboratory process such as for a gold crown or porcelain fused to metal (PFM) crown. Another option for utilization of the data file is to import it into a CAD/CAM software program and computer graphically design copings or full contour restorations for the case. The processed casts may or may not be used to finish the case such as would be done for a veneered zirconia crown (Fasbinder, 2009).

Accuracy of digital impressions

Several studies have shown digital impressions to be at least as accurate as conventional impressions. One study compared the accuracy of casts made from full arch conventional and digital impressions (Ogledzki et al., 2011). Three master casts were scanned three times with the Lava COS and impressed three times with polyvinylsiloxane impression material and casts were fabricated from each scan and impression. The accuracy of the casts was measured with a commercial graphic analysis program. There was no significant difference in accuracy of the casts compared to the master casts with either impression technique. Another study evaluated the accuracy of full arch digital and conventional impressions. Conventional monophase polyether impressions of a master cast were compared to digital impressions made with the CEREC AC BlueCam and Lava COS systems. There was no significant difference in the trueness and precision of the full arch casts made with either the conventional or digital impression techniques (Ender and Mehl, 2011). One *in vitro*

study compared the accuracy of full ceramic crowns fabricated from intraoral scans using Lava COS, CEREC AC, and iTero digital impressions with two different conventional impression techniques (Seelbach et al., 2013). The mean margin fit of crowns was $48 \pm 25 \, \mu m$ for Lava COS, $30 \pm 17 \, \mu m$ for CEREC AC, $41 \pm 16 \, \mu m$ for iTero, $33 \pm 19 \, \mu m$ for single-step putty wash technique, and $60 \pm 30 \, \mu m$ for the two-step putty wash technique. The mean internal fit was $29 \pm 7 \, \mu m$ for Lava COS, $88 \pm 20 \, \mu m$ for CEREC AC, $50 \pm 2 \, \mu m$ for iTero, $36 \pm 5 \, \mu m$ for single-step putty wash technique, and 35 ± 7 for two-step putty wash technique. There was no significant difference in the margin fit or internal adaptation of the crowns using any of the techniques.

A number of other studies report that digital impressions have improved accuracy compared to conventional impressions. One study compared the fit of crowns fabricated using both an intraoral digital impression and a conventional impression (Syrek et al., 2010). Two zirconia crowns were fabricated for each of 20 patients on the same tooth preparation. One crown was fabricated from a digital impression using the Lava COS system and the other crown from a conventional silicone impression. The margin fit was measured using a replica technique at the time of crown cementation. The crowns fabricated using a digital impression had a significantly better margin fit (49 μm) than those fabricated from a conventional impression (71 μm). A clinical study compared the fit of Lava DVS zirconia crowns fabricated using digital impressions from the Lava COS system and Vita Rapid Layering Technique crowns using digital impressions with the CEREC AC system (Brawek et al., 2013). Fourteen patients requiring a posterior crown had two crowns fabricated using each digital impression technique. A replica technique was used to measure the clinical adaptation and fit for both crowns on each preparation. The Lava COS crowns had a significantly better mean marginal fit ($51 \pm 38 \, \mu m$) compared to the CEREC crowns ($83 \pm 51 \, \mu m$); however, the difference in fit may not be clinically relevant because both were well below the accepted clinical threshold of $100 - 120 \, \mu m$.

Intraoral digital impressions with the Lava COS and True Definition scanners have clinical research demonstrating consistent accuracy (Ender and Mehl, 2011; Kugel *et al.*, 2008; Ogledzki *et al.*, 2011). One clinical study measured the accuracy of zirconia crowns on 37 crown preparations made from digital impressions using the Lava COS system (Scotti *et al.*, 2011). Silicon replicas were used to measure the internal adaptation and margin fit of the crowns. The mean margin gap was reported as $48.65 \pm 29.45\,\mu m$ and the mean axial wall gap was $112.03 \pm 54.45\,\mu m$ with no significant difference in fit between anterior and posterior crowns. Another randomized clinical study compared the accuracy of two types of zirconia crowns made with conventional impressions and digital impressions using the Lava COS (Fasbinder *et al.*, 2012b). Both a digital and conventional impression was made for each preparation for 25 zirconia crowns made with a hand layered veneer and 25 zirconia crowns made with a digital veneering process. Both crowns were measured intraorally for margin fit and internal adaptation on the clinical preparation using a replica technique. There was no significant difference in the internal fit of the two types of zirconia crowns; however, the crowns made with a digital impression had a better margin fit ($51.45 \pm 18.59\,\mu m$) than those made with a conventional impression technique ($78.62 \pm 24.62\,\mu m$).

Chairside CAD/CAM systems

The CEREC OmniCam (Sirona Dental Systems) and the E4D Dentist system (Planmeca E4D Technologies) are the two currently available complete chairside CAD/CAM systems (Levine, 2009; Mormann, 2006). Chairside CAD/CAM systems rely on accurate digital impressions similar to digital impression systems discussed in Chapter 2. However, they also include computer software for designing full contour restorations as well as a milling chamber for fabrication of the restoration in the dental office. Chairside CAD/CAM systems can produce inlays, onlays, veneers, and crowns for both natural teeth and implants. They also have the ability to fabricate short-span fixed partial dentures as well as provisional restorations in the dental office.

Some clinicians may decide that designing full contour restorations on a computer is a greater learning curve than they may want to tackle, especially when they have been accustomed to having dental laboratory technicians fabricate restorations for them. The CEREC Connect system for the CEREC OmniCam and the E4D Sky network for the E4D Dentists system offer the opportunity to use the chairside systems as purely digital impression systems for cases desired to be fabricated in the dental laboratory.

Chairside CAD/CAM clinical workflow

The clinical workflow to fabricate a chairside restoration with either the CEREC OmniCam or the E4D systems are relatively similar with the differences primarily a function of the unique cameras, software, and milling chambers used by each system. Once the tooth preparation has been completed, the margins visualized for recording, and the area isolated from moisture, the tooth preparation and adjacent teeth can be scanned using the camera (Box 4.2). A scan of the facial surfaces of the dentition in maximum intercuspation is used to align the scanned opposing arches or quadrants. The margin of the preparation is drawn on the virtual cast to identify the limits of the restoration within the software program. The software program uses data from the prepared teeth, adjacent teeth, and opposing teeth to calculate and propose the initial design of the restoration on the cast. The software program also contains various evaluation tools and editing tools to refine the proposal based on the specific needs of the case and desires of the clinician. These include items such as the size and intensity of the proximal contacts, location, and intensity of the occlusal contacts as well as the contours of the proposal. The final restoration design is transmitted to the milling chamber where a previously manufactured block of the desired restorative material is milled to match the full contour design from the software program. Once the fit of the restoration has been verified on the tooth preparation, it is cemented with appropriate cement. Final contouring and polishing of the restoration is completed using a series of microfine diamonds and polishing instruments.

Box 4.2 Workflow chart #2: Chairside CAD/CAM Workflow (CEREC OmniCam/Sirona Dental).

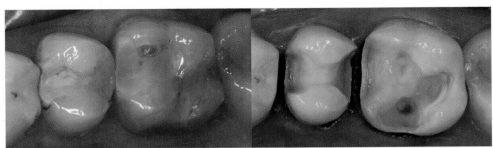

Pre-operative view of teeth #13-#14   Inlay #13 and Onlay #14 preparations

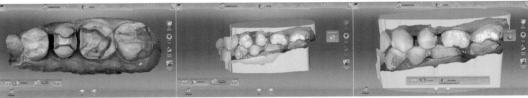

Scanned preparations   Buccal bite scan to align models   Mounted opposing models

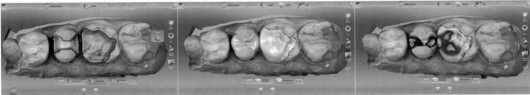

Identify the margin of the preparation   Initial biogeneric proposals   Edit the occlusal contacts and intensity

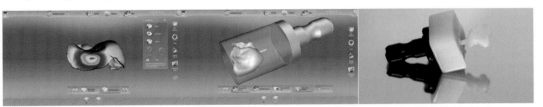

Edit the proximal contact size and intensity   Milling screen   Milled restoration in the block

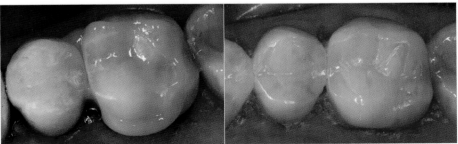

Onlay #14 cemented with dual cure resin cement   Post-operative view of Lava Ultimate inlay and onlay

Accuracy of chairside CAD/CAM systems

CEREC has over 25 years of both laboratory and clinical research confirming the accuracy of CEREC chairside CAD/CAM restorations (Martin and Jedynakiewicz, 2000; Estafan *et al.*, 2003). One *in vitro* study measured the fit of CEREC crowns compared to those fabricated using a variety of laboratory techniques (Ellingsen and Fasbinder, 2002). There was no significant difference in crown margin fit between the CEREC chairside CAD/CAM and laboratory fabricated techniques with CEREC crowns having a mean margin gap of 64.5 ± 24.7 μm for ceramic crowns and 66.0 ± 14.1 μm for composite crowns. One study evaluated the margin fit of CEREC CAD/CAM composite crowns using different margin designs. They reported 105 ± 34 μm for a beveled margin, 94 ± 27 μm for a chamfer margin, and 91 ± 22 μm for a shoulder margin using the CEREC 3 system (Tsitrou *et al.*, 2007). Another study reported on the influence of the degree of preparation taper and software luting space setting on the marginal fit of CEREC crowns. The mean marginal gaps ranged from 53 to 67 μm depending on the luting space setting and were not affected by the occlusal convergence angle of the abutment (Nakamura *et al.*, 2003).

The E4D system has been more recently introduced for chairside CAD/CAM restorations and to date, it has limited published research on margin fit and internal adaptation. One study measured the marginal fit of E4D fabricated crowns on typodont preparations completed by 62 different clinicians (Renne *et al.*, 2012). Each of the crown preparations was judged as good, fair, or poor by using both a replica technique and visual examination looking at common criteria for ceramic restorations. The quality of the preparation significantly influenced the accuracy of the margin fit (p <0.05). Ideal preparations had mean margin fits of 38.5 μm, fair preparations had mean margin fits of 58.3 μm, and poor preparations had mean margin fits of 90.1 μm. A second *in vitro* study measured the margin fit and internal adaptation of E4D fabricated e.Max CAD crowns (Plourde *et al.*, 2011). Mean margin fits varied from 79.32 ± 63.18 μm for buccal margins to 50.39 ± 34.98 μm for lingual margins.

Chairside restorative materials

Chairside CAD/CAM restorations are monolithic. This means that the entire restoration is composed of a single material rather than a bilayer restoration consisting of a coping and veneer layer. Monolithic restorations have several unique features. Dental manufacturers produce the monolithic materials resulting in a dense, homogeneous material without porosity or voids, which maximizes the material's physical properties. The restorative materials are delivered in a solid block form on a milling mandrel specific to the chairside CAD/CAM milling chamber. Current milling systems utilize a subtractive wet-grinding process to shape or mill the desired restoration contour from the preformed blocks based on the volumetric design created with the software program. These materials can be efficiently milled in a time period suitable for delivery at the same appointment the tooth is prepared, imaged, and designed. Post-milling handling time is a key consideration for the investment required for some of the restorative block materials.

There are a number of categories of restorative materials available for chairside CAD/CAM restorations (Fasbinder, 2010; Fasbinder *et al.*, 2012a) (Table 4.1). Each of these categories of materials offer unique features designed for their specific clinical applications. The chairside CAD/CAM system represents the process by which these materials are fabricated into a restoration, while the clinical outcome of the restoration is primarily determined by the choice of the restorative material. Esthetic ceramic materials contain a glass component and have very good translucency and moderate flexural strength. Vitablocs Mark II (Vident) and CEREC Blocs (Sirona Dental Systems) are feldspathic glass ceramics. Both materials are fine-grained, homogeneous feldspathic porcelain with an average particle size of 4 μm. The small particle size allows for a high gloss finish and minimizes abrasive wear of the opposing dentition. IPS Empress CAD (Ivoclar) is a 35–45% leucite-reinforced glass-ceramic similar to IPS Empress 1 but with a finer particle size of 1–5 μm. The presence of the glass component in these materials permits them to be etched with hydrofluoric acid, treated with a silane coupler, and adhesively bonded to the tooth using resin

Table 4.1   Chairside CAD/CAM restorative materials.

Material	Brand	Surface Preparation
Adhesive ceramic leucite-reinforced	IPS EmpressCAD (Ivoclar)	60 sec HFI acid etch; silanate
Adhesive ceramic feldspathic	Vita Mark II (Vident) Sirona Blocs (Sirona)	60 sec HFI acid etch; silanate
High-strength ceramic lithium disilicate	IPS emaxCAD (Ivoclar)	20 sec HFI acid etch; silanate
Hybrid ceramic	Enamic (Vident)	60 sec HFI acid etch; silanate
Nano-ceramic	Lava Ultimate (3M ESPE)	Air abrasion 30–50 μm silica; silanate
Composite	Paradigm MZ100 (3M ESPE)	Air abrasion 30–50 μm silica; silanate
Temporary acrylic	TelloCAD (Ivoclar) Vita CAD-Temp (Vident)	Air abrasion 30–50 μm silica; silanate

All materials are available for both E4D and CEREC systems expect Vita materials that are restricted to the CEREC system.

cement. Adhesive bonding of these materials is critical to their long-term success, as they do not have sufficient strength to permit conventional cementation with either resin modified glass ionomer or traditional glass ionomer cements. The adhesive bonding not only provides retention for the restoration but also contributes to the clinical strength of the restoration to resist fracture.

IPS e.Max CAD (Ivoclar) offers a substantial increase in flexural strength and fracture toughness compared to esthetic ceramic materials. It consists of 0.2–1.0 μm lithium metasilicate crystals with approximately 40% crystals by volume. This partially crystallized "soft" state allows the block to be easily milled without excessive diamond bur wear or damage to the material. After the lithium disilicate restoration is milled, it must undergo a two-stage firing process in a porcelain oven under vacuum to complete the crystallization of the lithium disilicate. This creates a glass ceramic with a fine grain size of approximately 1.5 μm and a 70% crystal volume incorporated in a glass matrix.

Recently introduced nanoceramic and hybrid ceramic materials purport to offer the benefits of easy handling similar to composite materials, with the strength and surface finish of ceramics. Lava Ultimate (3M ESPE) contains silica particles of 20 nm, zirconia particles of 4–11 nm, and agglomerated nano-sized particles of silica and zirconia all embedded in a highly cross-linked polymer matrix. The aggregated clusters are comprised of 20 nm silica and 4–11 nm zirconia particles, with approximately an 80% ceramic load. Vita Enamic (Vident) is comprised of a dual-network structure where ceramic and polymer are merged together. The manufacturer claims that this material incorporates the benefits of ceramic and composite materials in one product offering both strength and elasticity; therefore, it is being advocated for its crack prevention capability. In addition, the polymer network may contribute to reduced brittleness in comparison to a pure dental ceramic.

Two types of composite resin blocks are also available for use in chairside CAD/CAM applications. One type is designed for final restorations, and the other type is used for long-term provisional restorations. Paradigm MZ100 (3M/ESPE) is a composite block based on the Z100 composite chemistry and relies on a proprietary processing technique to maximize the degree of cross-linking (Rusin, 2001). Paradigm MZ100 has zirconia-silica filler particles and is 85% filled by weight with an average particle size of 0.6 μm. It is radiopaque and available in six shades and is recommended for definitive composite restoration applications. CAD/CAM provisional blocks are available for chairside fabrication of long-term crowns and fixed partial dentures. The CAD/CAM process avoids an air-inhibited layer on conventional self-cure or VLC acrylics as well as polymerization shrinkage. Vita CAD-Temp blocks (Vident) is a highly cross-linked, microfilled polymer that is available in extended block sizes including 40 mm and 55 mm lengths to accommodate multiple unit FPDs. Telio CAD (Ivoclar) is a millable cross-linked polymethyl methacrylate (PMMA) block for provisional crowns and FPDs. The block is part of the Telio System that includes a self-curing composite, desensitizer, and cement. It is available in 40 and 55 mm size blocks and in six shades.

Clinical longevity

The clinical survival rate of chairside CAD/CAM generated restorations has been used as a measure of their clinical performance. Long-term randomized clinical trials are considered the most robust study design to properly address the state of the evidence in clinical research. The random allocation procedure used in those studies minimizes biases, therefore, balancing out both known and unknown confounders and assuring a fair distribution of treatments among patients. Alternatively, retrospective studies may generate large datasets in a short amount of time as they are generally done by collecting data from past records, rather than following patients (restorations) over time. However, these studies are unable to be standardized and therefore result in a great degree of inaccuracy and inherent biases. Irrespective of the type of study, the most common clinical evaluation methods used to access the status of the restorations are the United States Public Health Service (USPHS) criteria or a modified version of them. Several restoration characteristics are evaluated and followed over time, including shade match, margin discoloration, anatomic form, margin finish, margin adaptation, surface finish, recurrent caries, and tooth or restoration fractures.

A small percentage of chairside CAD/CAM generated restorations may develop postoperative sensitivity; however, most clinical studies report resolution of sensitivity after the initial observations without treatment. The sensitivity is generally mild and tends to be within the expected range for large cavity preparations. Irreversible pulpitis is a rare finding and can generally be attributed to extensive tooth damage preoperatively. Similarly, the reported incidence of recurrent caries around margins of chairside CAD/CAM generated restorations tends to be low. This may be attributed to the careful inclusion criteria used in those studies, generally selecting populations with a current need for large restoration replacements, but otherwise stable. Therefore,

most of the relevant data in the literature tends to focus on surface changes such as anatomic form retention, quality of the surface finish, and early signs of material chipping or fracture as well as margin characteristics such as increased margin detection and discoloration over time.

There is a plentitude of articles that report on the long-term clinical performance of CEREC restorations, which contrasts with a significant lack of clinical evidence on other chairside systems. This is partially due to the fact that the CEREC System has been available since the early 1990s, whereas other systems have been more recently introduced. Clinical studies of the earlier versions of the software have been previously reviewed and include papers published between 1991 and 2006 (Fasbinder, 2006). A systematic review of 29 clinical studies, which included a total of 2,862 CEREC ceramic inlays, reported a survival rate of 97.4% after a period of 4.2 years (Martin and Jedynakiewicz, 1999). The primary mode of failure was fracture of the ceramic restoration. Less common failure modes included fracture of the tooth, wear of the cement, and postoperative sensitivity. More recently another systematic review focused on survival rates of longer-term clinical trials (Wittneben et al., 2009). A total of 1,957 single-tooth restorations fabricated with CAD/CAM technology were followed for more than 3 years of functional service. Among the data of the 16 studies evaluated, 48% of the restorations were prospectively analyzed and 52% were studied retrospectively for a mean exposure time of 7.9 years. The calculated failure rate was 1.75% per year estimated per 100 restoration years (95% CI 1.22–2.52%), based on the reported survival rate of 91.6% after 5 years. The most common modes of failure reported were fractures of the restoration or tooth. Moreover, restorations fabricated with feldspathic porcelain had the highest 5-year survival rate, in contrast with the lowest 5-year survival rate calculated for glass-ceramic restorations.

Among the CEREC literature, several of the studies published data on CAD/CAM generated feldspathic porcelain or Vitablocs Mark II restorations. Posselt and Kerschbaum conducted a study of 2,328 inlays and onlays for 794 patients in a private practice and they reported 35 failures over 9 years (Posselt and Kerschbaum, 2003). The

Kaplan–Meier survival probability reported was 97.4% at 5 years and 94.5% at 9 years. Another study reported a Kaplan–Meier survival probability of 90.4% after 10 years for 200 Vitablocs Mark II restorations placed in 108 patients in private practice (Otto and De Nisco, 2002). In a follow-up report of that study, the authors reported an 88.7% success rate at 17 years (Otto and Schneider, 2008). From 1991 to 2006, a series of papers reported the clinical status of 1,011 CEREC restorations for up to 18 years (Reiss and Walther, 1991; Reiss and Walther, 2000; Reiss, 2006). After 5 years, the survival probability was 95% and after 7 years, it was 91.6%. At 10 years, the survival probability was 90% and it declined to 84.9% at 16.7 years. Federlin and colleagues published 2- and 3-year data on the clinical performance of 29 Vitabloc Mark II CEREC onlays paired against cast gold onlays in a split-mouth study design (Federlin et al., 2006). Only one ceramic onlay fractured and two presented small porcelain chipping by the 2-year follow-up. Even though the 3-year failure rate of ceramic onlays increased to 6.9%, no significant differences were found in survival rates between onlays fabricated with either Vitabloc Mark II or cast gold. The only significant difference reported was in margin adaptation, but the authors concluded that chairside ceramic onlays meet the American Association Acceptance Guidelines criteria (10% failure) for posterior tooth-colored restorative materials (Federlin et al., 2006; Federlin et al., 2007). Similar survival rates were reported in a clinical study in which dental students placed 60 Vitabloc Mark II CEREC inlays after instruction and training that included 15 hours of an interactive computer-based CEREC course. Four failures were reported after 2 years (6.7% failure rate) as follows: two teeth needed endodontic treatment (within the first 6 months), one onlay fractured and one inlay received a failing score due to insufficient marginal adaptation. Additionally, no secondary caries was observed and no statistically significant changes were recorded for color match, surface texture, and anatomic form. Another common finding between this and similar studies was the gradual and not statistical significant increase of "bravo" ratings for marginal adaptation and marginal discoloration over time (Wrbas et al., 2007). Slightly higher failure rate was reported when dental students with minimal experience

fabricated 20 CEREC endo-crowns using Vitablocs Mark II. Failures were recorded at 12 month (tooth and restoration fracture) and at 18 months (localized insufficient porcelain thickness) and amounted to 10% of the restorations. Margin discoloration and insipient margin gap formation increased in proportion to observation time. The calculated Kaplan–Meier survival rate of CEREC endo-crowns was 96% at 12 months and 90% after 2 years (Bernhart et al., 2010). In contrast, a longer-term study evaluated the longitudinal performance of 310 CEREC onlays. One operator placed all restorations and special attention was given to keep preparation margins within enamel whenever possible. After 8 years of follow-up, 286 paired onlays were available for evaluation and the calculated survival probability was 99.3%. The only two fractures observed in this study were on maxillary premolars of one patient with occlusal parafunction (Arnetzl and Arnetzl, 2012). Another study looked at the clinical performance of paired onlays fabricated by fourth-year dental students in a prospective randomized controlled clinical trial of Vitabloc Mark II onlays that were cemented with a self-adhesive cement (RelyX Unicem, 3M ESPE) (Schenke et al., 2012). The influence of selective enamel etching was also evaluated so each patient had one onlay cemented with the self-etch technique and the other one after selective etching. Statistically significant changes were observed for marginal adaptation and marginal discoloration between baseline and 2 years, but no statistically significant difference was recorded between the two different cementation groups. The authors concluded that selective enamel etching did not significantly influence the results (two onlays de-bonded, one from each group; two onlays fractured from the self-etch group). Two long-term clinical trials indicated that failures tend to continue to happen at a slow rate over time. In the first study, there was no intent to standardize the preparations, as the purpose was to evaluate the long-term clinical performance of extensive chairside all-ceramic restorations in general (Roggendorf et al., 2012). Therefore several restoration designs were included such as onlays, crowns (standard, reduced, implant, and endo-crowns) and veneers using two different CAD/CAM block materials (Vitablocs Mark II and

ProCAD). At the 7-year follow-up, 59 of the original 78 restorations were available for evaluation using modified USPHS criteria. A total of eight failures resulted in a 7-year survival rate of 86.9% and a calculated annual failure rate of 1.9%. No significant influence of the extension of the restorations or type of ceramic material was reported. The second long-term study was a randomized clinical trial designed to access the longitudinal performance of 80 inlays milled with either a composite block material (Paradigm MZ100, 3M ESPE) or feldspathic ceramic (Vitablocs Mark II) cemented with a dual-cured resin cement (RelyX ARC, 3M ESPE) after total etch technique (Fasbinder *et al.*, 2013b). At the 10-year recall, 71 inlays were available for evaluation. No significant difference in margin adaptation between the two materials was evident after 10 years; however, a significant decrease in margin adaptation was noted when both materials were compared to baseline due to margin wear of the adhesive luting cement. Fewer fractures were noted in the composite group with a calculated survival rate of 95% for Paradigm MZ100 inlays versus 87.5% for Vitablocs Mark II. Given the length of the observation, the calculated annual failure rates were 0.5% for composite inlays and 1.25% for ceramic inlays, thus reflecting continued but low failure rates for CAD/CAM inlays over time.

A few published clinical studies are available specifically on leucite-reinforced CAD/CAM restorations. Guess *et al.* reported a prospective clinical investigation on the survival rate and long-term behavior of IPS e.Max Press and Pro-CAD molar onlay restorations (Guess *et al.*, 2009). The Kaplan–Meier survivability at 3 years was 97% for the ProCAD onlays and 100% for the IPS e.Max Press onlays. Only one ProCAD onlay fractured and authors concluded that wear of the resin cement at the occlusal margin was a critical factor in the long-term success of the restorations. Another randomized clinical study that included leucite-reinforced and feldspathic CEREC onlays cemented with a self-etching, self-adhesive resin cement reported no significant differences in the clinical performance between the two materials at 3 years (Fasbinder *et al.*, 2011). This trend continued to be observed at the 5-year follow-up (Fasbinder *et al.*, 2013a). According to USPHS criteria, there was no significant difference in

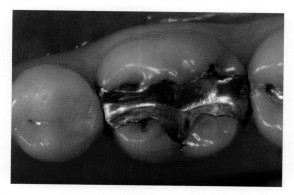

Figure 4.3 Preoperative view of tooth #30.

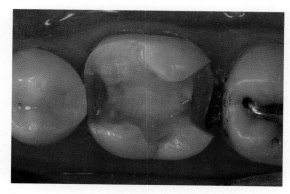

Figure 4.4 Onlay preparation for chairside CAD/CAM onlay #30.

margin adaptation between the two materials at 5 years or when results were compared to baseline values (Figures 4.3–4.7).

A more discriminative criterion was then applied for margin adaptation in an attempt to capture early trends in margin wear. Alpha-1 was used when margins were nondetectable, alpha-2 when the detectable margins were noted in less than 50% of the occlusal margin and alpha-3 when a significant catch was recorded in more than 50% of the occlusal margin. An increased trend for localized crevice formation was noted over time and a significant difference was found between baseline and 5-year data for both materials when the more discriminative criterion was applied.

There are few clinical studies on IPS e.Max CAD. A previously mentioned study by Guess and colleagues on the survival rate and long-term

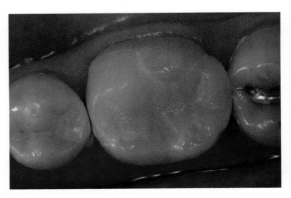

Figure 4.5 Immediate delivery of leucite-reinforced chairside ceramic onlay (Paradigm C) at preparation appointment.

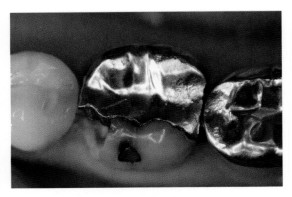

Figure 4.8 Preoperative view of tooth #19.

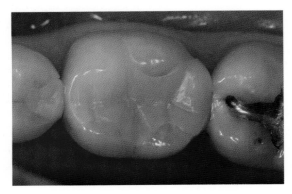

Figure 4.6 Three year recall of the leucite-reinforced chairside ceramic onlay (Paradigm C) for #30.

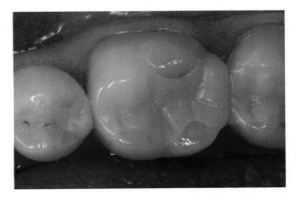

Figure 4.7 Five year recall of the leucite-reinforced chairside ceramic onlay (Paradigm C) for #30.

behavior of IPS e.Max Press and ProCAD molar onlay restorations reported a Kaplan–Meier survivability at 3 years of 100% for the IPS e.Max Press onlays (Guess *et al.*, 2009). Reich and coworkers reported a clinical study on the performance of chairside-generated CAD/CAM e.max CAD crowns (Reich *et al.*, 2010). A CEREC system was used to deliver 41 e.Max CAD full-contour crowns in 34 patients. After 2 years, one crown exhibited secondary caries and two crowns received root canal treatment. An ongoing longitudinal clinical study is evaluating the clinical performance of 100 IPS e.Max CAD full-contour crowns (Fasbinder *et al.*, 2010; Fasbinder *et al.*, 2012a). The first 62 crowns were delivered with a self-etching bonding agent and resin cement or a self-adhesive resin cement. A second group of 38 crowns was placed at a later time using a newer self-etching, self-curing cement. Each of the full-contour crowns was placed in a single treatment appointment with the CEREC system. There were no reported crown failures after 2 years (100% survival rate) and no chipping or cracking were clinically visible. Five-year data is currently being gathered in this study and these trends continue to be observed (Figures 4.8–4.11).

Summary

In summary, the current state of the evidence on the clinical performance of CAD/CAM generated restorations is favorable and indicates that these restorations perform predictably well in the clinical setting. Adhesive retention of these

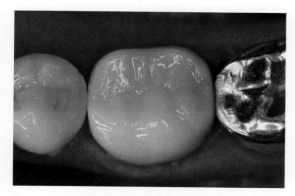

Figure 4.9 Immediate delivery of chairside CAD/CAM lithium disilicate crown (IPS e.MaxCAD) at the preparation appointment.

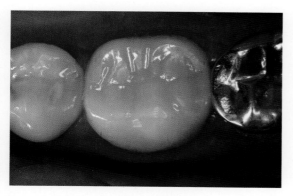

Figure 4.10 Three year recall of the chairside CAD/CAM lithium disilicate crown (IPS e.MaxCAD) for tooth #19.

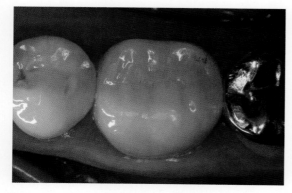

Figure 4.11 Five year recall of the chairside CAD/CAM lithium disilicate crown (IPS e.MaxCAD) for tooth #19.

restorations does not seem to be a significant issue when careful luting technique is followed. The incidence of postoperative sensitivity and recurrent caries is generally an insignificant finding. Margin adaptation is initially very good; however, there is a tendency for increase in margin discontinuity and discoloration over time as a function of the wear of the resin luting cement. A small tendency for material chipping and fracture may happen over time but failures tend to be within the acceptable range according to the American Association Acceptance Guidelines criteria.

The clinical application of computerized technology is one of the most significant developments for restorative dentistry in recent years. Laboratory and clinical evidence confirms the accuracy of the digital process. And a number of clinical studies have documented the clinical success and durability of the restorations. Ongoing developments of computerized systems continue to expand the clinical applications to multiple unit restorations and implants. Success with digital impressions is still dependent on mastering similar skills required for conventional impressions, such as achieving optimal soft tissue retraction and moisture control, which enable accurate image acquisition and data recording.

References

Arnetzl, G.V. & Arnetzl, G. (2012) Reliability of nonretentive all-ceramic CAD/CAM overlays. *International Journal of Computerized Dentistry*, **15**, 185–197.

Bernhart, J., Bräuning, A., & Altenburger, M.J., *et al.* (2010) Cerec3D endocrowns–two-year clinical examination of CAD/CAM crowns for restoring endodontically treated molars. *International Journal of Computerized Dentistry*, **13**, 141–154.

Beuer, F., Schweiger, J., & Edelhoff, D. (2008) Digital dentistry: an overview of recent developments for CAD/CAM generated restorations. *British Dental Journal*, **204**, 505–511.

Brawek, P.K., Wolfart, S., & Endres, L., *et al.* (2013) The clinical accuracy of single crowns exclusively fabricated by digital workflow–the comparison of two systems. *Clinical Oral Investigations*, **17**, 2119–2125.

Ellingsen, L.A. & Fasbinder, D.J. (2002) In vitro evaluation of CAD/CAM ceramic crowns. *Journal of Dental Research*, (Special Issue A), 2640.

Ender, A. & Mehl, A. (2011) Full arch scans: conventional versus digital impressions--an in-vitro study. *International Journal of Computerized Dentistry*, **14**, 11–21.

Estafan, D., Dussetschleger, F., & Agosta, C., *et al.* (2003) Scanning electron microscope evaluation of CEREC II and CEREC III inlays. *General Dentistry*, **51**, 450–454.

Fasbinder, D.J. (2006) Clinical performance of chairside CAD/CAM restorations. *The Journal of the American Dental Association*, **137**(Suppl), 22S–31S.

Fasbinder, D.J. (2009) Digital workflow for the LAVA COS system. *Insite Dentistry*, 114–117.

Fasbinder, D.J. (2010) Materials for chairside CAD/CAM restorations. *Compend Contin Educ Dent*, **31**, 702–4. 706, 708

Fasbinder, D.J., Dennison, J.B., & Heys, D., *et al.* (2010) A clinical evaluation of chairside lithium disilicate CAD/CAM crowns: a two-year report. *The Journal of the American Dental Association*, **141**(Suppl 2), 10S–14S.

Fasbinder, D.J., Dennison, J.B., & Heys, D., *et al.* (2012a) Clinical evaluation of lithium disilicate chairside CAD/CAM crowns at 4 years. *Journal of Dental Research*, **91**, 645.

Fasbinder, D.J., Neiva, G.F., & Dennison, J., *et al.* (2011) Clinical evaluation of CAD/CAM-generated ceramic onlays. *Journal of Dental Research*, **90**, 378.

Fasbinder, D.J., Neiva, G.F., & Dennison, J.B., *et al.* (2013a) Clinical evaluation of CAD/CAM-generated ceramic onlays: 5-year report. *Journal of Dental Research*, **92**, 177.

Fasbinder, D.J. (2012b) Evaluation of zirconia crowns made from conventional and digital impressions. *Journal of Dental Research*, **91**, 644.

Fasbinder, D.J., Neiva, G.F., & Dennison, J.B., *et al.* (2013b) Clinical performance of CAD/CAM-generated composite inlays after 10 years. *Journal of Cosmetic Dentistry*, **28**, 135–144.

Federlin, M., Männer, T., & Hiller, K., *et al.* (2006) Two-year clinical performance of cast gold vs ceramic partial crowns. *Clinical Oral Investigations*, **10**, 126–133.

Federlin, M., Wagner, J., & Männer, K., *et al.* (2007) Three-year clinical performance of cast gold vs ceramic partial crowns. *Clinical Oral Investigations*, **11**, 345–352.

Guess, P.C., Strub, J.R., & Steinhart, N., *et al.* (2009) All-ceramic partial coverage restorations--midterm results of a 5-year prospective clinical splitmouth study. *Journal of Dentistry*, **37**, 627–637.

Kugel, G., Chaimattayompol, N., & Perry, R., *et al.* (2008) Comparison of digital vs. conventional impression systems for marginal accuracy. *Journal of Dental Research*, **87**, 1119.

Levine, N. (2009) To the sky and beyond. *Dental Products Report*, 116.

Martin, N. & Jedynakiewicz, N.M. (1999) Clinical performance of CEREC ceramic inlays: a systematic review. *Dental Materials*, **15**, 54–61.

Martin, N. & Jedynakiewicz, N.M. (2000) Interface dimensions of CEREC-2 MOD inlays. *Dental Materials*, **16**, 68–74.

Mormann, W.H. (2006) The evolution of the CEREC system. *The Journal of the American Dental Association*, **137**(Suppl), 7S–13S.

Nakamura, T., Dei, N., & Kojima, T., *et al.* (2003) Marginal and internal fit of Cerec 3 CAD/CAM all-ceramic crowns. *The International Journal of Prosthodontics*, **16**, 244–248.

Ogledzki, M., Wenzel, K., & Doherty, E., *et al.* (2011) Accuracy of 3M-Brontes stereolithography models compared to plaster models. *Journal of Dental Research*, **90**, 1060.

Otto, T. & De Nisco, S. (2002) Computer-aided direct ceramic restorations: a 10-year prospective clinical study of Cerec CAD/CAM inlays and onlays. *The International Journal of Prosthodontics*, **15**, 122–128.

Otto, T. & Schneider, D. (2008) Long-term clinical results of chairside Cerec CAD/CAM inlays and onlays: a case series. *The International Journal of Prosthodontics*, **21**, 53–59.

Plourde, J., Harsono, M., & Fox, L., *et al.* (2011) Marginal and internal fit of E4D CAD/CAM all-ceramic crowns. *Journal of Dental Research*, **90**, 638.

Posselt, A. & Kerschbaum, T. (2003) Longevity of 2328 chairside Cerec inlays and onlays. *International Journal of Computerized Dentistry*, **6**, 231–248.

Poticny, D. & Fasbinder, D.J. (2011) Accuracy of digital model articulation. *Journal of Dental Research*, **90**, 131.

Reich, S., Fischer, S., & Sobotta, B., *et al.* (2010) A preliminary study on the short-term efficacy of chairside computer-aided design/computer-assisted manufacturing- generated posterior lithium disilicate crowns. *The International Journal of Prosthodontics*, **23**, 214–216.

Reiss, B. (2006) Clinical results of Cerec inlays in a dental practice over a period of 18 years. *International Journal of Computerized Dentistry*, **9**, 11–22.

Reiss, B. & Walther, W. (1991) Survival analysis and clinical evaluation of CEREC restorations in a private practice. In: International Symposium on Computer Restorations, p. 214. Quintessence, Berlin.

Reiss, B. & Walther, W. (2000) Clinical long-term results and 10-year Kaplan-Meier analysis of Cerec restorations. *International Journal of Computerized Dentistry*, **3**, 9–23.

Renne, W., McGill, S.T., & Forshee, K.V., *et al.* (2012) Predicting marginal fit of CAD/CAM crowns based on the presence or absence of common preparation errors. *The Journal of Prosthetic Dentistry*, **108**, 310–315.

Roggendorf, M.J., Kunzi, B., & Ebert, J., *et al.* (2012) Seven-year clinical performance of CEREC-2 all-ceramic CAD/CAM restorations placed within deeply destroyed teeth. *Clinical Oral Investigations*, **16**, 1413–1424.

Rusin, R.P. (2001) Properties and applications of a new composite block for CAD/CAM. *The Compendium of Continuing Education in Dentistry*, **22**, 35–41.

Schenke, F., Federlin, M., & Hiller, K.A., *et al.* (2012) Controlled, prospective, randomized, clinical evaluation of partial ceramic crowns inserted with RelyX Unicem with or without selective enamel etching. Results after 2 years. *Clinical Oral Investigations*, **16**, 451–461.

Scotti, R., Cardelli, P., & Baldissara, P., *et al.* (2011) Clinical fitting of CAD/CAM zirconia single crowns generated from digital intraoral impressions based on active wavefront sampling. *The Journal of Dentistry*, In Press.

Seelbach, P., Brueckel, C., & Wostmann, B. (2013) Accuracy of digital and conventional impression techniques and workflow. *Clinical Oral Investigations*, **17**, 1759–1764.

Syrek, A., Reich, G., & Ranftl, D., *et al.* (2010) Clinical evaluation of all-ceramic crowns fabricated from intraoral digital impressions based on the principle of active wavefront sampling. *Journal of Dentistry*, **38**, 553–559.

Tsitrou, E.A., Northeast, S.E., & van Noort, R. (2007) Evaluation of the marginal fit of three margin designs of resin composite crowns using CAD/CAM. *Journal of Dentistry*, **35**, 68–73.

Wittneben, J.G., Wright, R.F., & Weber, H.P., *et al.* (2009) A systematic review of the clinical performance of CAD/CAM single-tooth restorations. *The International Journal of Prosthodontics*, **22**, 466–471.

Wrbas, K.T., Hein, N., & Schirrmeister, J.F., *et al.* (2007) Two-year clinical evaluation of Cerec 3D ceramic inlays inserted by undergraduate dental students. *Quintessence International*, **38**, 575–581.

5 Digital Fixed Prosthodontics

Julie Holloway

Introduction

The introduction of CAD/CAM technology for simple intraoral imaging and restoration milling has exploded far beyond its initial application. Development of milling machines that could mill both complex external and internal geometries has broadened the scope of CAD/CAM technology from simple inlays/onlays to the entire realm of fixed prosthodontics. Since multi-axis milling was introduced for dental applications, development of high-strength materials specifically designed for CAD/CAM manufacturing of full coverage and multiunit restorations has not been far behind. In addition, the resolution and ease of use of intraoral cameras have now evolved so that an entire arch, rather than only a few teeth, can be scanned in a matter of minutes.

However, for dentists already skilled in analog techniques, the move to digital technologies comes at a cost in equipment, software, and time for training. The increased efficiencies gained in dental treatment by a move to digital processes can offset the costs, both for practitioners and for dental laboratories. In addition, the practitioners have many options in how they incorporate these technological advances into their practice's workflow (Figure 5.1).

Intraoral scans are made into physical casts or left as digital casts for computer-assisted modeling of future restoration(s) (Figure 5.2a, b). The final restoration is milled directly from ceramic or alloy for single restorations or milled from presintered/pattern materials that allow for more complex multiunit restorations to be indirectly fabricated (Figure 5.3). For dental laboratories, CAD/CAM technology allows increased standardization of the design and fabrication process. The wide variety of materials and techniques allow practitioners and laboratory technicians to choose the best method and best material to suit the functional and esthetic requirements of each patient.

CAD/CAM materials for the production of fixed restorations

Materials available for the fabrication of fixed restorations can be categorized in several different ways: by strength, composition, purpose, and fabrication method. There are basically three

Clinical Applications of Digital Dental Technology, First Edition. Edited by Radi Masri and Carl F. Driscoll.
© 2015 John Wiley & Sons, Inc. Published 2015 by John Wiley & Sons, Inc.

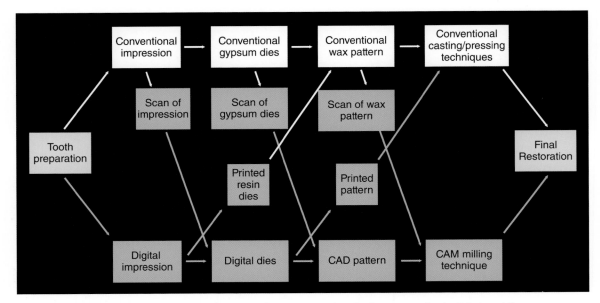

Figure 5.1 Possible workflow combinations from entirely conventional methods to a completely digital workflow.

applications for CAD/CAM materials: die materials, pattern materials, and restoration materials.

Die materials

Dies for the fabrication of fixed restorations must fulfill the following requirements:

- They must be an exact reproduction of the prepared tooth's geometry,
- They must be free from voids and distortions,
- They must capture the entire tooth preparation, as well as the area 0.5–1.0 mm apical to the finish line,
- They must allow adequate access and visualization of the margin.

Definitive dies are conventionally fabricated from gypsum poured into elastomeric impressions of prepared teeth. They have the advantages of being inexpensive, quick and easy to produce, and dimensionally accurate. However, dies fabricated from gypsum materials possess relatively poor abrasion resistance and care must be taken to avoid incorporation of air during mixing to avoid voids in the final die. Dies can also be fabricated from a digital impression, the advantage of which

being able to digitally manipulate, store, and share them easily with other dental professionals and laboratories (Figure 5.4). If there is a desire to convert a digital impression in to an analog die, there are currently two methods: computer-aided machining of resin and printing of resin. Either method can produce dies that possess high strength and good abrasion resistance.

Pattern materials

Patterns for cast alloy and pressed all-ceramic fixed restorations are usually formed free hand from wax. Wax is a weak material that is prone to distortion due to handling and temperature variations. Patterns can be fabricated from digital data as well, designed on a computer and then either milled from wax (Figure 5.5) or resin blanks or printed in resin. Large blanks can allow several patterns to be milled in one milling session (Figure 5.6a, b). The advantage of resin CAD/CAM patterns is that they are strong and insensitive to temperature variations. They can be useful for fabrication of large or complex frameworks, where small distortions in a connector could affect the fit of the entire framework. They can also be used as CAD/CAM patterns for

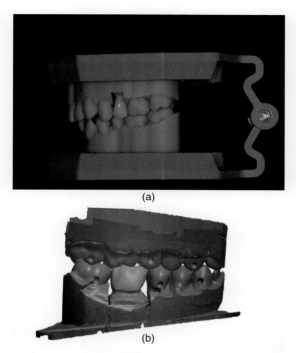

(a)

(b)

Figure 5.2 (a) Printed resin cast with CAD/CAM ceramic crown. (Courtesy Dr. David G. Gratton.)
(b) Digital cast with virtually designed crown.

veneering frameworks when pressable ceramics are pressed onto CAD/CAM substructures.

Restorative materials

Materials for fabrication of fixed restorations solely by the CAD/CAM process are produced by milling blocks of commercially produced material. Compared to restorations fabricated by hand in a dental laboratory, the blanks are produced under controlled conditions to increase the materials' homogeneity and reduce voids and inclusions, which weaken the material. The types of materials for CAD/CAM production of definitive restorations include:

- Composite
- Composite/ceramic hybrids
- Ceramics
- Glass-ceramics
- Alloys

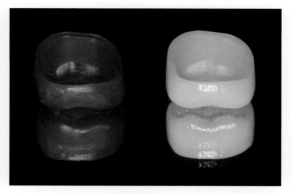

Figure 5.3 CAD/CAM wax pattern to be used with a conventional casting technique and CAD/CAM full contour zirconia crown.

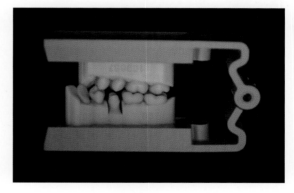

Figure 5.4 Printed resin die for fixed prosthodontics. (Courtesy Dr. David G. Gratton.)

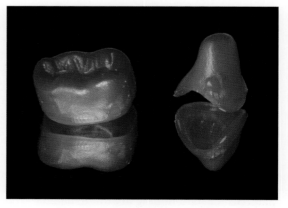

Figure 5.5 Milled wax patterns, full contour (left) and coping (right).

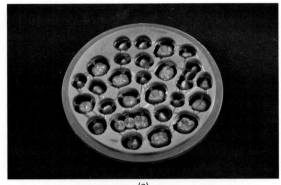

(a)

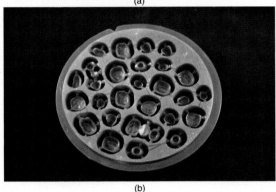

(b)

Figure 5.6 (a) Milled wax patterns, occlusal aspect. (b) Milled wax patterns, intaglio aspect.

Materials for CAD/CAM fixed restorations can be produced by either hard milling or soft milling. Hard milling is described as the milling of a restoration from a blank of material that is already in its final microstructural form. Once the milling is complete, the final restoration need only be polished or glazed prior to cementation. Soft milling refers to milling of a material in a "green" form that must undergo further heat treatments in order to produce its final microstructure and mechanical properties. This usually requires additional laboratory support for heat treatment and staining or layering with additional ceramics.

Hard milling

Materials for hard milling are those materials that are milled in their final state, no further heat treatments are necessary to transform the material into its final hardness and strength. They are generally milled at full contour, and the only treatments necessary after milling are polishing and/or staining and glazing. The types of hard milled materials consist of composites, composite/ceramic hybrids, and some ceramics. These materials are most often employed for the fabrication of single unit restorations using a dental milling machine (Figure 5.7a, b) see also Chapter 3.

Composites

Composites are resins reinforced with particles of inorganic filler. They are soft and easy to mill. However, their disadvantages include: low wear resistance, propensity for marginal microleakage, and questionable long-term color stability compared to ceramics. Newer composites for CAD/CAM applications are being produced with

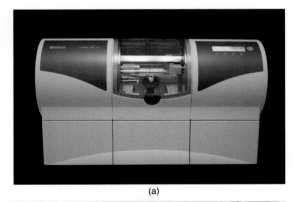

(a)

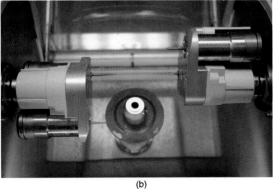

(b)

Figure 5.7 (a) Dental milling machine. (b) Milling chamber of dental milling machine.

higher filler content, which improves mechanical properties and reduces the disadvantages listed earlier. These materials represent a low-cost alternative for limited use as a definitive single tooth, full-coverage restoration or as a durable provisional restoration. Recent introduction of very highly filled "resin nano ceramic" is garnering interest (Koller *et al.*, 2012), with the manufacturer even offering a 10 year warranty against breakage.

Ceramics

Ceramics produced for in office hard milling applications are generally low to medium in strength. They contain a high glassy matrix content, making them translucent and easy to mill. The high amount of glass renders them brittle and susceptible to fracture at relatively low loads and also makes them prone to chipping in thin areas (margins) during milling, requiring careful examination for flaws prior to cementation. Once the milling is complete, the final restoration should be polished or submitted to a glazing heat treatment prior to cementation to reduce the external surface roughness caused by the milling process. Existing materials for in office hard milling (Figure 5.8) can be classified into three groups by composition of their crystalline phase:

- Feldspar containing ceramics
- Leucite containing ceramics
- Zirconia-reinforced lithium silicate

Feldspar (Figure 5.9) and leucite containing ceramics are the weakest materials (~140 MPa) for full coverage restorations and should be limited to restoration of anterior teeth. Their high glassy content imparts a translucency similar to tooth structure, and therefore, they are also candidates for ceramic veneers. These materials can be etched and silanated prior to luting with a resin cement to provide a strong bond to tooth structure (enamel).

A new type of dental ceramic composition, "zirconia-reinforced lithium silicate," has been recently introduced. It is purported to contain around 10% fine-grained zirconia dispersed within a lithium silicate glass-ceramic (Figure 5.10). The unique property of one manufacturer's version of this material is that it can either be luted

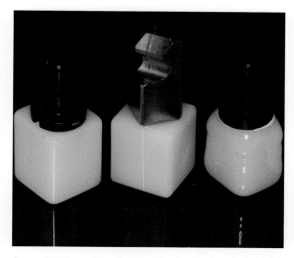

Figure 5.8 Examples of materials for hard-milled restorations (left to right): composite, leucite-reinforced ceramic, zirconia-reinforced lithium silicate ceramic.

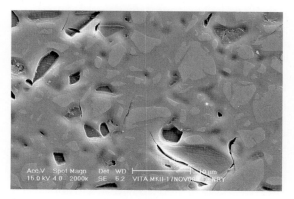

Figure 5.9 Micrograph of a feldspar-containing ceramic. Note the large amount of glassy matrix surrounding the crystalline phase. (Courtesy Dr. Isabelle Denry).

in the as-milled state or after an additional strengthening heat treatment. The material in the as-milled state has reportedly high translucency and low strength (~200 MPa), whereas after a 30 minute heat treatment, the strength increases to around 370 MPa (Larson, 2013). More data will be needed to investigate its properties and clinical performance.

Zirconium oxide (zirconia) ceramics can be fabricated by milling a block of densely sintered

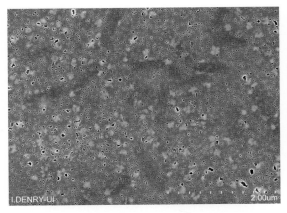

Figure 5.10 Micrograph of a new "zirconia-reinforced lithium silicate" ceramic. (Courtesy Dr. Isabelle Denry.)

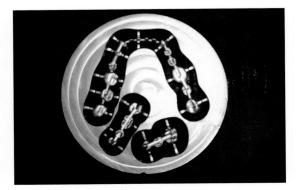

Figure 5.11 Blank of alloy containing milled FDPs. (Courtesy Dr. David G. Gratton.)

material, but are most commonly milled in the soft, partially sintered "green" stage. Hard milling of fully sintered zirconia ceramics was attempted early in their introduction to dentistry; however, it required much more robust milling machines than the "in office" type. The proponents of hard-milled zirconia claimed that margins were more accurate, as the sintering shrinkage had already taken place. Critics of hard-milled zirconia claimed that hard milling could induce flaws and cracks into the material, leading to failure. Tool wear was also an issue when trying to machine such a hard substance, and so explains the decline of hard milling and increasing popularity of soft machining in commercial laboratories. Hard milling of dental zirconia is only mentioned here in a historical context. Hard milling could regain popularity with the advent of advanced milling technologies, such as rotary ultrasonic machining (rotary diamond milling accelerated by piezoelectric ultrasonic vibration).

Alloys

Hard-milled alloys are generally produced by laboratories, utilizing large blanks of alloy to mill out crowns or fixed dental prostheses (FDP) frameworks (Figure 5.11). Titanium and titanium alloy blanks are routinely used for milling out implant abutments and superstructures; however, they have not been routinely used for complete veneer

crowns or FDPs. CAD/CAM milling of titanium and chromium cobalt alloys gives them new popularity, as it overcomes the main issue with cast base metal alloys; poor castability and marginal accuracy. Advantages of base metal alloys are that they are inexpensive relative to gold alloys, have low density but high stiffness and can be conventionally veneered with ceramic. Given the price of gold worldwide, the popularity of base metal alloys is increasing. Noble alloy restorations are not typically milled, due to the initial high expense of the blank and the expense of the unrecovered scrap chips. Other methods for producing alloy restorations include: electric discharge machining (a type of spark erosion milling on a graphite die) and a newly introduced powder metallurgical method by which compressed Co-Cr alloy powder is milled and then sintered, a process similar to zirconia soft milling (Fasbinder *et al.*, 2010).

Soft milling

Materials for soft milling are generally those that cannot be cut easily with diamond burs in their final state, so they are milled prior to final densification. Dental laboratories can produce multiple restorations using automated mills that do not require diamond burs to cut the material (Figure 5.12a, b). The soft, partially sintered "green" or partially crystallized blank is then fully sintered or crystallized by a heat treatment after milling. The sintering of partially sintered green pieces is accompanied by significant (~20%)

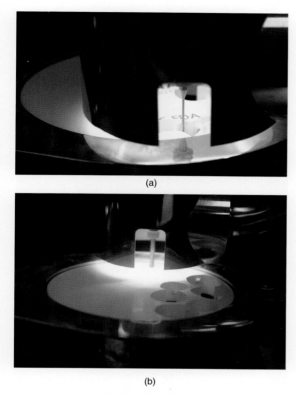

Figure 5.12 (a) Laboratory milling machine. (b) Soft milling of partially sintered zirconia.

shrinkage of the material, whereas crystallization of partially crystallized pieces does not. Due to their opacity, some of these materials may require the application of veneering ceramic to produce acceptable esthetics. These materials can be classified into three groups by composition of their crystalline phase:

- Lithium disilicate glass-ceramics
- Magnesium aluminum oxide-containing ceramics
- Aluminum oxide (alumina)-containing ceramics
- Zirconium oxide (zirconia)-ceramics

Lithium disilicate glass-ceramics are milled in an intermediate "blue" (metasilicate) (Figure 5.13) state then submitted to a tempering heat treatment that completes the (disilicate) crystallization process and almost triples the strength (~360 MPa)

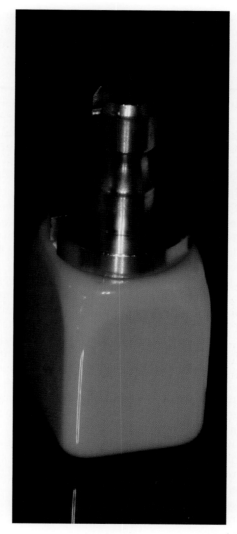

Figure 5.13 Block of pre-crystallized or "blue stage" lithium disilicate.

(Figure 5.14). Lithium disilicate glasses are produced in high and low translucencies (Figure 5.15a, b). This material possesses enough translucency to be suitable for full coverage crowns in the anterior regions. Lithium disilicate possess enough strength for posterior regions (the exception being perhaps second molars). Moreover, there is a block produced for limited 3-unit FDP applications, the most distal abutment should be anterior to the molar region as recommended by the manufacturer (Ivoclar Vivadent).

Magnesium aluminum oxide ceramics (Inceram Spinell) are fabricated by milling a framework in the partially sintered state, sintering at high temperature, infiltrating the porous framework with a low-fusing glass, then veneering with conventional ceramics. The fact that it is the weakest of the soft-machined materials (~280 MPa) is only indicated for production of copings for full coverage restorations and should be limited to restoration of anterior teeth. The glass infiltration step content imparts a translucency similar to lithium disilicate ceramics (Figure 5.16). The advantage of this material is that extensive intrinsic coloration can be achieved when the veneering porcelains are applied. This material can be bonded to tooth structure with Panavia 21 cement.

Aluminum oxide (alumina) ceramics can be fabricated by several methods, by milling:

A framework in the partially sintered state, sintering at high temperature, infiltrating the porous framework with a low-fusing glass, then veneering with conventional ceramics (Inceram Alumina).

A digitally enlarged refractory die, isostatically pressing a coping of alumina powder onto the die, sintering, then veneering with conventional ceramics (Procera Alumina), or a digitally enlarged restoration or framework from a partially sintered blank, then veneering with conventional ceramics.

Alumina-based ceramics are not used without adding an esthetic veneer of porcelain, as they are rather opaque (see Figure 5.16-right). These materials have high strength (~600 MPa) and the advantage of employing extensive intrinsic coloration methods when the veneering porcelains are applied.

An increasingly popular material, soft-milled zirconium oxide (zirconia) ceramics can be fabricated by two methods, by either:

- Milling a digitally enlarged refractory die, isostatically pressing a coping of zirconia powder onto the die, sintering, then veneering with conventional ceramics (Procera Zirconia) or;
- Milling a digitally enlarged restoration or framework from a partially sintered blank.

This requires either the dies or the restoration itself be milled at an increased size to compensate for the sintering shrinkage (Figure 5.17a, b). This

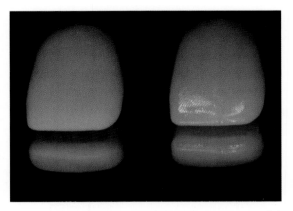

Figure 5.14 Milled "blue stage" lithium disilicate crown (left) and crystallized final crown (right).

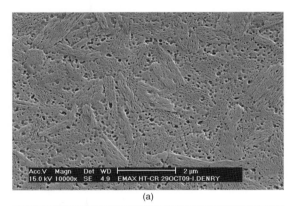

(a)

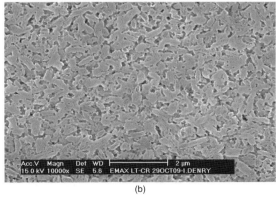

(b)

Figure 5.15 (a) Micrograph of a high-translucency lithium glass-ceramic ceramic. Note the large, but few crystals compared to the low-translucency form. (Courtesy Dr. Isabelle Denry.) (b) Micrograph of a low translucency lithium glass-ceramic ceramic. Note the smaller, but more numerous crystals. (Courtesy Dr. Isabelle Denry.)

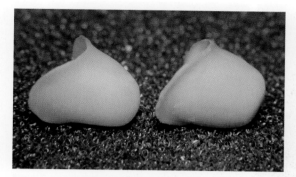

Figure 5.16 Copings made of magnesium aluminum oxide (left) and aluminum oxide (right), note the difference in translucency.

compensation can only be achieved by digital manipulation of the data, so that shrinkage is uniform and volumetrically controlled. Zirconia is a rather opaque material, usually supplied to dental laboratories as chalky white blanks (Figure 5.18 a–d).

Once they are milled to their designed shape, the restoration or framework is either soaked in or painted with in a dyeing liquid to approximate the shade (Figure 5.19). After the milled crown has been shaded with the coloring solution, it is sintered in a high-temperature furnace for several hours (Figure 5.20a, b).

During the sintering process, the zirconia shrinks and becomes much more dense. Since this material has no glassy phase, it is rather opaque (Figure 5.21). Varying the composition and/or sintering temperature can manipulate the translucency of zirconia dental ceramics. Depending on the selected translucency of the zirconia, full contour restorations are now possible for the posterior region without application of an esthetic ceramic veneer. The driving factor in developing more translucent zirconia for full contour zirconia restorations has been the high incidence of chipping associated with veneered zirconia frameworks. Full contour zirconia restorations also save a fabrication step, as no veneering porcelain need be applied and contoured.

In summary, a range of materials can be used to digitally produce restorations without conventional laboratory fabrication methods. These materials vary in their strength and esthetic properties, therefore knowledge of the range

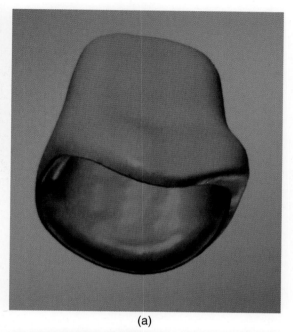

(a)

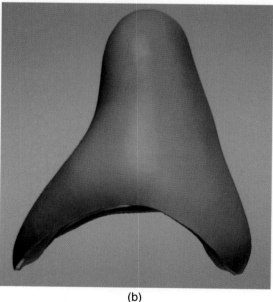

(b)

Figure 5.17 (a) Digital design of enlarged coping for soft milling of zirconia. (b) Digital design of enlarged coping for soft milling of zirconia.

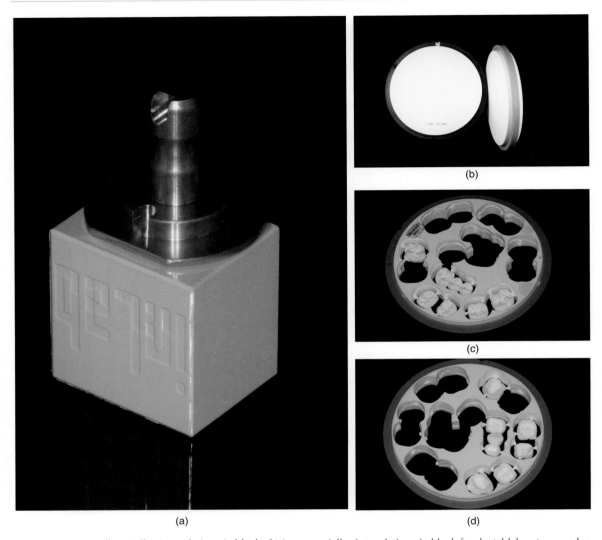

Figure 5.18 (a) Small partially sintered zirconia blank. (b) Large partially sintered zirconia blank for dental laboratory production of multiple units. (c) Milled partially sintered zirconia restorations, occlusal aspect. (d) Milled partially sintered zirconia restorations, intaglio aspect.

of materials and their appropriate application is necessary for longevity and clinical success (Figure 5.22).

Provisional restorations

Provisional crowns or fixed partial dental prostheses where once essential to prosthodontic therapy. Definitive restorations made by conventional laboratory techniques often require a minimum

of 2 weeks to fabricate, causing a delay between tooth preparation and delivery of the final restoration. The period needed for restoration fabrication necessitates placing a provisional crown for maintenance of patient comfort, esthetics, and pulpal health. Now that simple restorations can be fabricated the same day as tooth preparation, provisional crowns are not necessarily fabricated for each prepared tooth as has been done customarily. However, not all clinical situations are amenable to treatment using

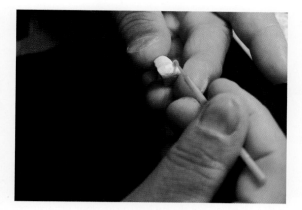

Figure 5.19 Presintering coloration of "green" zirconia.

same-day CAD/CAM restorations and therefore require the use of provisional restorations, such as large reconstructions, evaluation of the effects of changes in occlusion in the presence of a temporomandibular disorder, a planned change in occlusal vertical dimension, or while waiting for healing of pontic or implant sites. For these uses, the use of provisional restorations for a period of time can be extremely useful for patient comfort and feedback prior to fabrication of the restoration(s).

The word provisional prosthesis refers to "a fixed or removable dental prosthesis … designed to enhance esthetics, stabilization and/or function for a limited period of time, after which it is to be replaced by a definitive dental … prosthesis" (Rosenstiel *et al.*, 2006). A former lay term for this type of restoration, a "temporary," can give the impression to the patient that the restoration has little value and does not really serve a purpose. However, if the provisional crown becomes dislodged, the patient may experience pain, inability to chew, and esthetic compromise. If the patient is not bothered by any of the previous signs and symptoms, further complications such as adjacent tooth movement, opposing tooth movement, and pulpal pathosis may complicate or even preclude the delivery of the final prosthesis. A lack of communication with the patient about the purpose of a provisional restoration may reduce treatment efficiency and quality. In addition, lack of attention on the practitioner's part to the requirements of a provisional fixed restoration may also lead to unnecessary repairs, recementation appointments, unnecessary endodontic therapy, and gingival

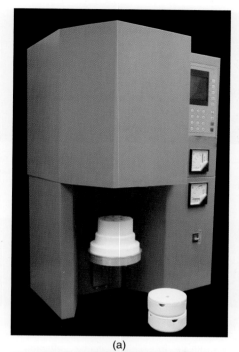

(a)

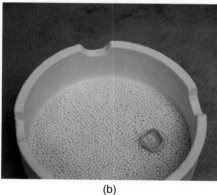

(b)

Figure 5.20 (a) High-temperature laboratory furnace for sintering zirconia restorations. (b) Colored "green" zirconia restoration in a saggar tray ready for sintering.

inflammation, all of which may prevent final impression procedures.

Provisional restorations must fulfill three requirements: biologic, mechanical, and esthetic. Biologic requirements of a provisional fixed prosthesis include protection of the pulp from thermal and bacterial insult, preservation of gingival health with easy access for hygiene procedures, and occlusal compatibility and stability. All of

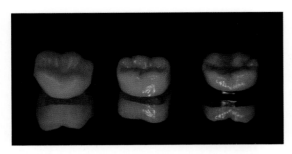

Figure 5.21 Crowns fabricated from CAD/CAM ceramic materials (left to right: Lithium disilicate monolithic ceramic, low-translucency zirconia core veneered with ceramic, conventional metal-ceramic restoration).

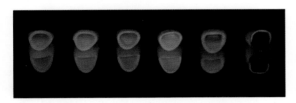

Figure 5.22 Crowns fabricated from CAD/CAM ceramic materials (right to left: Leucite-reinforced monolithic ceramic, Lithium disilicate monolithic ceramic, alumina ceramic core veneered with ceramic, low-translucency zirconia core veneered with ceramic, high-translucency tinted zirconia core veneered with ceramic, conventional metal-ceramic restoration).

these requirements are the responsibility of the dentist to manage appropriately. If a provisional restoration marginal fit does not adequately cover the prepared dentinal tubules, pulpal irritation already begun by the tooth preparation process can continue resulting in pulpitis and possibly endodontic therapy. Marginal and axial contours that impinge upon gingival tissues can cause ischemia or inhibit plaque removal, resulting in gingivitis that can thwart attempts of making an acceptable traditional impression. Recognition and control of compatible occlusal contacts, both static and dynamic, are required to control supereruption of opposing teeth. Supereruption will result in excessive occlusal adjustment of the definitive restoration, reducing clinical efficiency and also resistance to fracture. Improper location, size and/or tightness of proximal contacts can cause movement of adjacent teeth that will also require excessive proximal adjustment and possibly complications due to close root proximity with adjacent teeth. Provisional restorations must be

mechanically durable, maintaining all the biologic and esthetic requirements as well as protecting the tooth preparation itself.

Traditionally, provisional restorations have been formed chairside from auto-polymerizing or light-polymerized resins. This requires the joining of two pieces of information: the internal surface form and the external surface form. The internal surface form is representative of the geometry of the tooth preparation, allowing the inside (intaglio) surface of the provisional restoration to fit the prepared tooth. The external surface form is representative of the desired shape of the outside of the restored tooth, including proper emergence profile, contours, and occlusal and proximal contacts. When these two surfaces are joined, the space inside forms a mold cavity. Conventionally, the internal surface form may be the prepared tooth itself or a cast of the prepared tooth. External surface forms are either custom or preformed. Custom external surface forms include: a duplication of the tooth prior to tooth preparation (impression or vacuum-formed/putty matrix) or a proposed form obtained by a preoperative evaluation (impression or vacuum-formed/putty matrix of a diagnostic waxup). Preformed external surface forms include the wide variety of premade resin and metal crown forms available on the market and are limited to single unit restorations. The mold cavity between the internal and external surface forms is filled with auto-polymerizing or light-polymerizing resin to fabricate a provisional resin crown.

Provisional restorations can be made by one of three techniques: direct, indirect, and indirect/direct combination technique. The direct method uses the patient's own tooth preparation as the external surface form. The direct method has many disadvantages: such as poorer marginal fit and patient exposure to the heat and chemicals of unpolymerized resins. The indirect method uses a cast or digital analog of the tooth preparation as the internal surface form, avoiding the disadvantages of the direct method. However, it is time consuming to make an impression of the tooth preparations and then pour in gypsum prior to beginning the provisional restoration itself. The indirect/direct method first uses a diagnostic tooth preparation as the internal surface form to prepare a shell for later relining

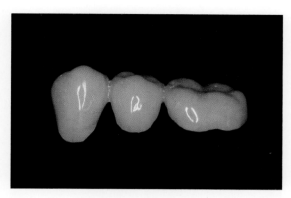

Figure 5.23 Indirect/direct combination technique - shell for later relining milled and polished prior to tooth preparation.

directly in the patient's mouth (Figure 5.23). The advantage of the indirect/direct combination method is that most of the time consuming steps are done prior to the patient appointment and the shell is only relined in the patient's mouth (Figure 5.24).

Using a digital workflow, the internal surface form consists of a 3D virtual image of the prepared tooth and a 3D virtual image of the intended tooth prior to preparation, a scan of a preoperative diagnostic waxing or a virtual shape proposal generated by computer. The digital information is sent to a milling machine at the time of tooth preparation and the internal and external surface forms are milled from solid blocks/discs of resin [(poly)methylmethacrylate (PMMA) or composite], thereby eliminating the need to have analog

representations of the internal and external surface forms and then fill a mold cavity (Figure 5.25). This reduces the patient exposure to chemicals dramatically, as the commercially produced blanks from which provisional restorations are milled contain only around 1% residual free monomer. Therefore, the digital method of fabricating a provisional crown is an entirely indirect method.

Given that provisional restorations must be formed efficiently at the time of tooth preparation, digital technologies also allow fabrication of large multiunit composite or PMMA external surface forms in advance. A preoperative evaluation (diagnostic waxup) and/or diagnostic tooth preparations are provided to the dental laboratory, digital design software is used to virtually "prep" the tooth with a margin near the gingival margin and/or design the external contours, and then the provisional shell is milled for later relining in the mouth at the time of tooth preparation. When multiunit restorations are planned, the dentist will likely need to recruit the assistance of a dental laboratory possessing a large commercial mill, as the blanks for in-office mills are generally too small for multiunit restorations larger than 5 units. Moreover, the practitioner must inquire about the appropriate materials for relining a milled provisional so that delamination, separation, or leakage does not occur between the milled material and the relining material.

Milled provisional restorations can be milled from a blank of resin of one color or layered colors. When using a monocolor blank, the crown or all the units of a fixed dental prosthesis will all be

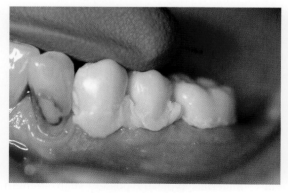

Figure 5.24 Indirect/direct combination technique – shell relined directly in the patient's mouth

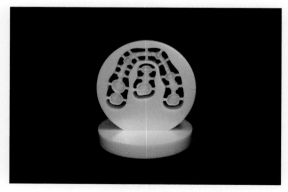

Figure 5.25 Milled provisional multiunit restoration, occlusal aspect. (Courtesy Dr. David G. Gratton.)

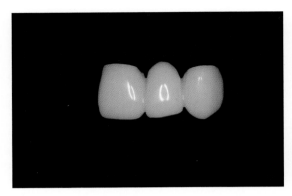

Figure 5.26 CAD/CAM Provisional – note the monocolor appearance, a disadvantage for provisionals in the anterior region.

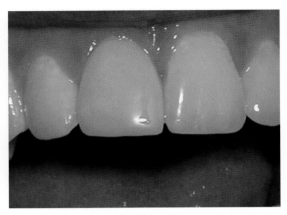

Figure 5.27 The monochromatic appearance of a milled ceramic crown is rarely acceptable for single teeth in the anterior region, despite good color match and polishing.

the same shade (Figure 5.26). All milled materials need to be highly polished prior to cementation in the mouth. Depending on the composition of the milled blank, adjustment of color and characterization may be possible using matching materials.

It is important to use matching materials for long-term color stability and adhesion. Please note that in office mills often require additional software and/or a modified tank or coolant filler system to avoid clogging of the cooling and lubricating circulation system caused by ground polymer particles.

Given that not all clinical situations can be restored the same day as tooth preparation, CAD/CAM provisional restorations have many advantages. The composite-based materials in particular are sufficient in their mechanical properties, wear resistance, color stability, and bonding ability to warrant their use as long-term provisional restorations (Table 5.1).

Single unit ceramic restorations

Chairside

One advantage of the materials used for "hard" milling of full contour definitive restorations is that they are typically translucent due to a high amount of glassy phase. Unfortunately, the high amount of glassy matrix in materials designed for chairside milling conversely means a relatively low amount of strengthening crystalline phase.

These materials typically possess lower strength, some only being recommended for anterior restorations. Ceramics for chairside production of full coverage restorations can be moderately esthetic due to their translucency but lack the ability for complex intrinsic characterization and can only be polished to bring the milled surface to an acceptable gloss (Figure 5.27). Newer blocks are being produced with enamel/dentin gradients, but would also require additional extrinsic staining in the anterior esthetic zone (Figure 5.28a–c). The other advantage is that these materials can be etched, silanated, and bonded to tooth structure, which also increases their fracture resistance slightly. This is also an advantage for restoration of conservative preparations (inlays, onlays, and veneers) or short preparations where adhesive luting may be of benefit for retention. They represent the weakest of the CAD/CAM materials, so their selection for molar teeth should be done with caution. Their production is entirely in the dentist's hands so adherence to the manufacturer's handling precautions, such as avoidance of air-abrasion and thorough polishing, should be strictly followed.

Laboratory fabricated

These materials typically possess high strength and are suitable for single units, as well as large multiunit FDPs. Unfortunately an increase in

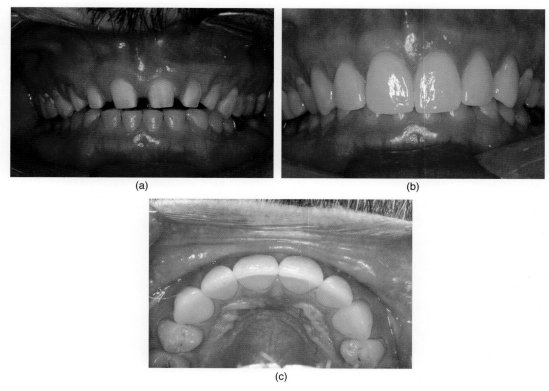

Figure 5.28 (a) Conservative tooth preparations. (b) The monochromatic appearance has been improved by surface staining and application of glaze. (c) The lack of staining on the palatal surfaces of the crowns points out the monochromatic nature of most ceramic blanks.

strength is usually accompanied by an increase in opacity. Some of these materials can only be used as frameworks that are veneered with more translucent, esthetic ceramics. More recently, formulations with increased translucency have been developed that are esthetic enough to use as full contour restorations in the posterior region (Figure 5.29). Table 5.1 outlines the manufacturer recommendations for clinical application of various ceramics for single unit restorations.

Ceramics for multiunit complex restorations

All-ceramic FDPs have had a history of unpredictable clinical performance. The failure of all-ceramic FDPs can be categorized as: fracture of the veneering ceramic, fracture through a connector, or fracture through the material at an abutment. It has only been recently that modern materials and production techniques have yielded products that possess the strength suitable for large multiunit FDPs. Many of these materials are opaque and can only be used as frameworks that

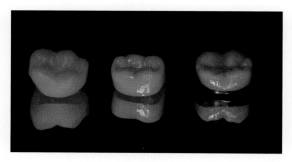

Figure 5.29 Molar restorations: lithium disilicate (left), full contour zirconia (middle), conventional metal-ceramic (right).

Table 5.1 Materials for fixed prosthodontic restorations and provisional restorations and their properties.

Composition	Strength	Milling stage	Full contour	Heat treatment needed	Application:	Etchable
Acrylate polymer	80 MPa	Hard	Yes	N/A	Interims	N/A
Composite	140 MPa	Hard	Yes	N/A	Interims	N/A
Feldspar ceramic	150 MPa	Hard	Yes	No	Single unit, anterior	Yes
Leucite ceramic	160 MPa	Hard	Yes	No	Single unit, anterior	Yes
Zirconia-reinforced Lithium silicate	210 MPa/ or 370 MPa	Soft	Yes	No, but possible	Single unit	Yes
Lithium disilicate	360 MPa	Hard	Yes	Yes	Single and Multiunit (4 unit posterior)	Yes
Glass-infiltrated $MgAl_2O_4$	280 MPa	Soft	No	Infiltration glass needed and layering ceramic	Single, anterior	Slightly
Glass-infiltrated Al_2O_3	600 Mpa	Soft	No	Infiltration glass needed and layering ceramic	Single- and multiunit (Anterior FDP up to 3 units)	No
3Y-TZP	800–1200 MPa	Soft	No	Presinter colorant, layering ceramic possible	Single- and multiunit (FDP up to 16 units)	No

are veneered with more translucent, low-strength ceramics, requiring laboratory support and time for fabrication (Figure 5.30a, b). It is not surprising that the most common failure historically seen has been chipping of the veneering ceramic. Understanding of the stresses that accumulate due to differences in thermal diffusivity during cooling has changed laboratory protocols and reduced the incidence of chipping in zirconia restorations veneered with ceramic. Fracture through connectors has been documented, likely due to either clinical situations, where interocclusal space is limited or defects produced in the laboratory by grinding the tissue surface of a connector. The "Law of Beams" states that when a connector for an FDP is reduced to 1/2 its original width, the resistance to deformation is likewise decreased by 1/2. However, when the height of the connector is reduced by 1/2, it has 1/8 the strength of the original connector. Another example of this law involves the edentulous span length (deflection of

an FDP). The deflection of an FPD is proportional to the cube of its length.

The force on 1 pontic is 1x the M-D distance;
The force on 2 pontics is 8x the M-D distance;
The force on 3 pontics is 27x the M-D distance.

Brittle materials such as ceramics have a very high elastic modulus. That is to say that these materials do not tend to bend before they reach the breaking point. Therefore, when applying the Law of Beams to all-ceramic FDPs, the concern is not about deflection but about stress concentration that could lead to fracture. Manufacturers prescribe the recommended dimensions for connectors when fabricating an FDP from their material using these same guidelines (Table 5.1 and Figure 5.31a, b). Most dental zirconia manufacturers limit the number of posterior pontics to three teeth with a cumulative mesial-distal span of 25 mm between abutments (Figure 5.32).

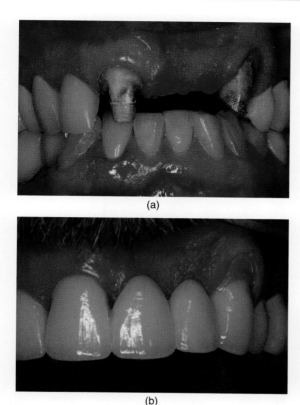

(a)

(b)

Figure 5.30 (a) Edentulous area with tall tooth preparations provides for adequate connector size and shape. (b) Veneered zirconia 4-unit anterior FDP. Note to use of pink ceramic to improve esthetics.

These recommendations are to reduce stress concentrations that develop at the thinnest areas, the connectors. Indeed, fractographic evaluations of all-ceramic bridges have reported that failures typically originate from flaws within the connector region due to the stress concentration.

A sharp radius of curvature on the tissue surface of a connector strongly increases the chance of fracture due to stress concentration at the flaw (Rekow et al., 2011) (Figure 5.33a, b). It is easy to see that areas of limited interocclusal space that encroach on the recommended connector size should not be attempted with all-ceramic materials.

More recently, zirconia formulations with increased translucency have been developed that are esthetic enough to use as full contour restorations in the posterior region. These full-contour restorations should allow connectors to be larger

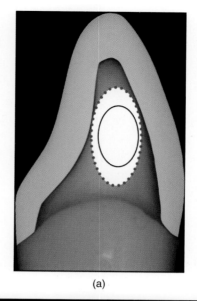

(a)

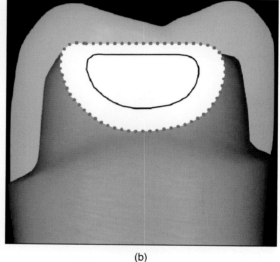

(b)

Figure 5.31 (a) and (b) Connector location and cross-sectional area – the dotted line denotes the size needed for most ceramic connectors as compared to conventional (smaller) metal one.

since it is not necessary to provide cutback of the framework to allow for veneering porcelain (Figure 5.34). Table 5.1 outlines the manufacturer recommendations for clinical application of various ceramics, including for multiunit restorations.

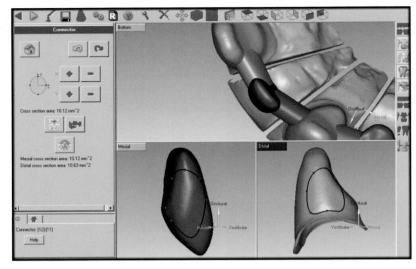

Figure 5.32 Computer planning of connectors for an all-ceramic (zirconia) FDP. (Courtesy Dr. David G. Gratton.)

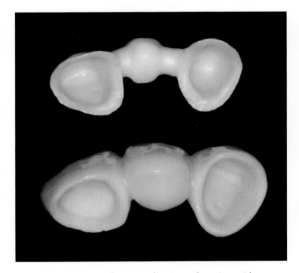

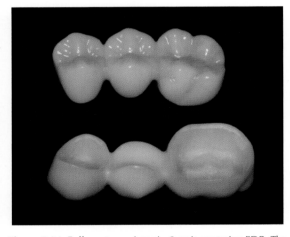

Figure 5.34 Full contour zirconia 3-unit posterior FDP. The connector size is the minimum allowed and the tissue surface is rounded.

Figure 5.33 Zirconia framework prior to layering with veneering porcelain (above). Note the connector size and placement to the facial due to opposing incisal contacts. The completed, veneered zirconia 3-unit anterior FDP is shown below.

Tooth preparation design

Tooth preparations for CAD/CAM produced all-ceramic crowns vary little compared to those made to receive all-ceramic crowns fabricated by other techniques. The strength and opacity of the ceramic itself determines the recommendation for the amount of tooth reduction. Typically, monolithic materials can be used with more conservative tooth preparation than the layered systems. A basic rule is that the restoration should have relatively even thickness circumferentially. Compared to metal-ceramic restorations, adequate reduction for fracture resistance usually requires more reduction on occlusal and incisal edges and rounded internal line angles (Figure 5.35a, b).

Sharp internal angles inside the restoration may lead to stress concentration and fracture. For many ceramics that can be milled chairside, the recommended minimum thicknesses are as follows: minimum axial wall thickness = 1.0 mm; minimum thickness under a cusp = 1.5 mm (anterior), 2.0 mm (posterior); minimum thickness under a groove = 1.5–2.0 mm. Depth cuts are beneficial in ensuring adequate reduction, self-limiting burs are helpful in obtaining consistent reduction. Incisally and occlusally, a greater ceramic thickness of 2 mm is usually required for esthetics and strength, respectively (Figure 5.35c). Only minor differences in tooth preparation design exist for the various ceramic systems, they all must exhibit tapered walls, smooth margins, and rounded internal line angles and cusps/incisal edges.

Margin design

Compared to preparations for metal-ceramic restorations, the amount of tooth reduction is generally more for all-ceramic restorations due to the need for a uniform 1 mm wide rounded shoulder or wide chamfer margin design (Figure 5.36a–c). To allow for an even thickness for adequate strength, the tooth must be prepared more proximally and lingually than for conventional metal-ceramic restorations. The shoulder should be rounded internally to reduce stresses within the tooth and ceramic, but should have a 90° angle

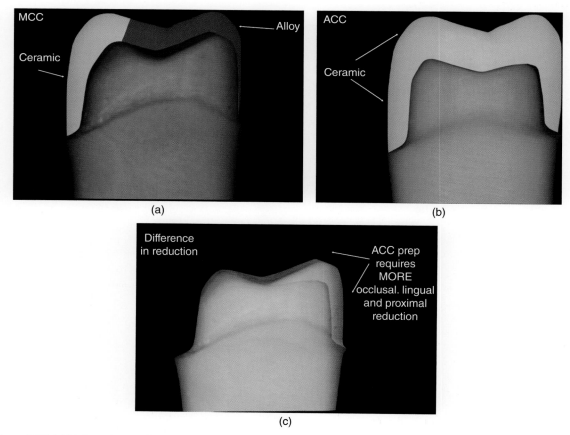

Figure 5.35 (a) Molar reduction for a meta-ceramic crown with metal occlusal. (b) Molar reduction for an all-ceramic crown. (c) Reduction differences: the reduction is drastically more in the posterior region, due to strength requirements.

at the external cavosurface margin (Donovan, 2008). If the shoulder preparation has a sharp axiogingival internal line angle, as in a conventional metal-ceramic preparation, the scanning device may not be able to capture the area of the axiogingival internal line angle accurately (Donovan, 2008). Increasing the convergence angle (taper) of tooth preparations has been reported to improve the internal and marginal adaptation of zirconia-based crowns (Beuer *et al.*, 2008). Knife-edge margins, thin chamfers, and sloped shoulders are not indicated for all-ceramic restorations due the likelihood of fracture of thin areas of unsupported ceramic. Conversely, using a bur with a small diameter or over-preparation may leave a lip of unsupported enamel at the margin. This lip of unsupported enamel is difficult for a digital impression to register, difficult to

mill accurately and may break off at crown try-in, leaving an open margin.

Milling considerations for tooth preparation

Regardless of the milling system used, the bur that is responsible for milling the intaglio surface of the restoration has the potential to influence preparation guidelines. A bur responsible for milling only the occlusal surface has little impact on the preparation guidelines. Given the size restrictions of chairside milling systems, the geometry of the burs should be considered when preparing teeth for milled restorations. The length of the intaglio-milling bur determines the depth that can be milled, as measured from the lowest point of the

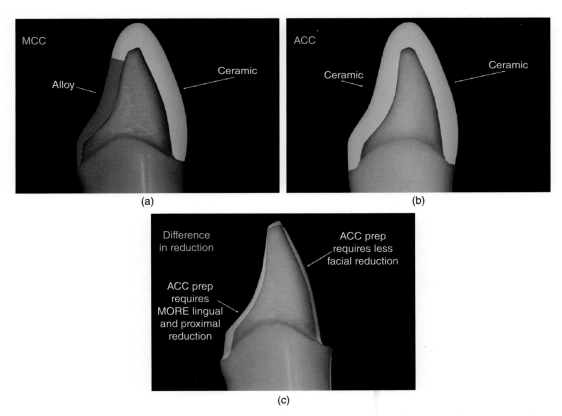

Figure 5.36 (a) Incisor reduction for a metal-ceramic crown with metal palatal surface. (b) Incisor reduction for an all-ceramic crown. (c) Reduction differences: the reduction is drastically more for ACCs on the palatal and proximal, however slightly less facially.

margin to deepest part of the intaglio surface. For most molar preparations the diameter of the bur is inconsequential if the precautions for rounded occlusal cusp reduction are observed. Anterior tooth preparations, however, are generally smaller in diameter and taller incisogingivally. Some milling burs are stepped, becoming wider about halfway down their shank. When milling tall parallel preparations, such as mandibular incisors, the wider part of the bur may inadvertently mill away the margin when trying to mill the depth of the incisal edge. Therefore, a minimum 6° taper or greater is recommended for tall preparations. Moreover, incisal edges that are thinner than the tip of the milling bur will cause the inside of the crown to be overmilled, (Figure 5.37) causing a thin weak restoration. The width of the burs varies according to the milling system and some systems contain several bur sizes that can more accurately mill the intaglio surface of thin incisal edges.

For optimal digital impressions, tooth preparations should follow the long axis of the tooth. Deviation from this can cause ditching at the margin and nonuniform axial reduction. This can be especially difficult if the practitioner wants to "correct" tooth position restoratively. In addition, making the digital impression at a path of withdrawal different from the rest of the teeth can lead to poor CAD designs and/or require increased editing of the design.

Single restoration design

The design of all-ceramic crowns is dependent on the material intended for fabrication of the restoration. For those ceramics that are produced as full contour, monolithic restorations, the tooth preparation, and external contours determine the design. Areas of under-reduction will compromise the strength of the restoration, especially in load bearing areas such as the occluding surfaces. Consequently, the importance of strict adherence to tooth reduction guidelines cannot be understated. In comparisons of milled versus pressed ceramics of the same composition, milling appears to reduce the strength of some ceramics by about 10%. This reduction in strength is likely due to small flaws that are created during the milling process. Marginal chipping is still a concern for some ceramics, as this directly affects marginal accuracy and fit.

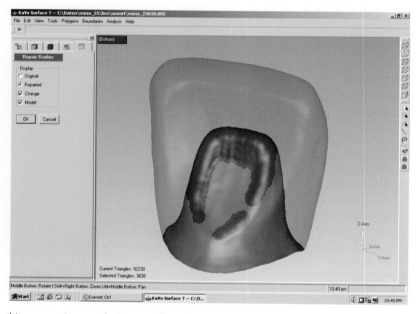

Figure 5.37 Sharp, thin preparations results in overmilling due to the diameter of the bur crown. (Courtesy Dr. David G. Gratton.)

The design of frameworks for layered all-ceramic crowns is typically a coping of uniform thickness over the preparation. However, chipping of the layering ceramic in unsupported areas such as the marginal ridges can occur in load bearing regions of the mouth. Chipping that results in loss of proximal contact can result in food impaction and tooth migration, requiring the restoration be remade. Some authors recommend all-ceramic framework designs that more closely resemble metal-ceramic frameworks, where an even thickness of the layering ceramic rather than the framework is planned. There is still debate about whether the design of layered all-ceramic restorations should mimic the guidelines for metal-ceramic frameworks.

Multiunit design

Before the introduction of zirconia for dental applications, all-ceramic multiunit restorations have been plaqued by unpredictable longevity. Fracture through connectors has been an issue, due to the size requirements for such a brittle material and also due to the sensitivity of ceramic connectors to sharp geometries and flaws induced by laboratory manipulation. Most ceramics that are strong enough for multiunit applications recommend minimum connector dimensions that should be strictly adhered to by the technician. Most ceramic manufacturers state the recommended application (anterior, posterior), connector size, and number of pontics possible for their material(s). Most manufacturers do not recommend posterior cantilevers in areas of reduced interocclusal space.

As the trend for stronger materials keeps developing, it is likely that the amount of tooth reduction will become more conservative. But as with any other indirect restoration, the predictability of CAD/CAM restorations is contingent upon a proper preparation design and reduction, a detailed impression (whether elastomeric or an optical/digital scan), and knowledge of restoration design. All these considerations must come together to produce a restoration that will satisfy dentist and patient expectations and long-term dental health.

Longevity and prognosis

It is generally accepted that fracture is the most common mode of failure of all-ceramic restorations, regardless of method of production. Many reports of low restoration fracture rates document the clinical durability of most milled all-ceramic restorations. Similar to other ceramic restorations, ceramic fracture and tooth fracture account for the primary failure mechanisms (Wittneben et al., 2009). Translucent ceramics are weaker than more opaque types of ceramics (Denry, 2013) meaning that the ideal ceramic for all applications is still not a reality. Another factor that would adversely affect prognosis of a CAD/CAM restoration is poor marginal fit. The marginal accuracy is influenced by: errors involved capturing a digital impression, error introduced during designing the virtual restoration, the limitations of the mechanical milling process, and material chipping during milling (Figure 5.38). Marginal gaps of 53– 67 μm have been found in studies and marginal gap tends to increase when tooth preparations become more tapered (Nakamura et al., 2003; Santos et al., 2013).

Clinical evaluations of single CAD/CAM crowns are often classified and reported according to the restoration material. The first materials that emerged on the market have the most reports

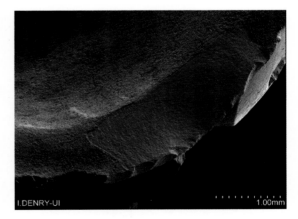

Figure 5.38 Large chip (highlighted in green) at margin of leucite-reinforced ceramic. (Micrograph courtesy Dr. Isabelle Denry.)

in the literature regarding clinical longevity. Feldspathic blocks were one of the first crown materials introduced to the market for chairside milling. One study compared milled feldspathic crowns with In-Ceram Spinell crowns over a period of 4 years and found no significant survival rate (Wassermann *et al.*, 2006). A material with similar properties, leucite-containing ceramics, has demonstrated an overall survival rate of 95.2 % at 11 years; 98.9% survival for crowns in the anterior region and 84.4 % survival in the posterior region (Della Bona and Kelly, 2008). The decrease in survival in the posterior region is likely due to the higher loads exerted by the masticatory system, shorter overall tooth height, and increased loading resulting in fatigue (Figure 5.39). In addition, high-glass-containing ceramics are particularly sensitive to stress corrosion, the corrosive effect of the wet oral environment that drives slow crack growth (Shenoy and Shenoy, 2010).

The current formulation of lithium disilicate for CAD/CAM restorations has only been on the market since the late 2000s. One study of 2 year survival data of machined lithium disilicate crowns showed no cases of crown fracture or surface chipping. Some margin discoloration was found in three crowns cemented with a self-etching, dual-curing cement. All other data indicated no appreciable change in the crowns during the two-year study (Fasbinder *et al.*, 2010).

Polished full-contour zirconia restorations have been shown to have better light transmission than glazed or layered zirconia frameworks. Polish of full contour zirconia may cause less wear of the restoration itself, but has been shown to increase wear of the opposing dentition (Beuer *et al.*, 2012).

Despite the differences in their crystalline phase, processing method, and loading (anterior or posterior), most clinical trials have reported survival rates of greater than 90%. Only a few systems have been successful for the restoration of molars, and additional clinical factors such as adequate occlusal thickness of material and type of cementation can outweigh materials considerations (Strub and Malament, 2013).

Damage

Damage to ceramic restorations can occur during milling, during laboratory fabrication, during the delivery phase, and during function. Flaws introduced into ceramics are particularly deleterious to the strength and clinical survival of a dental restoration. Milling using rotary instruments shapes a restoration by removal of small particles from the surface. The resulting surface often has defects caused by chipping of the material during milling (Figure 5.40). These small flaws can act as stress concentrators that initiate a crack in the material, eventually leading to fracture of the restoration (Figure 5.41).

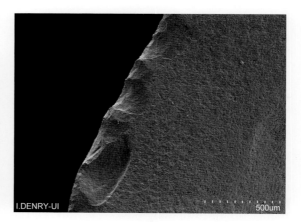

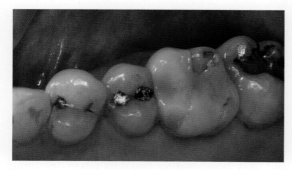

Figure 5.39 Fractured ML functional cusp of feldspathic ceramic onlay.

Figure 5.40 Chipping caused by milling. (Micrograph courtesy Dr. Isabelle Denry.)

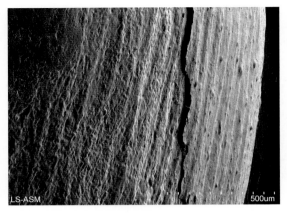

Figure 5.41 Crack emanating from chipping at margin. (Micrograph courtesy Dr. Isabelle Denry.)

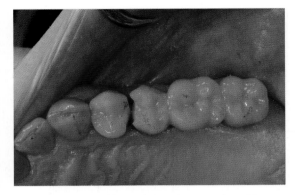

Figure 5.42 Fractured layered zirconia restorations. (Courtesy Dr. David G. Gratton.)

During fabrication, dental laboratories must fabricate restorations to fulfill a wide range of clinical situations. In adjusting restorations, the laboratory may air-abrade the surface to clean it prior to ceramic application of glazing. Damage from particle abrasion, not necessarily immediately apparent, has been shown to compromise the fatigue strength of zirconia and alumina ceramics in crown-like structures. In fatigue, small flaws introduced by particle abrasion can lead to fracture (Denry, 2013).

Fixed partial dental prostheses

One clinical study of posterior FDPs over a 5-year observation period reported only one fracture of the zirconia-based framework, which suggests a promising future for all-ceramic FPDs (Raigrodski *et al.*, 2012b). However, the overall survival rate was 73.9 % because of other complications, such as secondary caries (21.7%) and chipping of the veneering ceramic (15.2%) (Della Bona and Kelly, 2008). A recent systematic review on survival and complications of zirconia FDPs including 12 clinical studies concluded that clinical complications included chipping of veneering porcelain (Figure 5.42), abutment failure, and framework fracture (Raigrodski *et al.*, 2012a). The clinical survival of full contour zirconia FDPs is

as yet unknown, but results on full arch implant restorations are promising.

Occlusion

Accuracy

Clinical experience has shown that there are many confounding factors that affect occlusion in crowns prepared by conventional techniques. Even with meticulous attention to impression techniques, maxillomandibular records, and optimal laboratory procedures, discrepancies in occlusion are commonly noted at the clinical try-in appointment. Compared to full coverage restorations fabricated by conventional laboratory methods, there exist even more factors that affect accuracy of occlusal contact of CAD/CAM restorations. A recent study has shown that digital impressions produce an accurate replica of the teeth (Patzelt *et al.*, 2014). However, even in a well-controlled research environment, the steps of digitally "waxing" the proposed restoration and the actual milling itself introduce errors in occlusion. There can be as much as a 25% difference between a digital proposal and its milled crown in regard to the number, location, size, and shape of occlusal contacts (Figure 5.43). Capturing the dynamic eccentric movements of the patient and then incorporating that data when designing a crown can reduce possible interferences and

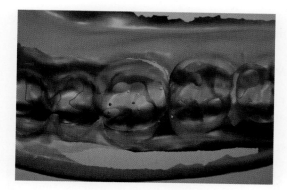

Figure 5.43 Digital proposal for all ceramic crown, the colored dots mark the planned occlusal contacts.

Oral region	Average occlusal forces
Incisors	112.7 – 149 N
Canines/Premolars	322.6 – 582.5 N
Molars	387.3 – 1647.5 N

Figure 5.44 Range and magnitude of human bite forces by region of the mouth.

Occlusal forces

Knowledge of the magnitude of masticatory forces can assist the practitioner in choosing an appropriate material for a particular restorative situation. Normal occlusal forces range from 2 to 40 pounds (9-180N) with a duration lasting 0.25–0.33 seconds during normal mastication (Larson, 2009a; Larson, 2009b). Maximum biting forces in young subjects has been found to average 115–120 pounds (516-532N) in the posterior region (Larson, 2009a; Larson, 2009b). Several factors can increase the amount of force that patients can exert upon their teeth beyond these recorded averages; male gender, low gonial angle, and parafunctional habits to name a few. Logically, occlusal forces are greatest the more posteriorly, with the second molar taking 55% of the maximum biting force and the incisors taking 20% of the total force (Larson, 2012). This explains the increased clinical incidence of full coverage all-ceramic crown failures seen in the molar region. When occlusal loads are delivered to one tooth, as in the case of loss of posterior support, it has been reported

reduce the number of static contacts. For materials that are easily adjusted in the mouth, this is likely not an overwhelming issue. However, for extremely hard materials such as zirconia, intraoral adjustment can be difficult and the polishing needed afterward can be tedious.

that the forces can be up to ten times greater on that tooth than when maximum biting forces are distributed over several teeth (Larson, 2012). Figure 5.44 shows the range and magnitude of biting forces in humans (Gibbs et al., 1981; Larson, 2012; Laurell and Lundgren, 1984; Lundgren and Laurell, 1986).

Single unit restorations

When these occlusal loads are delivered to a single tooth restoration, the resulting stresses within the restoration and within the tooth itself can also be magnified by several factors. Intracoronal MOD cavity preparations weaken remaining tooth structure, so much so that the outward deformation of the facial and lingual walls approaches about 0.15 µm/N of load applied (Larson, 2012). For full coverage restorations, inclined planes or slopes of cusps receive higher forces and it has been advised that maintaining points of occlusal contact, rather than areas of occlusal contact, will decrease the stress at the apical region of teeth (Larson, 2012). However, point contacts may actually increase stresses within full coverage restorations, a very real concern for all-ceramic CAD/CAM restorations since they have been shown to fracture under the site of loading. When occlusal loads are considered relative to the area that was loaded, as in pounds per square inch, kilogram per square centimeter, or Newtons per square meter, known as a Pascal. Therefore, it is enlightening to see that high bite forces can be directed over very small areas, thus dramatically increasing the stress within a restorative material (Figure 5.45).

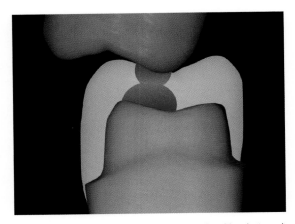

Figure 5.45 Stress concentration under occlusal loads (in red).

Broadening an occlusal contact would provide a "snowshoe effect" where the forces of mastication are distributed over a greater amount of crown material, thus reducing the stresses inside the restoration and hopefully reducing the chance of fracture. However, many natural teeth would have to be modified to provide such a contact and the chance of lateral loading and pressure to the tooth and supporting periodontium would increase. In addition, variables such as the geometry of the tooth preparation, whether the material can be adhesively luted to tooth structure and the deleterious effects of cyclic loading (fatigue) confound predictions of strength adequacy for any given material or region of the mouth. Laboratory testing can provide some ranges of material strength to guide the practitioner, but exact reproduction of the repeated loading and environment during mastication or accidentally biting on a hard object in food is not straightforward. If we apply a "safety factor" of 5, meaning the material should be five times the average load encountered, it appears that most ceramic materials are suitable for anterior teeth. Unfortunately, there does not seem to be a clinically proven all-ceramic crown choice for molars at this time, and CAD/CAM production of base metal restorations may be the treatment of choice when limited occlusal reduction is encountered on second molars. Full-contour zirconia may eventually prove to be suitable in the molar regions if adequate reduction guidelines are scrupulously followed, long-term

clinical trials will be needed to determine this material's long-term suitability.

Multiunit restorations

FDPs fabricated using CAD/CAM technology are relatively new, zirconia being the predominant material used. Failure of multiunit zirconia restorations has been either chipping of the layering ceramic or fracture through the connectors. Moreover, perhaps full contour zirconia may solve the veneer chipping issue as well as allow for larger connector cross-sectional area to prevent fracture. Close attention should be paid to the size of the connector and contour of the gingival aspect of the connector. When creating access for hygiene, the laboratory connector should employ a rounded, concave surface that is devoid of sharp angles. Once the prosthesis is milled and sintered, adjustment of this area with abrasives should be avoided to reduce the possibility of fracture through the connector (Figure 5.46).

Wear of opposing dentition

Abrasion of opposing teeth or restorations has long been a concern when employing ceramic materials to restore occluding surfaces. While some low-strength ceramics benefit from a glassy glaze fired into the surface to increase strength and reduce abrasion against opposing teeth, the opposite has been true of zirconia materials.

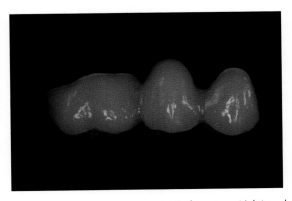

Figure 5.46 Correct connector gingival contour (right) and incorrect, sharp contour (left) that may lead to fracture.

Highly polished zirconia has been shown in laboratory tests to be less abrasive than both glazed zirconia and stained and then glazed zirconia or conventional ceramics (Janyavula *et al.*, 2013).

Esthetic limitations

Metal-ceramic restorations, still the most commonly fabricated type of full coverage and multiunit restoration, carry with them frequent esthetic complications of exposure of the metal margin and gingival discoloration. Classic metal-ceramic restorations require not only aggressive tooth reduction but also a skilled laboratory technician to achieve excellent esthetics. Outstanding esthetics can be achieved with high-strength all-ceramic materials, often with less aggressive tooth preparation.

As production of monolithic all-ceramic restorations switches from dental laboratory to chairside CAD/CAM methods, new esthetic challenges arise. The only surface modification most chairside hard-milled CAD/CAM restorations receive is polishing prior to (and after) cementation. This does not impart any color, but brings the restoration to acceptable level of surface luster. While acceptable in the posterior region and for intracoronal restorations, lack of color variation in the anterior region does not replicate natural tooth structure in the majority of patients. Since these types of restorations are milled from one blank of material, they are generally monocolor and not suitable for areas of high esthetic demand although newer blocks that contain an enamel as well as a dentin layer have been introduced. These are candidates for the rare patient whose natural teeth exhibit no intrinsic characterization (Figure 5.47). The quality of the final esthetics from machining alone is not acceptable for most patients. Most monochromatic CAD/CAM restorations require custom staining to modify the color of the restoration to ensure an esthetic match to a natural tooth. When compared to conventional metal-ceramic crowns that included intrinsic layering, one study found that patients and evaluators could not find a significant esthetic difference between translucent monolithic crowns that were only stained and glazed (Herrguth *et al.*, 2005). For teeth with low intrinsic characterization,

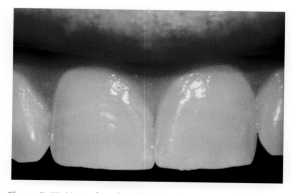

Figure 5.47 Natural teeth with little chromatic variation.

monolithic materials and surface staining can be acceptable. The practitioner only needs to select the correct shade and translucency prior to surface characterization (Figure 5.48a, b).

It is an inherently more difficult challenge when the intrinsic coloration of a tooth is complex and must be matched to adjacent natural teeth (Figure 5.49). Monolithic materials rarely succeed in achieving acceptability, even with surface staining. When such a complex esthetic situation exists, collaboration with a dental laboratory is required. Instead of milling a full contour restoration, a coping is produced that allows the laboratory technician to layer the rest of the crown with various colors and layers of ceramic to mimic the adjacent teeth. Skilled laboratory ceramists can provide the finishing artistic and esthetic touches required for the esthetic zone using the layering technique.

Teeth that are discolored also present a stimulating test of ability for both the practitioner and laboratory technician. Hemosiderin staining of teeth that have been traumatized is a difficult discoloration to overcome, even with a full coverage restoration. This should not be attempted with a translucent, monolithic material (Figure 5.50). The material of choice is a coping that is opaque, so as to cover the darkness and provide an undiscolored background for layering with dentin and enamel ceramics. An increased facial reduction of 1.2–1.4 mm is necessary for discolored teeth, and subgingival margins should be used to avoid darkness at the gingival margin (Figure 5.51a–c). Opaque materials are also the materials of choice

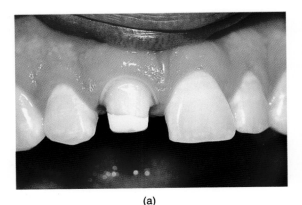

(a)

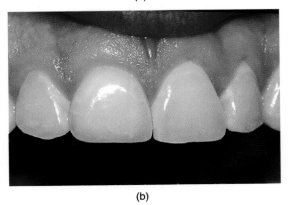

(b)

Figure 5.48 (a) Natural teeth with little chromatic variation, the tooth preparation has a zirconia post. (b) Restoration with monolithic leucite-reinforced ceramic, surface staining, and glazing has been performed.

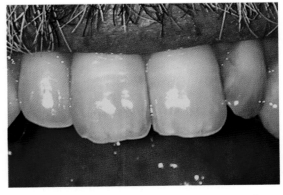

Figure 5.49 Natural teeth with extensive intrinsic characterization.

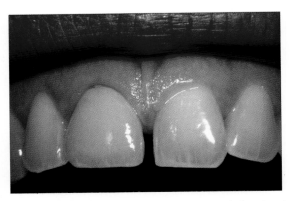

Figure 5.50 All-ceramic crown that does not mask discolored tooth preparation. The intrinsic characterization of the incisal edge is not replicated by a monolithic crown.

when the need arises to cover a metal post and core that cannot be removed.

It should be remembered that the degree of color match of an anterior single tooth restoration tends to decrease over time, owing to the shift in color and translucency of the adjacent teeth, not of the restoration.

Functional limitations

The correct selection of the material for the esthetic demand and region of the mouth will largely influence that restoration's prognosis. In order to select the correct material to withstand intraoral forces, knowledge of the magnitude of forces is necessary. Sensors have been used in dentistry to understand the mechanics of mastication and to provide reference values for studies on the biomechanics of dental prostheses. Investigators have found a wide range of maximum bite forces, because there is a wide range of anatomical and physiological variation in humans. Factors such as cranio-facial morphology, age, gender, periodontal support of teeth, signs and symptoms of temporomandibular disorders and pain, and state of dental health have been found to affect bite force. Reported values for bite forces in the incisor region are around 108–299 N, whereas it more than doubles in the molar region to 216–847 N (Fasbinder *et al.*, 2010; Lundgren and Laurell, 1986). A close correlation of masseter muscle size and bite force has been shown, short-faced subjects have thicker muscles and may exhibit stronger bite force than in normal or long-faced subjects (Koc *et al.*, 2010). Since weaker, more translucent materials are favored in the anterior region, functional limitations would be restorations in bruxers, cases of malocclusion, and occlusion in the palatal 1/3 of maxillary anterior teeth where reduction can be difficult and geometry complex.

From the results of several studies, Korber and colleagues surmised that posterior FDPs should be strong enough to withstand a mean load of 500 N (Korber *et al.*, 1982). Unfortunately, additional factors that accumulate damage over time, such as cyclic fatigue loading and stress corrosion fatigue caused by the oral environment, make predictions of whether a material will be strong enough to avoid failure difficult. Even if all the thickness and geometry requirements are met by providing adequate tooth reduction and proper connector design, some subjects will still be able to fracture single and multiunit all-ceramic restorations. At present, one of the most difficult material challenges is a unilateral, multiunit FDP in the anterior region, as it requires enough translucency to match the adjacent teeth, but also would require the strength of a relatively opaque material. It is prudent for the practitioner to follow manufacturers' recommended strength applications for each material and to be cautious when planning restorations in individuals with short faces or lack of mutually protected articulation. The table below summarizes the limitations and

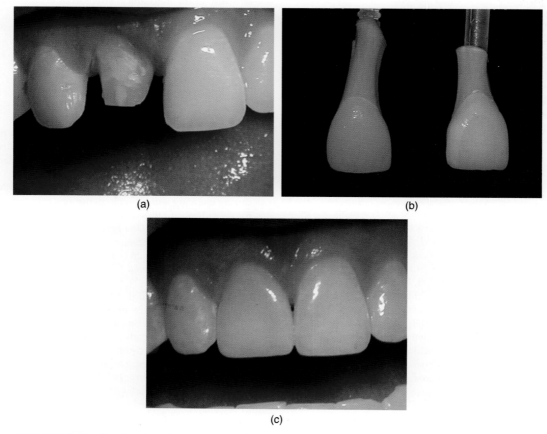

(a)

(b)

(c)

Figure 5.51 (a) Slightly discolored tooth preparation, adjacent teeth are opaque. (b) Two crowns of varying opacity: lithium disilicate (left) and layered zirconia (right). Even though they are the same shade, the difference in translucency is marked. (c) Due to the high value of the adjacent teeth, the zirconia crown was chosen as the definitive restoration.

materials recommendations for optimal esthetics and functional resistance to fracture (Table 5.1).

Summary

A paradigm shift in how fixed prosthodontics is performed has arrived. Technologies for digital impressions, manipulation of digital data for diagnosis and treatment planning, and production of CAD/CAM restorations are transforming how dentistry is provided to dental patients. New materials are being developed as an alternative to costly and unesthetic conventional alloys for fixed prosthodontics. The highest-strength materials are now suitable for high-stress applications, including FDPs. However, they are relatively new and still lack the support of long-term clinical experience and research. The beauty of technology incorporation for fixed prosthodontics is that the practitioner does not necessarily have to move to an entirely CAD/CAM workflow. Options exist to utilize digital technology for some aspects of patient treatment and conventional materials and methods for others. This allows the practitioner to progressively move toward digital methods as methods, equipment, training, and means provide.

References

Beuer, F., Edelhoff, D., & Gernet, W., *et al.* (2008) Effect of preparation angles on the precision of zirconia crown copings fabricated by CAD/CAM system. *Dental Materials Journal*, **27**, 814–820.

Beuer, F., Stimmelmayr, M., & Gueth, J.F., *et al.* (2012) In vitro performance of full-contour zirconia single crowns. *Dental Materials*, **28**, 449–456.

Della Bona, A. & Kelly, J.R. (2008) The clinical success of all-ceramic restorations. *Journal of the American Dental Association (1939)*, **139**(Suppl), 8S–13S.

Denry, I. (2013) How and when does fabrication damage adversely affect the clinical performance of ceramic restorations? *Dental Materials*, **29**, 85–96.

Donovan, T.E. (2008) Factors essential for successful all-ceramic restorations. *Journal of the American Dental Association (1939)*, **139**(Suppl), 14S–18S.

Fasbinder, D.J., Dennison, J.B., & Heys, D., *et al.* (2010) A clinical evaluation of chairside lithium disilicate CAD/CAM crowns: a two-year report. *Journal of the American Dental Association (1939)*, **141**(Suppl 2), 10S–14S.

Gibbs, C.H., Mahan, P.E., & Lundeen, H.C., *et al.* (1981) Occlusal forces during chewing and swallowing as measured by sound transmission. *The Journal of Prosthetic Dentistry*, **46**, 443–449.

Herrguth, M., Wichmann, M., & Reich, S. (2005) The aesthetics of all-ceramic veneered and monolithic CAD/CAM crowns. *Journal of Oral Rehabilitation*, **32**, 747–752.

Janyavula, S., Lawson, N., & Cakir, D., *et al.* (2013) The wear of polished and glazed zirconia against enamel. *The Journal of Prosthetic Dentistry*, **109**, 22–29.

Koc, D., Dogan, A., & Bek, B. (2010) Bite force and influential factors on bite force measurements: a literature review. *European Journal of Dentistry*, **4**, 223–232.

Koller, M., Arnetzl, G.V., & Holly, L., *et al.* (2012) Lava ultimate resin nano ceramic for CAD/CAM: customization case study. *International Journal of Computerized Dentistry*, **15**, 159–164.

Korber, K.H., Ludwig, K., & Huber, K. (1982) Experimental study of the mechanical strength of bridge frameworks for metalloceramics. *ZWR*, **91**(50), 53–61.

Larson, T.D. (2009a) Tooth wear: when to treat, why, and how. Part One. *Northwest Dentistry*, **88**, 31–38.

Larson, T.D. (2009b) Tooth wear: when to treat, why, and how. Part One. *Northwest Dentistry*, **88**, 31–38.

Larson, T.D. (2012) The effect of occlusal forces on restorations. *Northwest Dentistry*, **91**(25–7), 29–35.

Larson, T.D. (2013) Cementation: methods and materials. Part two. *Northwest Dentistry*, **92**, 29–35.

Laurell, L. & Lundgren, D. (1984) A standardized programme for studying the occlusal force pattern during chewing and biting in prosthetically restored dentitions. *Journal of Oral Rehabilitation*, **11**, 39–44.

Lundgren, D. & Laurell, L. (1986) Occlusal force pattern during chewing and biting in dentitions restored with fixed bridges of cross-arch extension.I. Bilateral end abutments. *Journal of Oral Rehabilitation*, **13**, 57–71.

Nakamura, T., Dei, N., & Kojima, T., *et al.* (2003) Marginal and internal fit of Cerec 3 CAD/CAM all-ceramic crowns. *The International Journal of Prosthodontics*, **16**, 244–248.

Patzelt, S.B., Emmanouilidi, A., & Stampf, S., *et al.* (2014) Accuracy of full-arch scans using intraoral scanners. *Clinical Oral Investigations*, **18**(6), 1687–1694.

Raigrodski, A.J., Hillstead, M.B., & Meng, G.K., *et al.* (2012a) Survival and complications of zirconia-based fixed dental prostheses: a systematic review. *The Journal of Prosthetic Dentistry*, **107**, 170–177.

Raigrodski, A.J., Yu, A., & Chiche, G.J., *et al.* (2012b) Clinical efficacy of veneered zirconium dioxide-based posterior partial fixed dental prostheses: five-year results. *The Journal of Prosthetic Dentistry*, **108**, 214–222.

Rekow, E.D., Silva, N.R., & Coelho, P.G., *et al.* (2011) Performance of dental ceramics: challenges for improvements. *Journal of Dental Research*, **90**, 937–952.

Rosenstiel, S.F., Land, M., & Fujimoto, J. (2006) Contemporary Fixed Prosthodontics. Mosby. 4th edition.

Santos, G.C.J., Santos, M.J.J., & Rizkalla, A.S., *et al.* (2013) Overview of CEREC CAD/CAM chairside system. *General Dentistry*, **61**, 36–40.quiz 41

Shenoy, A. & Shenoy, N. (2010) Dental ceramics: An update. *Journal of Conservative Dentistry*, **13**, 195–203.

Strub, J.R. & Malament, K.A. (2013) Do zirconia ceramics have a future in restorative dentistry? *The International Journal of Periodontics & Restorative Dentistry*, **33**, 259.

Wassermann, A., Kaiser, M., & Strub, J.R. (2006) Clinical long-term results of VITA In-Ceram Classic crowns and fixed partial dentures: A systematic literature review. *The International Journal of Prosthodontics*, **19**, 355–363.

Wittneben, J.G., Wright, R.F., & Weber, H.P., *et al.* (2009) A systematic review of the clinical performance of CAD/CAM single-tooth restorations. *The International Journal of Prosthodontics*, **22**, 466–471.

6 CAD/CAM Removable Prosthodontics

Nadim Z. Baba, Charles J. Goodacre, and Mathew T. Kattadiyil

Introduction

Computer-based technology has an ever-expanding impact upon dentistry with enhanced data acquisition and fabrication capabilities. Recently, this technology has been applied to removable prosthodontics, and the purpose of this chapter is to present the current status of computer technology for the fabrication of complete dentures and removable partial dentures.

History of complete dentures and the development of CAD/CAM technology

Several materials and techniques have historically been used for the fabrication of complete dentures. The materials include wood, ivory, enameled metal, porcelain, gold, vulcanite, celluloid, Bakelite, and poly (methyl methacrylate (PMMA)) resin. Wooden dentures were hand carved and some were inlaid with human teeth. Tacks were placed posteriorly to enhance chewing by functioning like cusps. Ivory dentures were either hand carved in totality from a block or carved and inlaid with human teeth to improve their natural appearance. Vulcanized rubber (Vulcanite), a highly cross-linked hard rubber, was introduced as a denture base material in the mid-1800s. It became the primary material used for denture fabrication for nearly 80 years. The process of making vulcanite dentures was extremely technique sensitive in addition to producing dentures that had poor esthetics (dark brown to gray color), a bad taste and a foul smell (Rueggeberg, 2002). However, dentures made from vulcanite were the first functional and affordable dentures.

In 1907, a Belgian chemist LH Baekeland discovered a synthetic resin (phenol formaldehyde) that became known as "Bakelite." It was tried as a denture base but was not popular because of the lack of dimensional stability in the mouth, and by the time it was modified into an acceptable form, PMMA was discovered. PMMA, a heat-processed material, was introduced in 1936 by Dr. Walter Wright and within 4 years from its introduction, 90 to 95% of all dentures were made using this material (Peyton, 1975). The physical and esthetic properties along with the handling characteristics of PMMA were an improvement over the previous materials used for removable prosthodontics.

Clinical Applications of Digital Dental Technology, First Edition. Edited by Radi Masri and Carl F. Driscoll.
© 2015 John Wiley & Sons, Inc. Published 2015 by John Wiley & Sons, Inc.

However, PMMA has its own disadvantages: a net volumetric shrinkage of about 6–7% causing a lack of optimal fit of the intaglio surface of the denture to the underlying soft tissue, adherence of *Candida albicans* to the acrylic resin (Berdicevsky *et al.*, 1980; Budtz-Jörgensen, 1974), and the presence of residual methyl methacrylate monomer. PMMA does not fulfill all the requirements of an ideal denture base material (Murray & Darvell, 1993).

Traditionally, five-appointment visits, in addition to post-placement visits, have been required for the fabrication of conventional complete dentures. The high number of visits required is one of several limitations that cause some dentists to abstain from treating completely edentulous patients (Christensen, 2006). Attempts have been made to shorten the number of appointments needed in order to make the process faster and less costly while keeping the procedure precise and accurate (Ling, 2000; Ling, 2004). A recent study quantified the costs of complete dentures fabricated using a simplified technique compared with a conventional one (Vecchia *et al.*, 2014). They found that the fabrication of the CD using the simplified technique demanded less time and cost 34.9% less.

The successful use of computer-aided design and computer-aided manufacturing (CAD/CAM) in the fabrication of fixed, implant, and maxillofacial prostheses (Rekow, 1987; Wichmann & Tschernitschek, 1993; Sarment *et al.*, 2003; Al Mardini *et al.*, 2005; Mörmann, 2004) along with a shortage of qualified dental laboratory technicians (Christensen *et al.*, 2005) encouraged the application of CAD/CAM in the field of removable prosthodontics. In 1994, Maeda *et al.* published the first laboratory study investigating the development of a computer-aided system for designing and fabricating complete dentures. They used a three-dimensional (3D) laser lithography technique to fabricate plastic shells of the dentition and record bases of the denture from photopolymerizing resin. Tooth-colored composite resin material was used to form the teeth; the two segments were then connected together and filled with colored autopolymerizing composite resin and polished manually. In an effort to improve the esthetics of CAD/CAM dentures, a software program was developed to automatically detect and reconstruct anatomical structures (important for the setup of artificial teeth) and suggest an artificial tooth arrangement (Busch & Kordass, 2006).

Years later, Kawahata *et al.* (1997) worked on duplicating a complete denture using the CAD/CAM system. They milled the dentures out of modeling wax using a computerized numerical control (CNC) machine and ball-end mills. They acknowledged the need for further improvement in the fabrication process. Wu *et al.* (2010) integrated CAD/CAM technology and laser rapid forming system (LRF) for the fabrication of a titanium record base for a complete denture. They concluded that the fabrication time and cost involved in the fabrication of a metallic denture bases could be reduced with the use of this technology.

Following these early attempts, several instigators presented various techniques for CAD/CAM complete denture fabrication in an effort to improve and facilitate the CAD/CAM denture fabrication (Maeda *et al.*, 1994; Kawahata *et al.*, 1997; Goodacre *et al.*, 2012; Kanazawa *et al.*, 2011; Inokoshi *et al.*, 2012; Sun *et al.*, 2009). Kawahata *et al.* (1997), Kanazawa *et al.* (2011), and Goodacre *et al.* (2012) used subtractive manufacturing (such as CNC machining) for the fabrication of their dentures. Kanazawa *et al.* (2011) scanned a patient's preexisting complete denture and a set of artificial teeth using 3D cone beam computed tomography (CBCT) to acquire data of the mucosal surfaces and the jaw relationship records. A 3D CAD software was used to design the virtual dentures. CNC machining was then used to mill a complete denture base where the teeth were manually bonded. They also measured the fabrication accuracy between the 3D master image they obtained from scanning and the 3D data from the fabricated acrylic denture. They found that the occlusal surface presented a 0.5 mm average deviation from the 3D image. Goodacre *et al.* (2012) reported the first clinical trial placement of a CAD/CAM denture base milled from prepolymerized PMMA in which recesses were created into which denture teeth were bonded.

Other authors (Maeda *et al.*, 1994; Inokoshi *et al.*, 2012; Sun *et al.*, 2009) used additive manufacturing (such as rapid prototyping (RP) or 3D printing) to fabricate their CAD/CAM dentures. Sun *et al.*

(2009) designed a complete denture following the scanning of edentulous casts and occlusal rims. They developed a special program to aid them in virtual teeth arrangement and the fabrication of virtual flasks. The flasks were then printed using RP, the artificial teeth inserted into the printed flasks and the traditional laboratory procedures of packing, processing and polishing were used to finalize the complete dentures.

Clinicians have long realized the importance of the trial placement appointment in the fabrication of complete dentures (Stephens, 1969; Payne, 1977). Inokoshi *et al* (2012) evaluated the suitability of using a 3D CAD software loaded with prototype dentures to fabricate trial placement dentures. Trial dentures were fabricated using the RP technique and compared with the conventional method. They concluded that the digitally fabricated trial dentures were as accurate as the conventional ones. They concluded that the adjustments of trial dentures (i.e., arrangement of teeth) required significantly longer chair time than the conventional ones. However, both the patients and the treating prosthodontist rated esthetics and stability of the conventionally fabricated trial dentures significantly higher than the RP trial dentures.

Recently, Katase *et al.* (2013) evaluated the accuracy of a method that simulates the face after changing the artificial teeth arrangement in complete dentures fabricated by RP. They simulated the faces of 10 edentulous patients with integrated facial and denture data. They compared the facial data of a patient wearing dentures fabricated by RP to the simulated ones. No significant differences were found between simulated faces and actual faces with RP dentures. They concluded that their method could be useful for clinicians who design complete dentures with a computer.

The previously described techniques used for the fabrication of CAD/CAM dentures are promising. However, they still require impressions to be made or casts to be fabricated for the manufacturing process. Only one study (Patzelt *et al.*, 2013) evaluated, *in vitro*, the feasibility of using intra-oral scanners (IOS) to digitize edentulous jaws in order to eliminate the need of conventional impression making. IOS have been successfully used in fixed prosthodontics and studies (Ender & Mehl, 2013; Mehl *et al.*, 2009; Luthardt *et al.*,

2005) showed that they are accurate. Patzelt *et al.* (2013) verified the accuracies of the data sets obtained by scanning edentulous jaws with different commercially available IOSs. They concluded that digitizing the edentulous jaws was feasible. However, they did not recommend the use of IOS *in vivo* to digitize the edentulous jaws due to the high level of inaccuracy.

Advantages of CAD/CAM dentures

It is advantageous to be able to provide dentures in 2 visits. This reduction in the number of patient visits when fabricating a CAD/CAM denture is advantageous for older patients, those who live in nursing homes or assisted living facilities and have difficulty in commuting for multiple appointments to the dental office. The clinical information (impressions, interocclusal records, and tooth selection) is recorded in one appointment of approximately 1–2 hours depending on the clinician's experience and the dentures placed in a second appointment.

The fabrication fees can be comparable or even lower than the laboratory fees of conventional dentures. In addition, less clinical chair time involved allows the dentist to provide more economic dentures.

All 3D images and collected data involved in the CAD/CAM denture fabrication are saved digitally. The stored data can be used to produce a spare denture or a replacement denture if the patient loses their denture(s). These new fabricated dentures will have the same form as the previous dentures, thereby eliminating or minimizing adaptation time for the patient. A surgical or radiographic template can be constructed using the same data to facilitate the treatment planning and placement of dental implants in the future.

The prepolymerized acrylic resin used for the fabrication of the denture base provides a superior fit and strength when compared to conventionally processed bases. The prepolymerized acrylic resin, since it is milled undergoes no polymerization shrinkage, which usually eliminates the need for incorporating posterior palatal seal especially for those patients with firm residual ridges.

Research at the University of Buffalo describes some favorable properties for prepolymerized acrylic resin. The material appears to contain less residual monomer and to be more hydrophobic than the conventionally processed acrylic resin which will result in a more bio-hygienic denture. Microorganisms such as *C. albicans* adhered less to the denture base, which reduces the potential for infections.

Disadvantages of CAD/CAM dentures

1. As the two commercially available CAD/CAM complete denture systems cannot provide the clinician with balanced dentures, a clinical remount will be required to adjust the denture teeth.
2. Even though the CAD/CAM denture fabrication process facilitates denture fabrication and reduces the appointment visits, there is a learning curve for the inexperienced clinician initially that could lead to unsatisfactory results.
3. The dentist needs to use a dimensionally stable and temperature resistant impression material to resist distortion during shipping.
4. The lack of trial placement appointment could create an increased chance for less than an ideal outcome and missed opportunity for minor adjustments. However, a 3-appointment process can be used whereby a trial denture is fabricated using either a milled base with the teeth set in wax or a completely milled prototype using a tooth-colored resin.

Commercially available CAD/CAM complete dentures

Currently, two commercial manufacturers are available for the fabrication of CAD/CAM dentures. Both manufacturers allow the fabrication of dentures in 2 appointments. The first appointment consists of data gathering (impressions, jaw relations, occlusal plane orientation, tooth mold, and shade selection) and the second appointment consists of denture placement and adjustments.

AvaDent™ Digital Dentures (Global Dental Science LLC., Scottsdale, AZ) uses subtractive manufacturing for the fabrication of their dentures. The dentures are milled from a prepolymerized block of acrylic resin and the denture teeth are

bonded to the base. Recently, they have developed the process of milling their own teeth, thereby creating a prosthesis where the teeth and base are a single unit (a monolithic prosthesis). Their current system offers the following products: (i) complete over complete dentures; (ii) single-arch complete dentures; (iii) implant-supported overdentures; (iv) immediate complete dentures; (v) provisional dentures; (vi) record bases; (vii) scanning guides; (viii) verification jigs; (ix) bone reduction guides; (x) conversion dentures; and (xi) definitive fixed complete dentures (fixed-detachable or hybrid prostheses).

Dentca™ (Dentca Inc., Los Angeles, CA) uses additive manufacturing (such as RP or 3D printing) to fabricate trial dentures and then the definitive denture(s) is/are processed conventionally using 3D printed flasks. The system allows for the fabrication of complete over complete dentures and single-arch dentures.

Step-by-step procedures for the fabrication of complete dentures using the AvaDent system.

AvaDent dentures can be fabricated using the following 3 methods: 1) Duplicate a patients existing denture for use in making a reline impression and interocclusal record. The duplicated denture and impression are then scanned along with the interocclusal record to fabricate a denture; 2) Use of Good Fit denture trays for impressions and records; 3) Use of anatomic measuring device (AMD). The following section describes the use of the AMD technique.

1. AvaDent has an introductory kit that contains the required impression trays and materials, anatomic measuring device (AMD) and adjustment instruments, thermometer, and tooth size templates. The AvaDent thermoplastic impression trays can be selected comparing the dimensions of the arch with the caliper provided and they can be molded to fit the edentulous arch (Figure 6.1). However, if the patient presents wearing existing dentures, the dentures are removed and laboratory putty is mixed and pressed into the dentures to form a base while molding the material around the

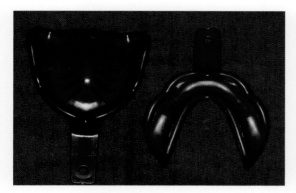

Figure 6.1 AvaDent Stock Trays.

denture. After the putty sets, the putty mold is trimmed, a flat land area created forming a putty cast on which the customizable trays can be adapted. Using the caliper, the putty cast is measured at the crest of the ridge to determine the appropriate size of the AvaDent trays to be used.

2. The selected trays are placed in a hot water bath (160–170 °F) until they become malleable. At such time they can be firmly adapted to the denture bearing areas on the putty casts and molded to create custom trays. They are then trimmed with an acrylic resin bur or shaped to the desired form to make sure they cover all the important anatomical structures to be captured in the impressions (soft palate up to or slightly beyond the vibrating line, pterygomaxillary fissures, retromolar pad areas, buccal shelf areas, available areas of the lateral throat form). When the putty cast does not cover the desired anatomic areas because the existing denture was deficient in coverage, the tray can be heated in the required area and stretched for appropriate coverage.

3. The trays are tried in the patient's mouth to confirm their accuracy and additional adjustments made as needed. Adhesive is applied to the tray and dried. An interocclusal registration material poly (vinyl siloxane) is applied on to the intaglio surface of the impression trays to form soft tissue stops (4 dabs for the maxillary and 3 for the mandibular tray) and then seated in the patient's mouth without excessive pressure, thereby leaving a space between the tray and the mucosa for the border molding and final impression material (Figure 6.2).

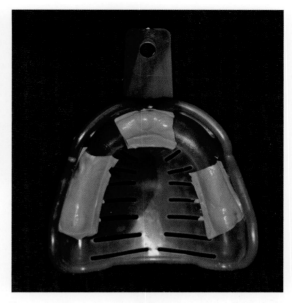

Figure 6.2 Impression material used to create stops in the intaglio surface of the stock tray.

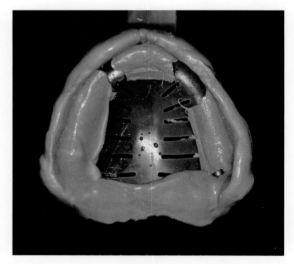

Figure 6.3 Border molding with Heavy-body impression material.

4. The border molding of the maxillary and mandibular trays is performed using the provided poly (vinyl siloxane) material, employing the conventional method of tissue manipulation (Figure 6.3). Adhesive is applied to the border molding impression material and a definitive impression is made after the

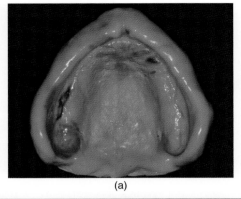

(a)

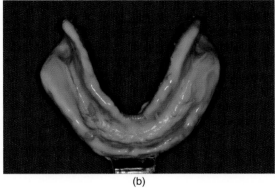

(b)

Figure 6.4 (a), (b) Maxillary and mandibular definitive impressions.

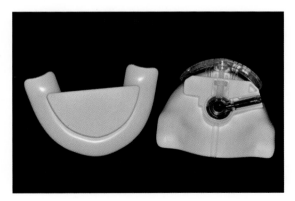

Figure 6.5 Mandibular and maxillary Anatomical Measuring devices.

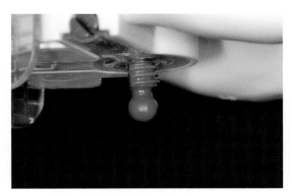

Figure 6.6 Stylus of the maxillary AMD device.

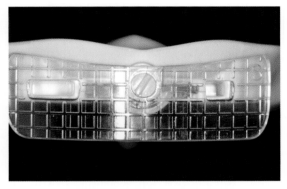

Figure 6.7 Adjustable lip support flange of the maxillary AMD.

application of a thin layer of a light-body wash poly (vinyl siloxane) impression material (Figure 6.4 a, b).

5. The jaw relation records are made using an AMD (Figure 6.5). The AMD is utilized to record: the occlusal vertical dimension (OVD), the maxillary lip support, the midline, the desired mediolateral orientation of the occlusal plane, centric relation (CR), teeth size, incisal edge position and location of the denture base resin around the necks of the prosthetic teeth.

The AMD consists of a maxillary and mandibular partial arch trays. The mandibular tray has a flat occlusal tracing plate and the maxillary tray has an incorporated centrally located adjustable stylus that serves as the central bearing pin for a gothic arch tracing (Figure 6.6). The maxillary tray also has an adjustable lip support flange (Figure 6.7).

The correct size of maxillary and mandibular AMD is selected from three available sizes using the provided caliper to measure the widest part of the patient's ridge utilizing the final impression or the putty cast made previously.

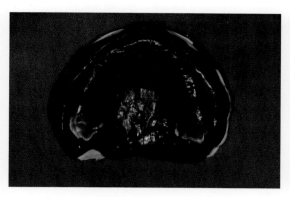

Figure 6.8 Relined intaglio surface of the maxillary AMD with heavy-body PVS.

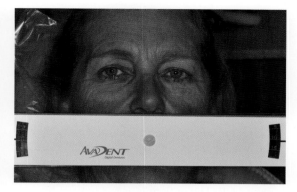

Figure 6.9 AvaDent ruler used to determine the appropriate occlusal plane.

6. The maxillary AMD is coated with tray adhesive. A heavy body poly (vinyl siloxane) impression material is expressed on the intaglio surface of the tray and the tray seated over the patient's edentulous ridge while aligning the adjustable lip support flange as parallel as possible to the interpupillary line. The maxillary AMD is then assessed for stability. It should ideally cover the ridge morphology of the maxillary arch as well as the portion of the palate to ensure accurate digital correlation of the AMD and the final maxillary impression, which will occur at the laboratory phase. Excess impression material causing unnatural contour is trimmed and the impression relined using light body poly (vinyl siloxane) (Figure 6.8).

7. An occlusal plane orientation ruler is then placed into specific recesses in the maxillary AMD tray and moved so it is aligned with the interpupillary line and the ruler number recorded. This process allows the occlusal plane to be aligned parallel with the interpupillary lines (Figure 6.9).

The number shown on the ruler is recorded onto the laboratory work authorization form. The mandibular tray is coated with the tray adhesive. A heavy body poly (vinyl siloxane) impression material is expressed on the intaglio surface of the tray and the tray seated over the patient's edentulous ridge. Care should be taken to ensure that the maxillary and mandibular AMDs are fairly parallel to each other and positioned so the maxillary stylus is located over the anterior aspect of the mandibular AMD. This allows sufficient

area for the stylus to navigate on the tracing plate during laterotrusive movements. The mandibular AMD impression is relined using light body poly (vinyl siloxane) (Figure 6.10).

1. The mandibular AMD is then assessed for stability. It should cover the ridge morphology of the mandibular arch to ensure accurate digital superimposition of the AMD and the final mandibular impression. Excess impression material causing unnatural contour is trimmed. With both maxillary and mandibular components of the AMDs in the patient's mouth, the lips should close comfortably around the AMD trays without any deformation of the lower third of the face.

2. The OVD is determined using conventional methods such as evaluating facial proportions and the modified Niswonger's technique. The

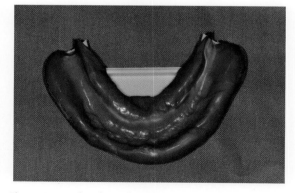

Figure 6.10 Relined intaglio surface of the mandibular AMD with heavy-body PVS.

existing CD can also be utilized as an excellent reference for determining the appropriate OVD. The OVD is recorded using the provided caliper, which measures two selected points on the nose and the chin. The slotted screw on the side of the maxillary AMD tray is used to increase or decrease the distance between the maxillary and mandibular AMD trays while the maxillary stylus maintains contact with the tracing plate of the mandibular AMD to establish the appropriate OVD (Figure 6.11).

3. An intraoral gothic arch tracing is made to record CR. The patient is asked to keep his jaws together and maintain the maxillary stylus in contact with the mandibular AMD. The patient is then instructed to move his jaw forward and backward, then left to make a laterotrusive movement from the CR position, and then to the contralateral side. This will cause the stylus to scribe a mark on the mandibular AMD creating a gothic arch tracing (Figure 6.12).

4. The AvaDent impression material adhesive can be applied to the mandibular tracing plate and the material dried. The movement of the stylus will then scribe a line in the adhesive. Alternately, articulating material can be rubbed on the tracing plate to help identify the lines scribed by the maxillary stylus. The apex of the recording denotes the CR position. The mandibular AMD is removed and a recess is made at the CR position using a round bur or acrylic resin bur at the apex of the gothic arch arrow point (Figure 6.13).

5. The maxillary lip support can then be adjusted by moving the lip support flange anteriorly

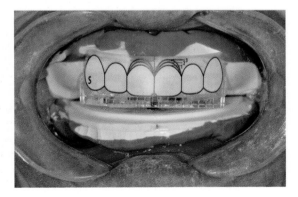

Figure 6.11 Establishment of the appropriate OVD with the selection mold tab cemented in place.

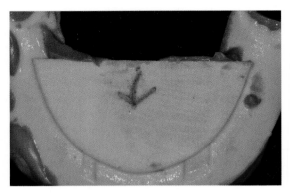

Figure 6.12 Gothic arch recording.

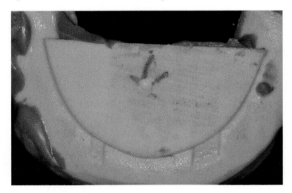

Figure 6.13 Recess created at the apex of the gothic arch recording.

or posteriorly until the desired lip support is obtained (Figure 6.14).

6. A thin permanent marker is used to mark the patient's maxillary midline on the lip support flange and the smile line can also be marked on the lip support flange. To determine the size of the denture teeth, three provided AvaDent Esthetic mold guides of different sizes are overlaid on the teeth of the patient's existing denture (Figure 6.15).

The position of the pink denture base resin around the necks of the teeth can also be selected from three numbered locations present on the template. The lip support flange is dried and the self-adhesive guide is oriented over the midline and smile line markings and pressed into position. The orientation of the guide is then assessed while the patient is at rest and smiling (Figure 6.16 a, b).

7. The mandibular AMD is reinserted in the patient's mouth and the mandible guided until

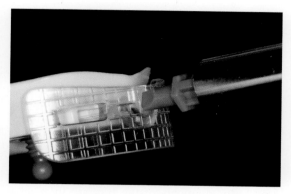

Figure 6.14 AvaDent wrench used to moved the maxillary AMD lip support flange.

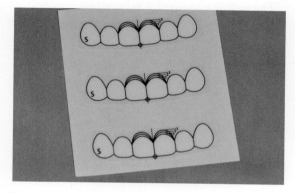

Figure 6.15 Self-adhesive teeth selection mold tabs.

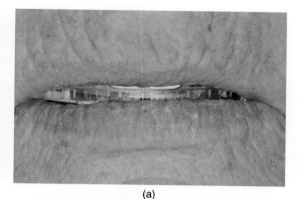

(a)

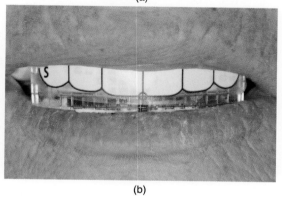

(b)

Figure 6.16 (a) Teeth selection mold tabs evaluated with lips at repose. (b) Teeth selection mold tabs evaluated with the patient smiling.

the stylus engages the CR recess located at the apex of the gothic arch tracing to ensure the patient is locked in CR. A generous amount of interocclusal registration material is injected into the space between the mandibular and maxillary AMDs so they are securely locked together (Figure 6.17). The firmly connected AMDs are removed from the mouth, disinfected, and mailed to Global Dental Science, LLC along with the final impressions, completed laboratory authorization form, and photographs of the smile and lips at rest.

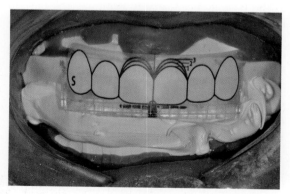

Figure 6.17 Injection of bite registration material to capture the centric relation.

Laboratory procedures

1. The disinfected complete arch impressions and the connected maxillary and mandibular AMDs are laser scanned.

2. A computer software program performs the following tasks: (i) builds the occlusal relationship of the maxillary and mandibular arches from the morphologic data obtained by scanning

the connected AMD trays and superimposing this data over the scans of the complete arch impressions; (ii) identifies and marks the denture borders; (iii) forms the intaglio surface of the denture base; (iv) virtually sets denture teeth so they occlude properly with the desired occlusal plane of orientation; and (v) forms the bases around the articulated denture teeth.

3. A digital preview of the prostheses is emailed to the clinician for approval (Figure 6.18 a–f). The denture bases are then milled from different choices of base material with recesses into which the requested denture teeth are bonded.

4. Prior to the fabrication of the final digital denture, the clinician can request an optional advanced try-in denture (ATI) (milled base with denture teeth set in wax rims) to allow for evaluation of esthetics, phonetics and functional components of the denture in the patient's mouth. Adjustments can be made to the trial denture by repositioning the teeth in the wax to meet the needs of the patient.

Denture placement and adjustments

The placement and post-placement adjustments of CAD/CAM complete dentures are similar to the placement of conventional dentures using pressure indicating paste and making adjustments to the base as necessary to optimize the base-to-mucosa contact (Figure 6.19). Intraoral occlusal adjustments are made as required. In the case of significant occlusal discrepancies, a clinical remount procedure can be performed.

Step-by-step procedures for the fabrication of complete dentures using the Dentca system

1. A Dentca system provides the clinician with a starter kit that contains stock trays of different sizes (S, M, L, and XL), a Dentca™ Lip ruler, a Dentca™ Jaw Gauge, and an EZ-Tracer™ (Figure 6.20).

2. The appropriate maxillary and mandibular trays are selected based on the patient's arch size. The Dentca trays are two-piece trays with detachable segments that need to be attached before making the definitive impression (Figure 6.21 a, b).

3. Adhesive is applied to the selected stock trays and the definitive impressions are made in the same manner used to make the definitive impressions for the AvaDent system.

4. After the definitive impressions are made, a #15C surgical blade is used to slice through the impression material on both the maxillary and mandibular impression following the demarcating borderline between the posterior and anterior parts of the trays. The anterior and posterior segments of the tray are then separated from each other using firm intermittent wiggling and pulling motions (Figure 6.22).

5. The gothic arch device is carefully attached to the anterior part of the mandibular definitive impression into slots located in the lingual surface of the tray (Figure 6.23). The flat occlusal tracing plate attached to the maxillary stock tray is covered with an aerosol indicator marking spray (Occlude®, Pascal International Inc., Bellevue, WA) or covered with EZ-Tracer™, a tracing material supplied by Dentca (Figure 6.24).

6. The anterior parts of the maxillary and mandibular impressions are then inserted in the patient's mouth and their stability checked. The OVD is determined in the traditional manner with the help of the Dentca Jaw Gauge and the stylus adjusted as needed making sure that it contacts the maxillary tracing plate (Figure 6.25). The gothic arch tracing is made as described previously for the AvaDent process. The maxillary tray is removed from the patient's mouth and a recess is made using a round bur or acrylic resin bur at the apex of the gothic arch arrow point (Figure 6.26).

7. The maxillary tray is reinserted in the patient's mouth and guided until the stylus engages in the recess to ensure the patient is locked in CR. An interocclusal recording material is injected into the space between the mandibular and maxillary trays. The connected trays are removed from the mouth and disinfected (Figure 6.27).

8. The length of the maxillary lip is measured with a Dentca Lip ruler. The measurement is made between the incisal papilla and the inferior border of the maxillary lip (Figure 6.28).

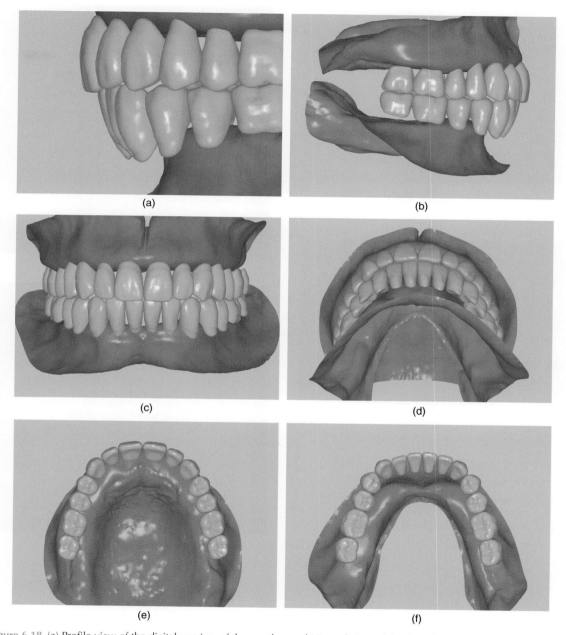

Figure 6.18 (a) Profile view of the digital preview of the prostheses. (b) Lateral view of the digital preview of the prostheses. (c) Frontal view of the digital preview of the prostheses. (d) Frontal below view of the digital preview of the prostheses. (e) Maxillary full arch view of the digital preview of the prostheses. (f) Mandibular full arch view of the digital preview of the prostheses.

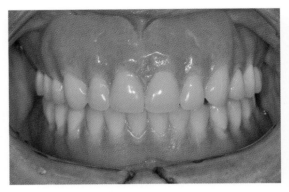

Figure 6.19 Placement of AvaDent digital complete dentures.

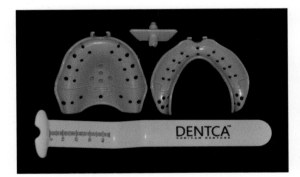

Figure 6.20 Maxillary and mandibular Dentca stock trays and lip ruler.

9. The disinfected trays with the bite registration material, the posterior detached parts of the impression trays, and a laboratory work authorization form are mailed to Dentca.

Laboratory procedures

1. The posterior segments of the trays are reattached to the anterior segments and the connected maxillary and mandibular definitive impressions are treated and laser scanned.
2. Virtual edentulous ridges are digitally articulated using a proprietary computer software.
3. The lip length measurement provided and the several anatomical landmarks are used to set the virtual teeth so they have a desired occlusal plane orientation and occlude properly.

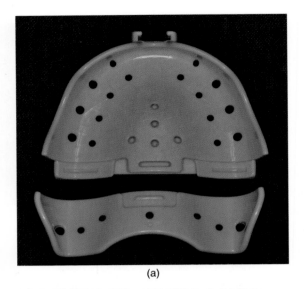

(a)

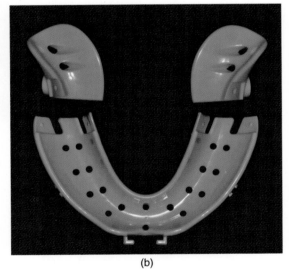

(b)

Figure 6.21 (a) Maxillary Dentca detachable tray. (b) Mandibular Dentca detachable tray.

4. The data is transferred to an RP machine that will fabricate stereolithographic analog of the digitally designed dentures. These trial dentures can also serve as surgical templates for implant placement and are provided at no charge if requested by the clinician. The trial dentures are similar in fit of the final dentures, approximate the proposed contours, and can

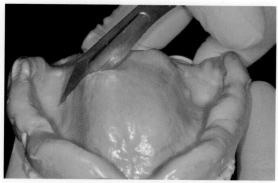

Figure 6.22 Surgical blade used to slice thru the definitive impression material (Courtesy of Dr. Ewa Parciak.)

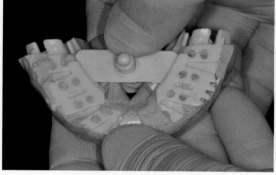

Figure 6.23 Stylus slotted into the mandibular Dentca tray (Courtesy of Dr. Ewa Parciak.)

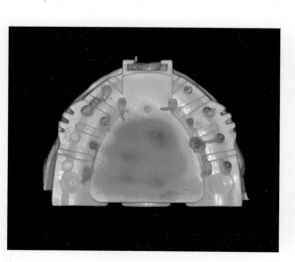

Figure 6.24 Aerosol indicator marking spray covering the maxillary occlusal tracing plate (Courtesy of Dr. Ewa Parciak.)

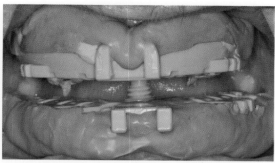

Figure 6.25 Establishment of the appropriate OVD (Courtesy of Dr. Ewa Parciak.)

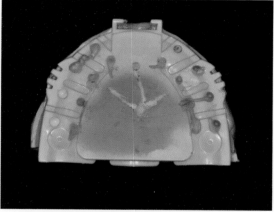

Figure 6.26 Gothic arch recording on the maxillary occlusal tracing plate (Courtesy of Dr. Ewa Parciak.)

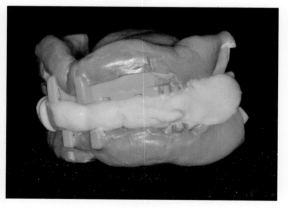

Figure 6.27 Dentca jaw relation record (Courtesy of Dr. Ewa Parciak.)

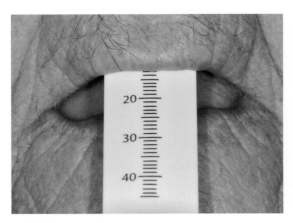

Figure 6.28 Dentca lip ruler used to measure the length of the maxillary lip (Courtesy of Dr. Ewa Parciak.)

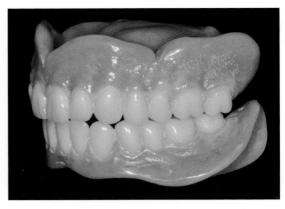

Figure 6.30 Definitive Dentca dentures (Courtesy of Dr. Ewa Parciak.)

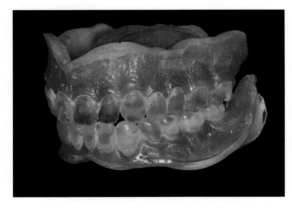

Figure 6.29 Dentca maxillary and mandibular stereolithographic trial dentures (Courtesy of Dr. Ewa Parciak.)

be used to evaluate the phonetics and the proposed occlusion of the denture in the patient's mouth. Unfortunately, the esthetic component cannot be evaluated giving the frosty appearance (no shade) of the teeth and modifications to teeth position are not possible (Figure 6.29).

5. The definitive denture is processed conventionally using 3D printed flasks (Figure 6.30).

Denture insertion and adjustments

The placement and post-placement adjustments of CAD/CAM complete dentures are similar to the placement of conventional dentures. Several applications of pressure indicating paste and adjustments might be necessary to achieve the desire result. An intraoral occlusal adjustment might be performed regardless of the precise nature of the digital denture fabrication. If significant occlusal discrepancies are noted, a clinical remount procedure can be performed.

AvaDent conversion denture for immediate loading of a complete arch implant prosthesis

It is possible to fabricate a digital conversion prosthesis that has an unique design for easy modification to an immediately loaded interim fixed complete denture on implants placed using a guided surgical protocol. The technique saves significant clinic time by allowing easy pick up and conversion of the digital denture to an interim fixed complete denture.

Clinical procedures

1. The first step in the conversion denture protocol is the fabrication of provisional dentures following the previously described steps involved in the fabrication of the digital complete dentures (Figure 6.31 a, b). The provisional monolithic dentures are fully milled (including both the denture base and teeth) using a proprietary technique.

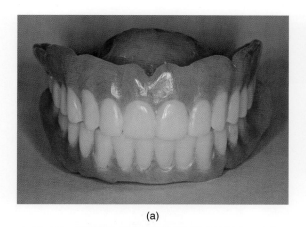

(a)

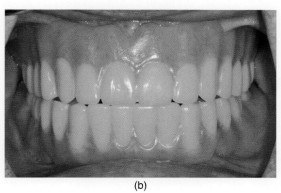

(b)

Figure 6.31 (a) AvaDent provisional digital complete dentures. (b) Trial placement of AvaDent provisional digital complete dentures.

2. A radiographic template is fabricated by AvaDent that is a duplicate of the mandibular provisional denture to which fiduciary markers (gutta percha placed into spherical indents made on the facial cameo surface) are placed (Figure 6.32). A CBCT scan is made of only the radiographic template and then the radiographic template is positioned intraorally using an index and a CBCT scan made of the patient following the NobelGuide™/NobelClinician protocol (Figure 6.33). The surgical planning for implant placement is performed using Nobel-Clinician software based on the orientation of the denture bases and teeth to the existing bone and vital anatomical structures so the most appropriate locations are identified for each implant (Figure. 6.34 a–d).

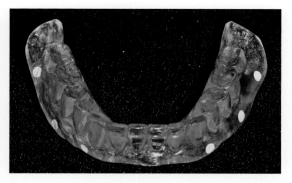

Figure 6.32 Radiographic template with fiduciary markers.

3. The virtually determined implant positions are finalized using the NobelClinician Software and the required data sent to Nobel Biocare for fabrication of a NobelGuide surgical template (Figure 6.35). The virtual implant positions are then used by Global Dental Science to fabricate an AvaDent conversion CD (Figure 6.36). This conversion denture has channels milled through the denture base at the appropriate positions where temporary copings would be located after their attachment to the implant abutments. It also has a pre-milled slot located around the denture base with a small number of struts that connects the peripheral denture base to the central portion of the conversion denture that will function as the immediate provisional fixed CD. The presence of the channels and slot facilitates easy conversion of the denture to a fixed prosthesis while using the positional stability of the peripheral denture base to accurately orient the prosthesis in the patient's mouth during attachment of the denture to the temporary copings.

4. The NobelGuide surgical template is then used to place the selected implants (NobelReplace® Conical Connection) as planned virtually (Figure 6.37 a, b). Nobel Biocare Multi-Unit abutments of appropriate height are attached to the implants and the abutment screws torqued to the manufacturer recommended values (Figure 6.38). Nobel Biocare Temporary Copings for Multi-Unit abutments are then attached to the Multi-Unit abutments (Figure 6.39).

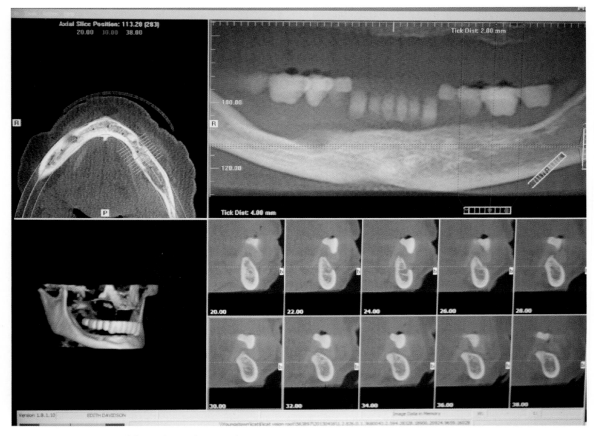

Figure 6.33 CBCT scan of the Radiographic template.

5. The AvaDent Conversion Denture is positioned over the temporary copings with the denture base and occlusion guiding the appropriate position (Figure 6.40 a–d). The denture is connected to the temporary copings by flowing autopolymerizing acrylic resin between the channels in the denture and the temporary copings and allowing the resin to polymerize (Figure 6.41). The temporary coping screws are then loosened and the prosthesis removed from the mouth (Figure 6.42).

The struts are sectioned to separate the peripheral section of the denture base from the central portion that will serve as the immediate fixed CD (Figure 6.43). Autopolymerizing resin is flowed as needed between the denture base and the temporary copings where voids were present to

attain a smooth transition between the denture base and copings (Figure 6.44). The converted mandibular provisional fixed CD is finished, polished and attached to the implant abutments using the temporary coping screws (Figure 6.45 and Figure 6.46). The occlusion is finalized against the previously fabricated maxillary provisional CD (Figure 6.47 a–c). Post operative medications and instructions are given to the patient followed by periodic reevaluation appointments.

Technique description for the fabrication of a digital definitive fixed complete denture

Once the implant healing phase is completed, the definitive phase for the fabrication of a mandibular

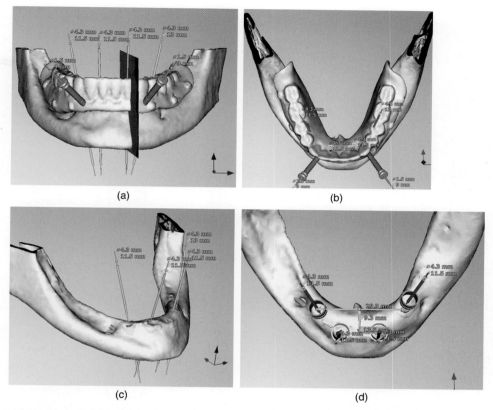

Figure 6.34 (a) Frontal view of the surgical planning with the virtual surgical template. (b) Occlusal view of the surgical planning with the virtual surgical template. (c) Lateral view of the most appropriate location of each planned implant. (d) Occlusal view of the most appropriate location of each planned implant.

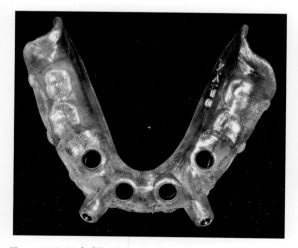

Figure 6.35 NobelGuide surgical template.

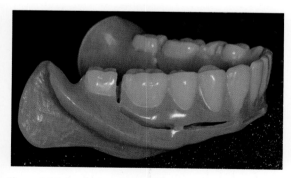

Figure 6.36 Avadent conversion denture.

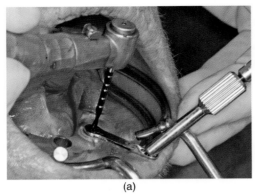

(a)

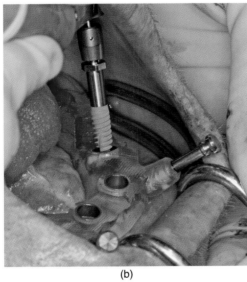

(b)

Figure 6.37 (a), (b) Implant placement using the NobelGuide surgical template.

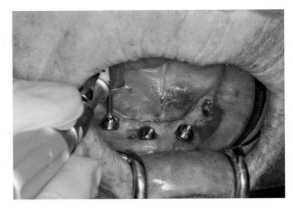

Figure 6.38 Placement of Nobel Biocare Multi-Unit abutments.

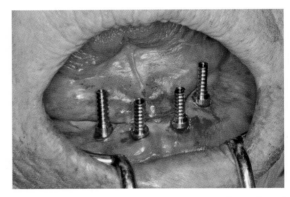

Figure 6.39 Placement of temporary copings for multi-unit abutments.

fixed complete denture begins. The steps involved in the fabrication include: *Final impressions and records*

Based on the information obtained from the Nobel Clinician software and the surgical guide used for the guided surgery, Global Dental Science provides an AvaDent implant record device (AIRD) (Figure 6.48) and AvaDent verification jig, (AVJ) which are designed to simplify the impression making process (Figure 6.49). The AIRD is a duplicate of the complete denture but has an occlusal opening that fits over the verification jig. It functions as an impression tray.

The resin AVJ fits simultaneously over and around either impression copings or temporary copings (Figure 6.50).

Either of these copings can be used for the final impression. The AVJ is positioned so there is a 2–3 mm space between the inferior surface of the jig and the mucosa. It is then secured to the copings by injecting flowable composite resin between the jig and the copings (Figure 6.51 a–c).

The Implant Record Device has an opening in the denture base that is large enough to fit around the AVJ that has been connected to the copings while also resting on the posterior edentulous

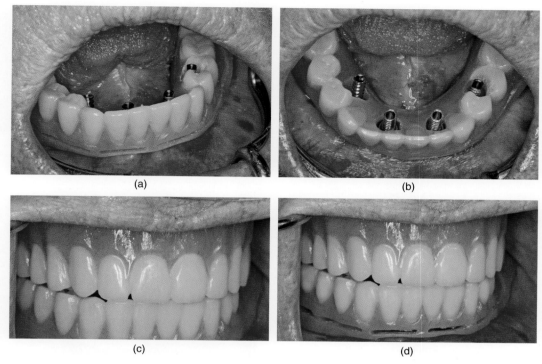

Figure 6.40 (a) Buccal view of the positioning of the Avadent conversion denture over the temporary copings. (b) Occlusal view of the positioning of the Avadent conversion denture over the temporary copings. (c) The occlusion guiding the position of the conversion denture. (d) Buccal view of the conversion denture in occlusion.

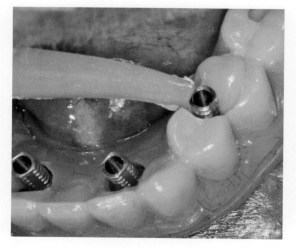

Figure 6.41 Autopolymerizing acrylic resin injected between the channels in the denture and the temporary copings.

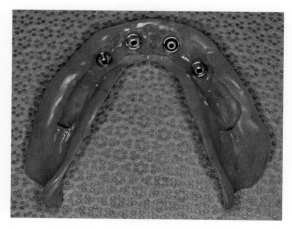

Figure 6.42 Intaglio surface of conversion denture.

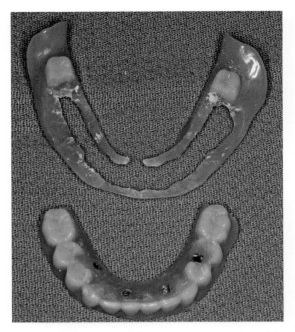

Figure 6.43 Sectioning of the struts and separation of the peripheral section of the denture base from the immediate fixed CD.

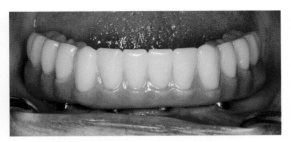

Figure 6.45 Frontal view of the provisional fixed CD.

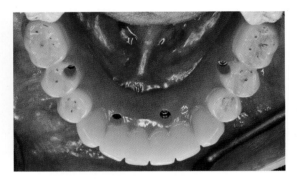

Figure 6.46 Occlusal view of the provisional fixed CD.

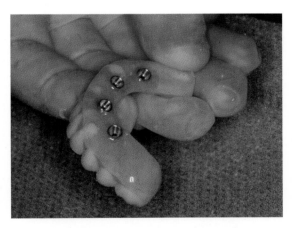

Figure 6.44 Voids between the denture base and temporary copings are filled with autopolymerizing resin.

ridge (Figure 6.52 a, b). If any portion of the device comes in contact with the AVJ, the device is adjusted sufficiently to remove the contact to allow easier and accurate placement.

The final impression is then made using the AIRD as an impression tray. Modeling base plate wax can be used to cover the open portion of the AIRD after it is coated with impression adhesive and then heavy-body impression material is placed in the device (Figure 6.53).

The wax will prevent the impression material from flowing out through the opening in the device prior to it being seated intraorally. Light-body impression material is expressed around the connected copings and underneath the AVJ. The AIRD which has been filled with the heavy body impression material is then seated over the AVJ (Figure 6.54 a, b).

The AIRD is oriented using the occlusion with the opposing provisional denture thereby capturing the impression at the correct OVD (Figure 6.55).

A finger or Q-tip is used to wipe across the occlusal opening in the AIRD to expose the occlusal aspect of the copings so they are located before polymerization of the impression material (Figure 6.56).

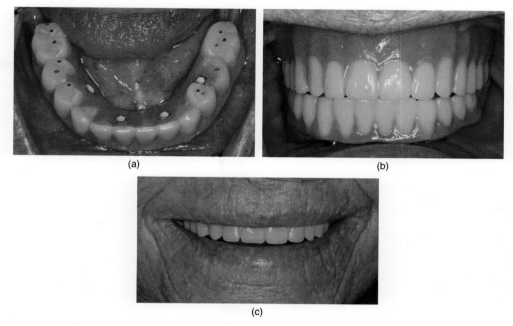

Figure 6.47 (a) Occlusal view of the finalized provisional fixed CD. (b) Frontal view of definitive dentures. (c) Frontal view of patient smile.

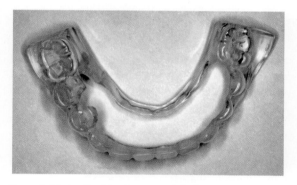

Figure 6.48 AvaDent implant record device.

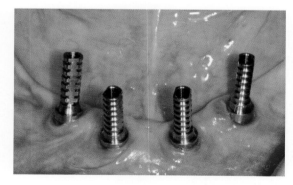

Figure 6.50 Placement of temporary copings for multi-unit abutments.

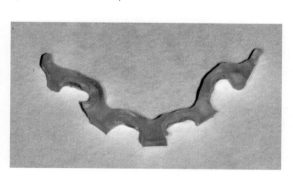

Figure 6.49 AvaDent verification jig.

After the impression material is properly polymerized, the screws in the temporary copings are loosened and the impression removed. The impression should have recorded the edentulous ridges and contain the AVJ with the connected impression copings. Excess impression material that would interfere with occlusal interdigitation of the AIRD with the maxillary denture is removed carefully and the impression

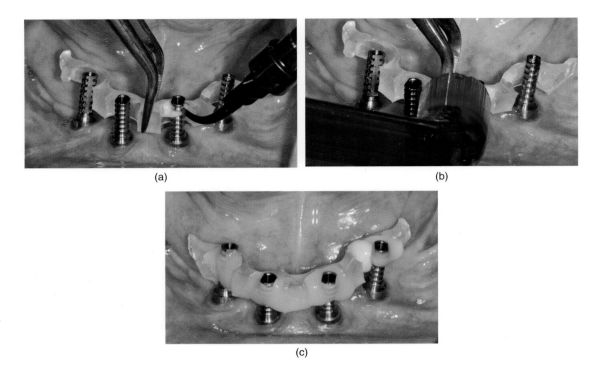

(a)   (b)

(c)

Figure 6.51 (a) Flowable composite resin syringed between the verification jig and the temporary copings. (b) Flowable composite resin light cured in place. (c) Verification jig secured to all temporary copings.

reseated and attached with a couple of screws (Figure 6.57 a–c).

An interocclusal record is made between the AIRD and the opposing provisional denture (Figure 6.58). The provisional fixed conversion CD is replaced and the screws tightened and the access holes sealed.

Laboratory phase

The final impression made with the AIRD is sent to Global Dental Science along with the interocclusal record made between the opposing AvaDent provisional maxillary complete denture and the AIRD for fabrication of the definitive complete denture and the AvaDent fixed complete denture that will have a milled titanium bar with pink acrylic resin and teeth utilizing a wrap around design. The digital data allows easy fabrication of a new definitive maxillary CD that is identical in morphology to the provisional maxillary CD. The maxillary denture can have commercially

available denture teeth placed into the milled recesses on the denture base or custom milled teeth. Using the already recorded digital data from the surgical phase and the information provided by the impression made with the AIRD and the new interocclusal records, Global Dental Science uses proprietary computer software to create a definitive maxillary CD and a mandibular fixed CD (Figure 6.59 a–d).

Placement of definitive maxillary denture and mandibular fixed CD

The Conversion Denture is removed and the definitive prostheses are placed and adjusted. The definitive fixed CD is torqued using the manufacturer recommended value. The access holes are sealed and post placement instructions given. The patient is shown how to maintain the prostheses and scheduled for periodic re-evaluations (Figure 6.60 a, b).

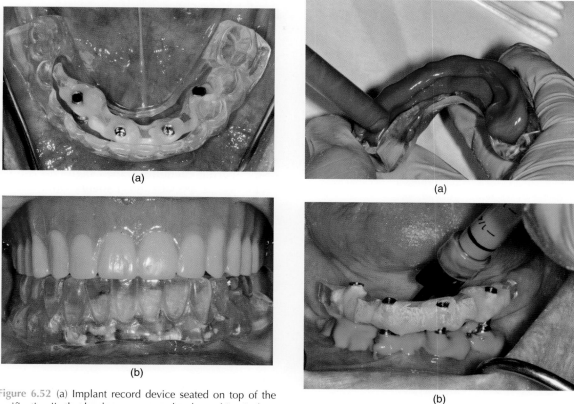

(a)

(b)

(a)

(b)

Figure 6.52 (a) Implant record device seated on top of the verification jig that has been connected to the multi-unit abutments. (b) Implant record device seated on top of the verification jig and resting on the posterior edentulous ridge.

Figure 6.54 (a) Heavy-body impression material placed in the record device. (b) Light-body impression material expressed around the connected copings and underneath the verification jig.

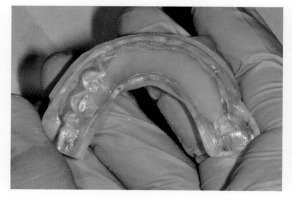

Figure 6.53 Implant record device covered with modeling base plate wax and coated with impression adhesive.

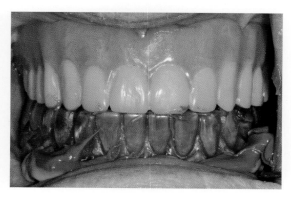

Figure 6.55 Use of the opposing provisional denture to orient the implant record device and capture the impression at the correct OVD.

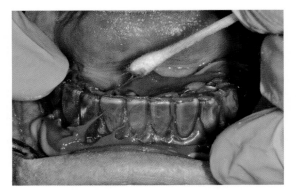

Figure 6.56 A Q-tip is used to expose the occlusal aspect of the temporary copings.

Computer-aided design of removable partial denture

The improvement in oral health and life expectancy of the elderly population has led to the retention of the patient's teeth for a longer period of time (Douglas & Watson, 2002). The decrease in the rate of tooth loss has lead to an increase in the need for removable partial dentures (RPD) (Ettinger *et al.*, 1984; Redford *et al.*, 1996). Even though osseointegrated dental implant-supported prostheses are excellent options to restore partial edentulism, their high cost can be prohibitive, especially for patients from a low

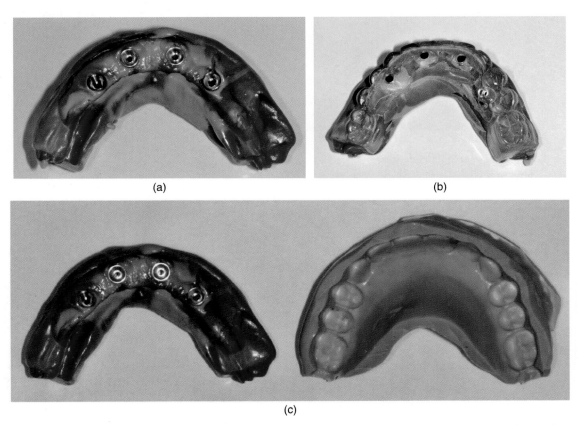

(a)

(b)

(c)

Figure 6.57 (a) Intaglio surface of the impression. (b) Cameo surface of the impression containing the verification jig with the connecting temporary abutments.

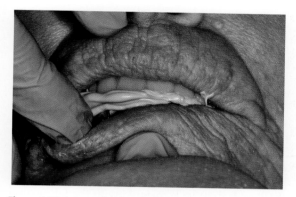

Figure 6.58 Interocclusal record between the implant record device and the opposing provisional denture.

socioeconomic situation (Dolan *et al.*, 2001). Several materials such as Type IV gold alloy, Cobalt Chrome (Co-Cr), Nickel-Chromium (Ni-Cr), and Ti-6Al-7Nb, a vanadium-free titanium (Ti), have been successfully cast for the fabrication of removable partial denture frameworks. Partials cast with gold alloys had a low modulus of elasticity and hence more susceptible to flexure and distortion under high occlusal forces. This resulted in the need for thick major connectors, a factor along with the inherent value of gold increased the laboratory costs. Chrome-based alloys became popular in the 1970s as a viable option to the gold alloys. During that period the majority of

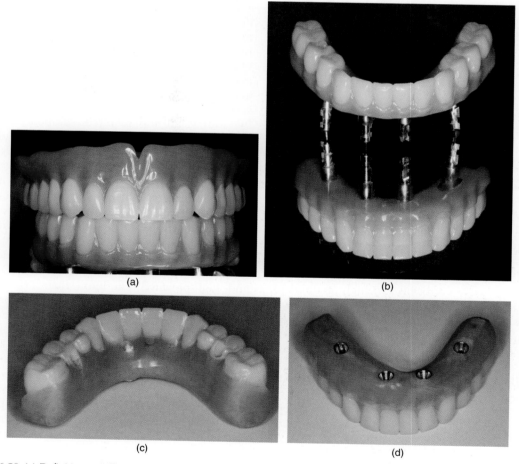

(a)

(b)

(c)

(d)

Figure 6.59 (a) Definitive maxillary CD and mandibular fixed complete denture. (b) Fixed complete denture showing a milled titanium bar with pink acrylic resin wrap around. (c) Lingual view of the definitive mandibular fixed complete denture. (d) Intaglio surface of the mandibular fixed complete denture.

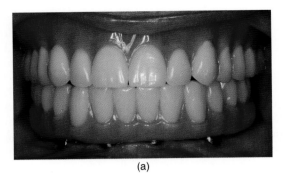

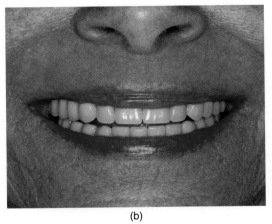

Figure 6.60 (a) Frontal view of the placement of the definitive denture and mandibular fixed CD. (b) Frontal view of patient smile.

dental laboratories switched to Co-Cr and Ni-Cr alloys. These alloys offered many advantages including (i) low cost, (ii) high strength, (iii) excellent resistance to corrosion, (iv) high modulus of elasticity, and (v) low density. Reports of adverse effects such as potential for toxicity and allergies encouraged the quest for safer materials leading to the introduction of titanium alloys (Covington *et al.*, 1985; Schmalz & Garhammer, 2002). A vanadium-free titanium alloy (Ti-6Al-7Nb) with excellent mechanical properties was introduced as an alternative for traditional casting alloys (Matsumura *et al.*, 2002). This alloy is biocompatible (Matsuno *et al.*, 2001), resistant to wear (Iijima *et al.*, 2003), strong (Iijima *et al.*, 2003; Kobayashi *et al.*, 1998), ductile (Kobayashi *et al.*, 1998), and resistant to corrosion (Khan *et al.*, 1996).

However, one of its main drawbacks is the casting porosity that can occur while fabricating the framework. Several studies evaluated the effect of design (Al-Mesmar *et al.*, 1999; Guttal & Patil, 2007), diameter and direction (Baltag *et al.*, 2002) of the sprue in an effort to minimize the porosity of titanium cast removable partial denture frameworks. Other difficulties and problems (Ohkubo *et al.*, 2006; Jang *et al.*, 2001; Sutton & Rogers, 2001) associated with casting of titanium motivated researchers to explore the possibility of using digital dentistry to avoid the disadvantages and challenges that are associated with the fabrication process of a removable partial denture. Recently, CAD software has been used to digitally design frameworks for an RPD prosthesis (Williams *et al.*, 2004; Eggbeer *et al.*, 2005; Han *et al.*, 2010). The design process comprises three steps: (i) the scanning of the definitive impression or a cast poured from the definitive impression, (ii) the exporting of the scanned information for digital preparation and surveying of the cast utilizing commercially available RPD computer aided design (CAD) software, and (iii) designing the 3D printed RPD by adding all the required components of a framework (minor and major connectors, guiding planes, rests, clasp assemblies, etc.). The design file data is then used to either print the framework in wax resin using an RP machine and then to invest the pattern and cast it using conventional methods (Williams *et al.*, 2004; Eggbeer *et al.*, 2005; Bibb *et al.*, 2006) or to fabricate the framework directly using a selective laser melting machine (Han *et al.*, 2010; Williams *et al.*, 2006). Selective laser melting (SLM) is a technology that uses 3D CAD data and high-powered ytterbium fiber laser beam to fuse high metallic powders together forming the previously designed 3D RPD framework. SLM has been widely and successfully used in metallurgical industries (Yadroitsev *et al.*, 2007).

In 2004, Williams *et al.* (2004) published the first laboratory study investigating the use of a CAD software to design the shape of a number of components for the RPD framework. The plastic patterns of these components were printed using a RP machine and successfully cast. Following casting of the plastic patterns they observed small fins on the divested casting suggesting an expansion of the plastic pattern. They then recommended the use of wax for the printing of future framework patterns to avoid this complication. Bibb *et al.* (2006) were the first to report trial fitting of a RPD framework designed with a CAD software and then printed using the RP technique. The framework was reported as clinically acceptable.

Advantages of digitally designed removable partial dentures

1. Reduced fabrication time and expenses; because there is no need for a refractory cast to wax, sprue and cast the RPD framework, multiple printed frameworks could be invested and cast simultaneously.
2. Increased profitability and productivity of the laboratory.
3. Increased communication and collaboration between the dental practitioner and the dental technician.
4. Less emphasis on conventional RPD fabrication process allows technician to focus on mastering the principles of digital RPD design.

Disadvantages of digitally designed removable partial dentures

1. Investment involved in purchasing the scanning software.
2. Investment in the purchase of the CAD software and printers.
3. Complications associated with the casting process such as the presence of surface porosities on the cast frameworks.
4. Increased labor cost for learning and perfecting the digital process.

Step-by-step procedures for the digital design and fabrication of a RPD using the RP technique

1. The definitive impression or the definitive cast is scanned in a high-speed scanner (Figure 6.61).
2. The scanned information is exported for digital preparation and surveying of the cast utilizing commercially available RPD CAD software.

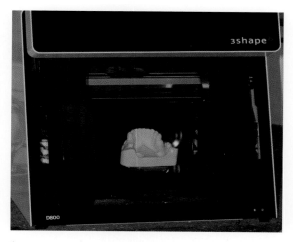

Figure 6.61 Definitive cast scanned in a high-speed scanner. (Courtesy of Dental Masters Laboratory.)

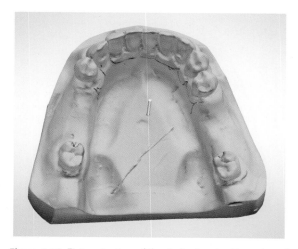

Figure 6.62 Determination of the desired path of insertion of the virtual cast (Courtesy of Dental Masters Laboratory.)

3. The virtual cast is prepared for the survey process. A blue directional rod in the center of palate assists in determining the desired path of insertion and is the virtual surveying tool (Figure 6.62). The cast is then oriented for the appropriate path of insertion.
4. The undercut blockout is completed next. Blocking out the undesirable undercuts and the location of the desired undercuts is completed (Figure 6.63).

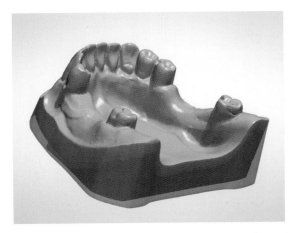

Figure 6.63 Blocking out of the undercuts (Courtesy of Dental Masters Laboratory.)

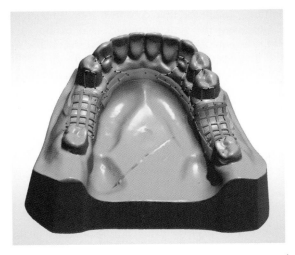

Figure 6.65 Addition of the major connector. (Courtesy of Dental Masters Laboratory.)

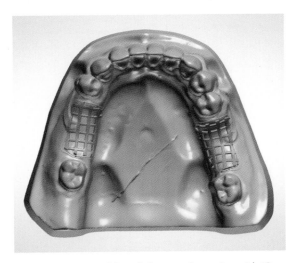

Figure 6.64 Design of the relief area and retention grids (Courtesy of Dental Masters Laboratory.)

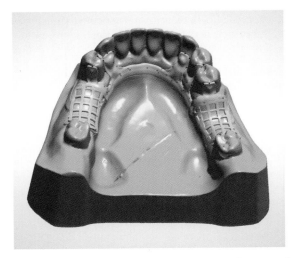

Figure 6.66 Outline of the minor connectors (Courtesy of Dental Masters Laboratory.)

5. The relief area and the retention grids (or mesh) are designed at this stage (Figure 6.64).
6. The next step is the addition of the major connector (Figure 6.65). The minor connectors are outlined with a connected blue dotted line and later added to the design (Figure 6.66).
7. The clasps are added at this stage by extending the blue dotted lines to the desired clasp shape and contour (Figure 6.67). The clasps thickness, width and contour can be properly designed for adequate strength of the framework.
8. The finish lines are virtually placed followed by the final sculpting and contouring of the digital waxing of the RPD framework (Figure 6.68).
9. The virtually designed framework is then inspected for internal finish lines (Figure 6.69), thickness of frame and prepared for printing

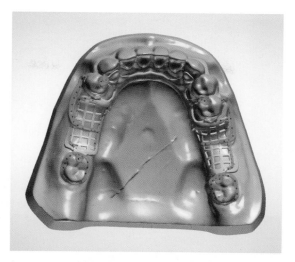

Figure 6.67 Addition of clasp to the design (Courtesy of Dental Masters Laboratory.)

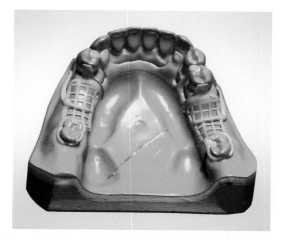

Figure 6.69 Virtual cast is inspected for internal finish lines (Courtesy of Dental Masters Laboratory.)

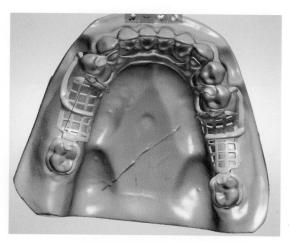

Figure 6.68 Placement of the finish lines followed by sculpting and contouring of the digital wax. (Courtesy of Dental Masters Laboratory.)

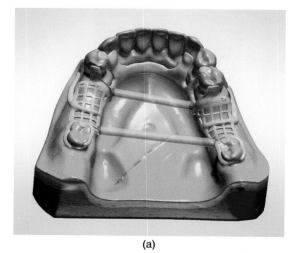

(a)

Figure 6.70 (a) Addition of cross arch support bars. (b) Virtual framework designed and ready for printing. (Courtesy of Dental Masters Laboratory.)

by adding cross arch support bars (Figure 6.70 a, b).

10. The file is then sent to the printer for the creation of wax or resin pattern (Figure 6.71 a–c).

11. The printed pattern is then sprued for investing.

12. The rest of the technical procedures for digital frameworks are the same as for the conventional partial fabrication process.

After the digital metal framework try in (Figure 6.72), conventional methods are used to fabricate the RPD which includes denture teeth setup and processing of the teeth and acrylic was done on the cast poured from the definitive impression. After processing, adjusting and polishing the completed RPD is placed and adjusted for comfort and function.

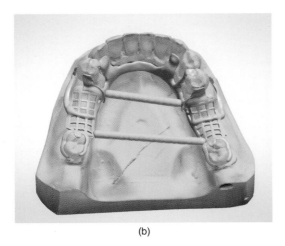

(b)

Figure 6.70 (*Continued*).

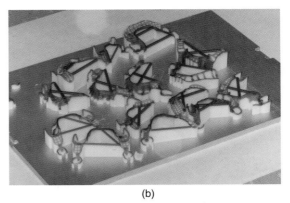

(b)

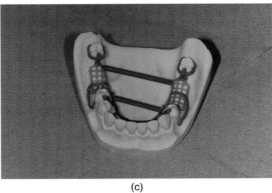

(c)

Figure 6.71 (*Continued*).

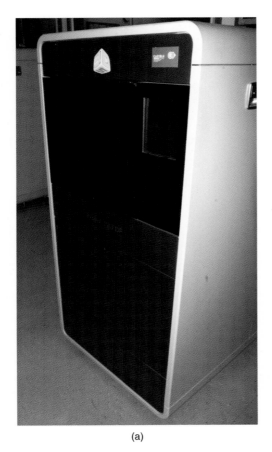

(a)

Figure 6.71 (a) 3D printer. (b) Printing of resin pattern. (c) Try-in and fitting of the resin pattern. (Courtesy of Dental Masters Laboratory.)

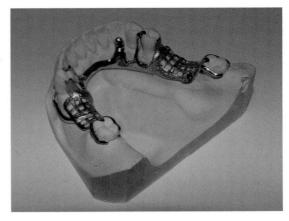

Figure 6.72 Polished RPD framework (Courtesy of Dental Masters Laboratory.)

Acknowledgments

The authors would like to thank Mr. Robert Kreyer, CDT, for his advice in the preparation of the section on computer-aided design of removable partial denture and the Dental Masters Laboratory for providing us with the laboratory pictures of the fabrication process of a CAD/CAM removable partial denture.

References

Al Mardini, M., Ercoli, C., & Graser, G.N. (2005) A technique to produce a mirror-image wax pattern of an ear using rapid prototyping technology. *Journal of Prosthetic Dentistry*, **94**, 195–198.

Al-Mesmar, H.S., Morgano, S.M., & Mark, L.E. (1999) Investigation of the effect of three Sprue designs on the porosity and the completeness of titanium cast removable partial denture frameworks. *Journal of Prosthetic Dentistry*, **82**, 15–21.

Baltag, I., Watanabe, K., Kusakari, H., & Miyakawa, O. (2002) Internal porosity of cast titanium removable partial dentures: influence of sprue direction and diameter on porosity in simplified circumferential clasps. *Journal of Prosthetic Dentistry*, **88**, 151–158.

Berdicevsky, I., Ben-Aryeh, H., Szagel, R., & Gutman, D. (1980) Oral candida of asymptomatic denture wearers. *International Journal of Oral Surgery*, **9**, 113–115.

Bibb, R.J., Eggbeer, D., Williams, R.J., & Woodward, A. (2006) Trial fitting of a removable partial denture framework made using computer-aided design and rapid prototyping techniques. *Proceedings of the Institution of Mechanical Engineers. Part H, Journal of Engineering in Medicine*, **220**, 793–797.

Budtz-Jörgensen, E. (1974) The significance of *Candida albicans* in denture stomatitis. *Scandinavian Journal of Dental Research*, **82**, 151–190.

Busch, M. & Kordass, B. (2006) Concept and development of a computerized positioning of prosthetic teeth for complete dentures. *International Journal of Computerized Dentistry*, **9**, 113–120.

Christensen, G.J. (2006) Removable prosthodontics: a forgotten part of dentistry. *The Alpha Omegan*, **99**, 26–28.

Christensen, G.J. & Yancey, W. (2005) Dental laboratory in crisis, part II: potential solutions to the challenges facing the industry. *Journal of the American Dental Association*, **136**, 783–786.

Covington, J.S., McBride, M.A., Slagle, W.F., & Disney, A.L. (1985) Quantization of nickel and beryllium leakage from base metal casting alloys. *Journal of Prosthetic Dentistry*, **54**, 127–136.

Dolan, T.A., Gilbert, G.H., Duncan, R.P., & Foerster, U. (2001) Risk indicators of edentulism, partial tooth loss and prosthetic status among black and white middle-aged and older adults. *Community Dentistry and Oral Epidemiology*, **29**, 329–340.

Douglas, C.W. & Watson, A.J. (2002) Future needs for fixed and removable partial dentures in the United States. *Journal of Prosthetic Dentistry*, **87**, 9–14.

Eggbeer, D., Bibb, R., & Williams, R.J. (2005) The computer-aided design and rapid prototyping fabrication of removable partial denture frameworks. *Proceedings of the Institution of Mechanical Engineers. Part H, Journal of Engineering in Medicine*, **219**, 195–202.

Ender, A. & Mehl, A. (2013) Accuracy of complete-arch dental impressions: a new method of measuring trueness and precision. *Journal of Prosthetic Dentistry*, **109**, 121–128.

Ettinger, R.L., Beck, J.D., & Jakobsen, J. (1984) Removable prosthodontic treatment needs: a survey. *Journal of Prosthetic Dentistry*, **51**, 419–427.

Goodacre, C.J., Garbacea, A., Naylor, W.P., Daher, T., Marchack, C.B., & Lowry, F. (2012) CAD/CAM fabricated complete dentures: concepts and clinical methods of obtaining required morphological data. *Journal of Prosthetic Dentistry*, **107**, 34–46.

Guttal, S.S. & Patil, N.P. (2007) Effect of sprue design on the castability an internal porosity in pure titanium castings. *Quintessence International*, **38**, e78–e82.

Han, J., Wang, Y., & Lü, P.J. (2010) A preliminary report of designing removable partial denture frameworks using a specifically developed software package. *International Journal of Prosthodontics*, **23**, 370–375.

Iijima, D., Yoneyama, T., Doi, H., Hamanaka, H., & Kurosaki, N. (2003) Wear properties of Ti and Ti-6Al-7Nb castings for dental prostheses. *Biomaterials*, **24**, 1519–1524.

Inokoshi, M., Kanazawa, M., & Minakuchi, S. (2012) Evaluation of a complete denture trial method applying rapid prototyping. *Dental Materials Journal*, **31**, 40–46.

Jang, K.S., Youn, S.J., & Kim, Y.S. (2001) Comparison of castability and surface roughness of commercially pure titanium and cobalt-chromium denture frameworks. *Journal of Prosthetic Dentistry*, **86**, 93–98.

Kanazawa, M., Inokoshi, M., Minakuchi, S., & Ohbayashi, N. (2011) Trial of a CAD/CAM system for fabricating complete dentures. *Dental Materials Journal*, **30**, 93–96.

Katase, H., Kanazawa, M., Inokoshi, M., & Minakuchi, S. (2013) Face simulation system for complete dentures by applying rapid prototyping. *Journal of Prosthetic Dentistry*, **109**, 353–360.

Kawahata, N., Ono, H., Nishi, Y., Hamano, T., & Nagaoka, E. (1997) Trial of duplication procedure for complete dentures by CAD/CAM. *Journal of Oral Rehabilitation*, **24**, 540–548.

Khan, M.A., Williams, R.L., & Williams, D.F. (1996) In-vitro corrosion and wear of titanium alloys in the biological environment. *Biomaterials*, **17**, 2117–2126.

Kobayashi, E., Wang, T.J., Doi, H., Yoneyama, T., & Hamanaka, H. (1998) Mechanical properties and corrosion resistance of Ti-6Al-7Nb alloy dental castings. *Journal of Material Sciences: Materials in Medicine*, **9**, 567–574.

Luthardt, R.G., Loos, R., & Quaas, S. (2005) Accuracy of intraoral data acquisition in comparison to the conventional impression (in English, German). *International Journal of Computerized Dentistry*, **8**, 283–294.

Ling, B.C. (2000) A practical three visit complete denture system. *Annals of the Royal Australasian College of Dental Surgeons*, **15**, 66–68.

Ling, B.C. (2004) A three-visit, complete-denture technique utilizing visible light-cured resin for tray and base plate construction. *Quintessence International*, **35**(4), 294–298.

Maeda, Y., Minoura, M., Tsutsumi, S., Okada, M., & Nokubi, T. (1994) A CAD/CAM system for removable denture. Part I: fabrication of complete dentures. *International Journal of Prosthodontics*, **7**, 17–21.

Matsumura, H., Yoneyama, T., & Shimoe, S. (2002) Veneering technique for a Ti-6Al-7Nb framework used in a resin-bonded fixed partial denture with a highly filled indirect composite. *Journal of Prosthetic Dentistry*, **88**, 636–639.

Matsuno, H., Yokoyama, A., Watari, F., Uo, M., & Kawasaki, T. (2001) Biocompatibility and osteogenesis of refractory metal implants, titanium, hafnium, nio- bium, tantalum and rhenium. *Biomaterials*, **22**, 1253–1262.

Mehl, A., Ender, A., Mörmann, W., & Attin, T. (2009) Accuracy testing of a new intraoral 3D camera (in English, German). *International Journal of Computerized Dentistry*, **12**, 11–28.

Mörmann, W.H. (2004) The origin of the Cerec method: a personal review of the first 5 years. *International Journal of Computerized Dentistry*, **7**, 11–24.

Murray, M.D. & Darvell, B.W. (1993) The evolution of the complete denture base. Theories of complete denture retention – a review. Part I. *Australian Dental Journal*, **38**, 216–219.

Ohkubo, C., Hosoi, T., Ford, J.P., & Watanabe, I. (2006) Effect of surface reaction layer on grindability of cast titanium alloys. *Dental Materials*, **22**, 268–274.

Patzelt, S.B., Vonau, S., Stampf, S., & Att, W. (2013) Assessing the feasibility and accuracy of digitizing edentulous jaws. *Journal of the American Dental Association*, **144**, 914–920.

Payne, S.H. (1977) The trial denture. *Dental Clinics of North America*, **21**, 321–328.

Peyton, F.A. (1975) History of resins in dentistry. *Dental Clinics of North America*, **19**, 211–222.

Redford, M., Drury, T.F., Kingman, A., & Brown, L.J. (1996) Denture use and the technical quality of dental prostheses among persons 18–74 years of age: United Sates, 1988–1991. *Journal of Dental Research*, **75**, 714–725.

Rekow, D. (1987) Computer-aided design and manufacturing in dentistry: A review of the state of the art. *Journal of Prosthetic Dentistry*, **59**, 512–516.

Rueggeberg, F.A. (2002) From vulcanite to vinyl, a history of resins in restorative dentistry. *Journal of Prosthetic Dentistry*, **87**, 364–379.

Sarment, D.P., Sukovic, P., & Clinthorne, N. (2003) Accuracy of implant placement with stereolithographic surgical guide. *International Journal of Oral and Maxillofacial Implants*, **18**, 571–577.

Schmalz, G. & Garhammer, P. (2002) Biologic interactions of dental cast alloys with oral tissues. *Dental Materials*, **18**, 396–406.

Stephens, A.P. (1969) Full denture try-in. *Journal of the Irish Dental Association*, **15**, 126–128.

Sun, Y., Lü, P., & Wang, Y. (2009) Study on CAD&RP for removable complete denture. *Computer Methods and Programs in Biomedicine*, **93**, 266–272.

Sutton, A.J. & Rogers, P.M. (2001) Discoloration of a titanium alloy removable partial denture: a clinical report. *Journal of Prosthodontics*, **10**, 102–104.

Vecchia, M.P., Regis, R.R., Cunha, T.R., de Andrade, I.M., de Matta, J.C., & de Souza, R.F. (2014) A randomized trial on simplified and conventional methods for complete denture fabrication: cost analysis. *Journal of Prosthodontics*, **23**(3), 182–191.

Williams, R.J., Bibb, R., & Rafik, T. (2004) A technique for fabricating patterns for removable partial denture frameworks using digitized casts and electronic surveying. *Journal of Prosthetic Dentistry*, **91**, 85–88.

Williams, R.J., Bibb, R., Eggbeer, D., & Collis, J. (2006) Use of CAD/CAM technology to fabricate a removable partial denture framework. *Journal of Prosthetic Dentistry*, **96**, 96–99.

Wichmann, M. & Tschernitschek, H. (1993) Quality assurance by x-ray structure analysis [In German]. *Deutsche Zahnärztliche Zeitschrift*, **48**, 682–686.

Wu, J., Gao, B., Tan, H., Chen, J., Tang, C.Y., & Tsui, C.P. (2010) A feasibility study on laser rapid forming of a complete titanium denture base plate. *Lasers in Medical Science*, **25**, 309–315.

Yadroitsev, I., Bertrand, P.H., & Smurov, I. (2007) Parametric analysis of the selective laser melting process. *Applied Surface Science*, **253**, 8064–8069.

7 Digital Implant Surgery

Hans-Peter Weber, Jacinto Cano, and Francesca Bonino

Introduction

Talk of digital technology in dentistry is nothing new. For years, new inventions have come out to the market in the digital world including dentistry, offering potentially better ways to treat patients. They have fascinated many dentists, especially of the younger generation, who are eager to try and explore the newest available concepts. However, the question should not be if digital technology works, but if it can really improve the quality and cost-effectiveness of dental treatment. As described in the early chapters in the book, the application of CAD/CAM systems to dentistry during the 1980s and 1990s (Duret and Preston, 1991; Mörmann et al., 1989; Andersson et al., 1996) has been one of the biggest revolutions in this field in the last 30 years. This technology consists of the digitized data of objects, which are transformed into a 3D construction file and transferred to a milling device. Thereby, the copy of the object is milled from a solid block of material such as metal or ceramic[s].

During the first decade, the dental applications of the CAD/CAM technology were restricted to ceramic restorations, such as inlays and crowns

(see Chapter 4 for more details). In implant dentistry, the fabrication of implant abutments and frameworks by means of the CAD/CAM technology was introduced in the early 1990s (Priest, 2005) and has greatly evolved since. The digital information of the product is obtained either by scanning a wax or acrylic resin pattern of the final design of the object or by virtually creating the final design of the object using a special software program (Kapos et al., 2009; Miyazaki et al., 2009). The digitized data are then transferred online to a production plant, where computer-controlled processing machines manufacture the scanned product. Finally, a dental technician refines the product sent back from the production plant to the dental laboratory.

In addition to the CAD/CAM technology, the development of 3D implant planning software has recently led to an evolution of novel treatment concepts in dental implant treatment. Computer tomography (CT) and 3D implant software provide clinicians with 3D information of a patient's bony structures. Furthermore, the combination of such images and the CAD/CAM technology allows the fabrication of surgical guides and implant-supported prostheses that are

Clinical Applications of Digital Dental Technology, First Edition. Edited by Radi Masri and Carl F. Driscoll.
© 2015 John Wiley & Sons, Inc. Published 2015 by John Wiley & Sons, Inc.

manufactured preoperatively based on the virtual treatment planning.

Today, computer-assisted surgery can be broadly divided into two groups: computer-guided (static) surgery, which this chapter focuses on, and computer-navigated (dynamic) surgery. According to the consensus statement published in 2009, the terms are defined (Hämmerle *et al.*, 2009) as follows:

- *Computer-guided (static) surgery.* The use of a static surgical guide that reproduces the virtual implant position directly from CT data and does not allow for intraoperative modification of the implant position.
- *Computer-navigated (dynamic) surgery.* The use of a surgical navigation system that reproduces the virtual implant position directly from CT data and allows for intraoperative changes in implant position.

The number of static surgery systems commercially available is greater than that of computer-navigated systems, and today, the static guided systems have become an established treatment (Jung *et al.*, 2009). It is estimated that about 20 planning programs for template-guided surgery (Table 7.1) are now available on the market (Neugebauer *et al.*, 2010). The majority of them rely on the use of an individually customized surgical guide, which is fabricated according to previously processed planning data. The manufacturers use either rapid prototyping or computer-driven drilling. The surgical guides can be categorized based on the type of the supporting form into bone-, tooth-, and mucosa-supported guides. It is important to mention that by means of tooth- and mucosa-supported surgical guides, it is possible to perform implant surgeries with a flapless surgical technique. Moreover, some systems allow immediate loading of implants, by providing a provisional or a definitive implant-supported prosthesis that is preoperatively created from the digital planning data using the CAD/CAM technique. In this chapter, an update of all the different systems available for computer-guided surgery, as well as important aspects such as accuracy, outcome, and clinical applications, will be discussed.

Prosthodontic plan and optimal 3D implant positioning

The optimal positioning of an implant in mesiodistal, corono-apical, and orofacial direction is essential for facilitating treatment success with implant-supported prostheses. Especially in indications with multiple missing teeth, in which landmarks from adjacent or contralateral teeth are missing, the use of a surgical guide, which is based on a prosthodontic plan and mock-up, is of utmost importance. The mock-up is tried in the patient to assess critical esthetic and functional parameters and will serve as the basis for the diagnostic guide, in which the planned tooth positions are visualized with the use of radiopaque material. Using implant planning software, digital implant selection and positioning can subsequently be performed, allowing to determine the best possible compromise between desirable implant position from a prosthodontic view and the surgical feasibility given by the anatomy and condition of the underlying alveolar structures. Thus, digital technology indeed enables prosthodontically driven implant placement in its best possible way and needs to be an integral part of computer-guided surgery.

Basics in computer-guided surgery

Radiographic imaging

Conventional radiology, such as intraoral radiographs and panoramic radiographic images, offers a two-dimensional view of the surgical site, whereas computer-assisted tomography (CT) provides information related to the buccolingual dimension and can be used to create a three-dimensional reconstruction. Since the first prototype was designed in 1967 by Hounsfield (Hounsfield, 1973), who then won the Nobel Prize for its development with Allan M. Cormack, the CT has undergone a gradual evolution up to six different generations. This classification is based on the organization of the various parts of the system and the physical displacement of the beam (Vannier, 2003), but the ability of the detector to capture an object by means of X-rays and to visualize multiple planes of it on a screen

Table 7.1   List of static implant planning software systems available on the market.

Software	Company
10 DR implant	10 DR Seoul, South Korea
Blue Sky Plan	Blue Sky Bio, Grayslake, IL, USA
coDiagnostiX	Dental Wings GmbH, Chemnitz, Germany
CTV (PraxisSoft)	M + K Dental, Kahla, Germany
DentalVox (Era Scientific)	Biosfera, Rimini, Italy
DentalSlice	Bioparts, Brasília, Brazil
DDent Plus I	AlloVision, Greenville, SC, USA
DigiGuide MDI	Imtec, Ardmore, OK, USA
Easy Guide (CAD Implant, Praxim)	Keystone Dental, Drilllington, MA, USA
Implant Location System	Tactile Technologies, Rehovot, Israel
InVivoDental	Anatomage, San Jose, CA, USA
Implant3D (Stent CAD); Implant3D Impla 3D Navi	Media Lab, La Spezia, Italy Schütz Dental, Rosbach, Germany
Implanner	Dolphin Imaging, Chatsworth, CA, USA
Implant3D CeHa; Implant IGS Monitor	med3D, Heidelberg, Germany C. Hafner, Pforzheim, Germany 2ingis, Brussels, Belgium
Implametric	3dent, Valencia, Spain
Nobel Guide (Litorim, Cath. Uni. Leuven, Belgium) (Oralim, Medicim)	Nobel Biocare, Göteborg, Sweden
Simplant/Surgiguide Facilitate ExpertEase	Materialize, Leuven, Belgium Astratech, Mölndal, Sweden Dentsply Friadent, Mannheim, Germany
Scan2Guide Implant Master	Ident, Foster, CA, USA Various
Sicat Implant Galileos Implant	Sicat, Bonn, Germany Sirona, Bensheim, Germany
Virtual implant placement (Implant Logic)	BioHorizons, Birmingham, AL, USA

remains a constant of this technology. Radiation exposure as well as space requirements and cost are disadvantages of CT. Nevertheless, CT image has become the "gold standard" of maxillofacial trauma cases (Finkle *et al.*, 1985), and it is used also for studying growth and development of the jaws, in oral pathology for the salivary glands, and for treatment planning in implant surgery.

Cone beam computer technology (CBCT) was introduced to the US market in 2001. CBCT differs from the CT image as the 3D volume of data is acquired during a single sweep of the scanner. The sensor and the radiation source rotate synchronously around the head of the patient, who is sitting or standing. Depending on the type of scanner used, the X-ray source rotates between 180° and 360° and creates a beam, which is conical in shape and gets a cylindrical or spherical volume of data. This volume is described as field of view (FOV). The FOV size is variable, but the most common ones are 6, 9, and 12 in. Among high-volume CBCT scanners, there are i-Cat™ (Imaging Sciences International, Hatfield, PA) and NewTom™ (QR, Verona, Italy). Another important variable is exposure time, which varies between 10 and 40 seconds. The CB Mercuray™ (Hitachi Medical Corporation, Tokyo, Japan) has a 10 second scan time for a 360° rotation, which can be combined with three different types of FOV. This implies a reduced risk of patient motion during image capture.

Compared to conventional CT, medical and craniofacial CBCT, the latter being specifically designed for implant dentistry, combine a relatively smaller exposure dose with a lower cost. The radiation source is composed of a conventional, low-radiation X-ray tube that produces a more focused beam, which is projected onto a specific detector. The scatter radiation is therefore considerably reduced (Danforth *et al.*, 2003; Mah *et al.*, 2003; Sukovic, 2003). The total radiation of CBCT devices is approximately 20% less than that of a helical CT and corresponds to the exposure of a full-mouth periapical series (Mah *et al.*, 2003). In addition, CBCT is smaller in size and less expensive (Winter *et al.*, 2005; Honda *et al.*, 2006; Hashimoto *et al.*, 2006). Another advantage of the CBCT technology over earlier generations of CT, which is critical for clinicians, is the low level of metal artifacts in primary and secondary reconstructions (Heiland *et al.*, 2005). As a consequence, the area around the metal object, such as an amalgam restoration or a porcelain fused to metal crown is usually of diagnostic quality. Finally, CBCT offers surface as well as radiographic view modes, the latter being similar to the traditional radiographs, which are easy-to-ready for the general practitioner. As a result, in the last 10 years, CBCT has become more readily as an alternative to conventional CT for imaging in the head and neck region. With that it has become extremely popular as a tool for the diagnosis and planning of implant surgery cases in conjunction with digital implant software programs. It has been recently pointed out, however, that the accuracy between different CBCT devices can vary (Eggers *et al.*, 2006). The geometric accuracy of a CBCT scanner is reported to be lower than that of a multislice CT scanner due to the inherent nature of this technology (Stratemann *et al.*, 2008). For example, it has been shown that the accuracy of the image intensifier system (Sirona® Galileos™) is adequate for linear measurements of the human mandible. Nevertheless, the measurements of geometric objects showed large deviations that resulted in the fabrication of surgical guides that were not reliable for guided implant placement (Weitz *et al.*, 2010). Similar findings were reported by other

authors, who stated that CBCT machines were not able to measure the distance between two points in the mandibular bone as accurately as CT, but on average provided satisfactory information about three-dimensional distances (Abboud *et al.*, 2013). In addition, both CBCT and CT scanners presented underestimations of uniform known measured objects, but only CBCT displayed overestimations that can lead to intrasurgical complications. Nevertheless, the author concluded that the geometric accuracy of most CBCT units was not comparable with that of the medical CT (Abboud *et al.*, 2013). Similarly, Sharpe and colleagues reported that the mechanical accuracy and the reproducibility of CBCT were about 1 mm (Sharpe *et al.*, 2006), which can be considered inadequate for guided surgery. It is believed that the lack of accuracy in CBCT is related to the inability of the system to localize correctly the so-called fiducial markers, which are reference points and can be identified with specific parts in the surgical field. There are various reasons for the error in the localization of fiducial markers in CBCT scanners. The cone beam technology lacks specific correction algorithms, which rectify the geometric errors closer to the circumference of the imaging field, especially in units with large apertures. The contrast of CBCT scanners is also lower, compared to that of CT. Furthermore, CBCT units can rotate with a slight wobble, providing an additional potential source of image distortion. Although a correction algorithm is used to remove this distortion prior to the image reconstruction, subsequent errors in the algorithm itself or changes in the wobble pattern over time may result in additional residual distortion. Studies discussing rotational displacement are, however, rare due to the inability of the hardware to adjust rotation in most cases (Oh *et al.*, 2007). Finally, the reconstruction time of a CBCT, which rotates around the patient's head, is longer than that of a medical CT. This implies a greater chance for the patient to move from the position it was occupied at the time that the CBCT started to capture data, resulting in another potential source of distortion.

Owing to these limitations, the indiscriminate use of CBCT might be a problem for implant planning systems, which base on geometric reference markers the planning of the implant position and the fabrication of surgical drilling guides. Therefore it is crucial for clinicians who employ guided surgery systems to ensure that fiducial markers are picked up accurately by the specific CBCT scanner used and that the CBCT scanner and the guided surgery system work together seamlessly to avoid large errors in the localization of the fiducial markers.

Dynamic versus static guided implant placement systems

As previously mentioned, guided implant placement systems can be classified into two different categories: dynamic and static. Dynamic systems were introduced in implant dentistry to minimize the risk of damaging intraoral critical anatomical structures. With dynamic surgery the current position of the surgical instruments in the surgical area is constantly displayed on a screen with a 3D image of the patient. In this way, the system allows real-time transfer of the preoperative planning and visual feedback on the screen (Widmann and Bale, 2006; Brief *et al.*, 2005). This type of systems relies on reference points present in the surgical field to track the position of the surgical instrument with the CT scan images of the patient projected on a screen. During implant placement, the handpiece is guided in real time, and the surgeon's direct view of the implant site is not limited. Image Guided Implantology™ (IGI; Image Navigation Ltd., New York, NY) and StealthStation Treon Navigation System™ (Medtronic, Minneapolis, MN) are two navigation systems marketed in USA. There is evidence suggesting that dynamic navigation systems are accurate (Wittwer *et al.*, 2007; Jung *et al.*, 2009) and can be a valid option for skilled surgeons, who want to perform a safe and controlled freehand implant placement. They are, however, very expensive and their applicability is limited to the surgical aspect of the implant therapy.

Static guided implant placement systems are more popular (see Table 7.2). A CT scan of the patient wearing a radiographic guide is taken and converted to a format that a specific software is able to read in order to digitally plan the implant placement. Based on that, a surgical guide is fabricated and used during the surgery to guide the implant placement. coDiagnostiX™ (Dental Wings, Montreal, Canada), Simplant™ (Materialise, Plymouth, MI), and Navigator™ (Biomet 3I, Palm Beach Gardens, FL) are some examples of static guided surgery systems.

In the review of Jung and coworkers (2009), a statistically significant higher mean precision was found with dynamic compared to static systems. However, this difference could be biased by the fact that there were more preclinical studies on accuracy for the dynamic systems and more clinical studies for the static systems. Nowadays, static systems are more commonly used in implant dentistry because dynamic systems have been found to be too complex and expensive. For this reason, only static guided surgery systems will be discussed in the following section and they will be referred to as computer-assisted or computer-guided implant systems.

Computer-assisted implant planning

There are many computer-aided implant surgery (CAS) systems available on the market. They can be classified as double-scan or single-scan protocols.

Double-scan protocol

The double-scan protocol software is characterized by the fact that both the patient wearing the radiographic guide and the radiographic guide alone, need to be separately digitalized by means of CT scanning. The two scans are matched, by using the presence of fiducial markers in the radiographic guide. The great advantage of this protocol is that the radiographic guide can be digitalized with high accuracy, irrespective of the patient scan and its eventually related artifacts. The disadvantage is that two different scans need to be taken. A single one is not sufficient as the gray values of the acrylic radiographic guide are almost the same as the ones of the soft tissue. The appliance should be up off the metal table or bar in the same orientation as it was in the patient's mouth. The radiologist obtains the Digital Imaging Communication of Medical Images (DICOM) files, reconstructs the scan and usually burns the CT scan data onto a CD. This CD is

Table 7.2   List of static systems and template fabrication methods.

Brand	Fabrication	Technology
Blue Sky Plan	Central/Local	3D-printing
coDiagnostiX	Local	Mechanical optical tracking; 3D-printing; CAM-milling
DentalVox	Central	CAM-milling
DentalSlice	Central	Stereolithography
DDent plus I	Local	Mechanical
Easy Guide	Central	CAM-milling
Implant Location System	Central	CAM temperature-forming
Implametric	Central	Stereolithography
Implant3D	Local	Mechanical
Implant3D (med3D)	Local	Mechanical optical tracking
Nobel Guide	Central	Stereolithography
Scan2guide	Central	Rapid manufacturing technology
Sicat Implant	Central	CAM-milling
Simplant	Central	Stereolithography
VIP Pilog Compu-Guide	Central	CAM-milling

sent to the company, which is able to match the two different scans and do the image processing and the segmentation, which allows for removing artifacts and separating objects such as teeth from the remaining dataset in 2D and 3D. After the central processing, the clinician receives from the company all the segmented data, and he is able to do the planning for the implant placement (Figure 7.1). The planning is sent again to the company, which finally provides the clinician with the surgical guide.

Since one of the key elements of the double-scan protocols is an accurate radiographic guide, the material to use and the steps to follow for its fabrication will be included. It is recommended to work on a validated diagnostic setup on a duplicated master cast. A 2.5–3 mm layer of resin material will cover the occlusal surfaces of the teeth, eventually the palate and 1–2 mm of the buccal aspect of the mucosa to provide a stable support. In particular, it is important to ensure an adequate representation of the soft tissue morphology in edentulous areas that will work as a planning reference and for repositioning purposes. The layer should be extended sufficiently also, to accommodate the fiducial markers and eventual anchor pins.

Single-scan protocol

The single-scan protocol allows the import of the 3D DICOM data set directly into the planning software and does not require a central processing. Unlike what occurs with double-scan systems, the clinician starts to work with the DICOM files without any kind of previous image processing. Most of the available software offers an easy-to-read 2D and 3D visualization and image editing functionalities, which are useful for diagnostics and planning. In particular, different anatomical structures can be visualized with different colors and transparency grades for the so-called segmentation (Figures 7.2 and 7.3). In summary, the main difference between single- and double-scan protocol is that the clinician, instead

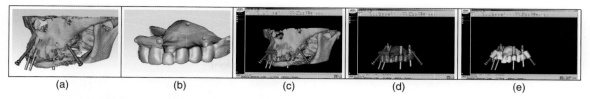

Figure 7.1 Double-scan protocol. (a) Patient scan. (b) Rx guide scan. (c) Overlapping both scans. (d) Implant placement driven by Rx guide. (e) Surgical guide.

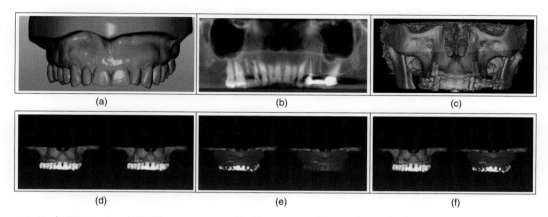

Figure 7.2 Single-Scan protocol. CBCT is not processed by the company. The masks need to be processed by the user. (a) Digitization of the waxup model. (b) Panoramic view with virtual implants placed. (c) 3D reconstruction. (d) Different masks for bone, teeth, and implants. (e) Different mask for bone, teeth, and digital waxup. (f) Different mask for bone, teeth, and implants.

of the company, carries out the image processing and the segmentation.

In single-scan systems, a radiographic guide made of barium sulfate mixed with acrylic is used to identify radiographically the teeth and eventually the various mucosal structures. A 20% barium sulfate mix will visualize the teeth that need to be restored in partially edentulous cases. The radiographic guide can have the same design as a treatment partial or an Essix appliance. If the patient is fully edentulous, the teeth are made with the same mix and the base with a 10% barium sulfate mix. In this way, both the teeth and the soft tissue will be easily identified in the CT (Rosenfeld and Mandelaris, 2006).

Surgical guides

Surgical guide fabrication methods

Computer-assisted surgery uses surgical guides that can be produced by the local laboratory technician or by the dentist, by using special mechanical positioning devices. Alternatively, they can be fabricated in a centralized facility with various types of CAD-CAM technology (Jabero and Sarment, 2006). The decentralized or local fabrication method uses software that provides the user with an information sheet that shows the coordinates of a positioning device (Mischkowski et al., 2006; Stein et al., 1998; Blanchet et al., 2004). The master cast and the scan guide need to be correctly located on the positioning device, by following the coordinates. In this way, the implant axes can be adequately simulated on the cast and a parallel milling system is able to reproduce them on the guide, by placing the surgical sleeves (Azari and Nikzad, 2008). The process of fixation on a milling system is quite precise and the coordinates can therefore be considered reliable (Varvara et al., 2003). To avoid higher deviation through the various production steps, direct fixation of the sleeves is preferred (Varvara et al., 2003).

For the systems with centralized fabrication, planning is performed on a standard computer by

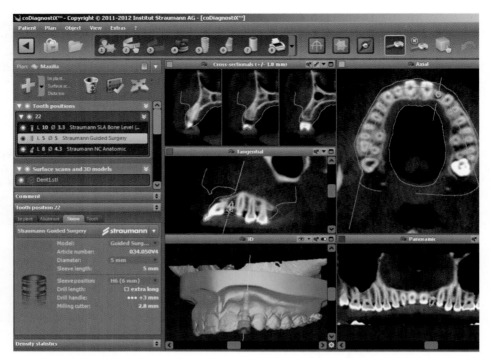

Figure 7.3 Screen shot of single-scan system software. In this particular case, the waxup has been digitized (STL files) and is overlapping the CBCT (DICOM files) on the 3D view.

the clinician, and the data are then transferred to the production center, which fabricates the surgical guides according to the data from the planning software. The surgical guides are produced mainly by means of stereolithographic technology. Particularly for large surgical guides, however, this technique is associated with high cost and long production time. Current developments are examining the concept of obtaining the surgical guide directly from the DICOM data, by using the patient scan and the scan of a conventional dental cast (Widmann *et al.*, 2007). As the fit is checked prior to the CT scan, a precise fit can also be expected after the placement of the sleeves, and there is no further need for adjustments (Oh *et al.*, 2007).

Another new concept is the use of 3D printing to generate 3D models and surgical guides, which can also be used for local fabrication in dental laboratories or dental offices. In the following sections, the characteristics of stereolithographic surgical guides and derived laboratory-based

surgical guides will be discussed. Moreover, a few comments will be made about 3D printed technology due to its promising preliminary results.

Stereolithographic surgical guides

The stereolithographic technology involves the reproduction of the surgical guide or model, by means of a laser beam that selectively solidifies an ultraviolet-sensitive liquid resin (Figure 7.4). As an example of this technique, the protocol of the NobelGuide™ system (Nobel Biocare AB, Zurich, Switzerland), which uses a double-scan software, will be presented in detail. A CT scan of the patient wearing a stable radiographic guide is taken. It is important to keep the occlusal plane parallel to the axial slices. Immediately after, a second scan of the radiographic guide itself is performed using the same CT scanner settings. The data are sent to the company where the two

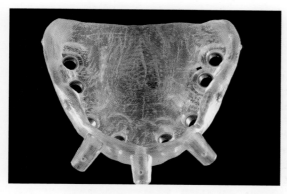

Figure 7.4 Stereolithographic surgical guide with eight sleeves (5 mm) and three fixations pins on the buccal aspect of the guide.

different scans will be combined using as a reference radiopaque gutta-percha markers (fiducial markers) in the radiographic guide. Only at this time can the clinician use the specific software and digitally plan the implant placement. In this user-friendly software, the shape of the implant will appear when the clinician indicates with a click of the mouse a point on top of the bone crest and another more apically. Its length, width, inclination, or position can be modified with different tools. Once the clinician is satisfied with his digital treatment plan, all the data is saved and sent to the NobelBiocare® workstation (Nobel Biocare AB, Zurich, Switzerland) for fabrication of a stereolithographic model. The surgical guide is produced in acrylic material using as a reference the stereolithographic model and the radiographic guide. The surgical stereolithographic guide includes metallic sleeves. During the surgery, the clinician will use a sequence of drill guides that match perfectly with the diameter of each surgical drill that needs to be used for the osteotomy. Finally, the implant will be placed using the same stereolithographic surgical guide. Several commercial systems are available in the market to fabricate stereolithographic guides.

One of the main disadvantages of stereolithographic materials fabrication is light sensitivity and lack of thermal stability of the material. However, according to D'haese *et al.*, (2010), it is unlikely that its production process has a major impact on the total accuracy of a mucosa-supported stereolithographic guide.

In the manual, it is recommended to keep the guide away from direct sunlight and not have it sterilized in an autoclave or with chemical sterilization.

Laboratory-made surgical guides

Dental laboratory-made surgical guides are fabricated on a dental cast (Figure 7.5). The guide is used for visualizing the subsequent idealized superstructures and its accurate fit can be checked intraorally and eventually adjusted before the CBCT. After CBCT acquisition, the radiological guide is converted into a surgical guide in the same laboratory-based setting.

Guided implant surgery requires several preoperative steps, starting with the fabrication of a radiographic guide, the CBCT acquisition of the guide in position, the computer-assisted implant planning and ending in the fabrication and use of a surgical guide for drilling and implant insertion. With such a complex sequence, during which every step is prone to errors, accuracy is of utmost importance.

The tooth-supported laboratory-based guides provide accuracy similar to or better than the aforementioned tooth-supported stereolithographic guides (Van Assche *et al.*, 2012). This may be explained by the fact that in the laboratory-based system, the same guide is used for both the radiographic examination and the surgery. Therefore, a stable and reproducible fitting position of the guide can be assured before the surgery. As a result, the operative steps during the drilling phase, performed with the same original guide, are very accurate (Van Assche *et al.*, 2007; Behneke *et al.*, 2011). As assessed by four recently published clinical studies with stereolithographic guides from NobelGuide™, SimPlant™, or StentCAD™ systems, mean horizontal deviations of 0.6–1.1 mm and maximum values between 1.4 and 1.8 mm are present at the entry point using the image fusion tool (Ersoy *et al.*, 2008; Ozan *et al.*, 2009; Arısan *et al.*, 2010; Van Assche *et al.*, 2010). In a clinical study published by Behneke *et al.*, (2011), the tooth-supported laboratory-based guides had mean deviations of 0.32 mm at shoulder level and 0.49 mm at the implant tip, and

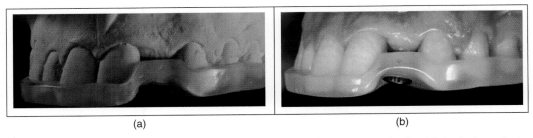

Figure 7.5 Laboratory made surgical guide. (a) Surgical guide is made on the master cast. (b) Good fitting in the patient mouth.

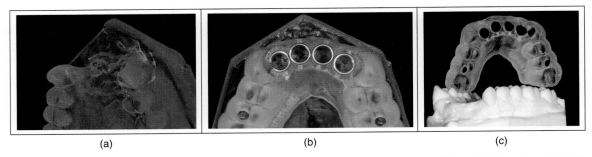

Figure 7.6 Printed model and printed surgical guide. (a) Printed model with teeth, soft tissue, and bone. (b) Printed surgical guide and printed model.

maxima of 0.97 mm and 1.38 mm at the same locations.

Digitally manufactured guides

DICOM datasets can be also utilized to produce models with a 3D printer technology (e.g., Spectrum Z510; Company Z Corporation, Aachen, Germany and the plaster powder ZP130). The principle of 3D print is to slice a digital object in cross sections that are printed in layers. Those layers are made of liquid, powder, or any sheet material and can be fused together and create objects with any different kind of shapes (Figure 7.6). To the contrary of the CAD/CAM, which is subtractive since material is removed from a block, this technique is additive and produces objects in layers. The print process is based on ink jet technology, where droplets of inks are projected from a small aperture to a surface to create an object (Stopp *et al.*, 2008). The accuracy requirements for anatomical models lie within a range of a tenth of a millimeter (Stopp *et al.*, 2007). By formulating

this method for model fabrication, treatment times and labor resource can be reduced. The guide could be produced on machined models or even produced by direct fabrication. This could potentially allow for treatment times to be ulteriorly reduced. However, Weitz *et al.* (2010) stated that the accuracy of a surgical guide-aided implant placement produced by rapid prototyping using a DICOM dataset from CBCT was not satisfactory. On the basis of CBCT scans (Sirona Galileos), a total of 10 models and 10 guides were produced using a rapid prototyping 3D printer. On the same patients, impressions were made and guides were fabricated on conventional models. To compare the fitting accuracy, the guides produced with both the rapid prototyping and the conventional laboratory-based method were checked in the patients' mouth. Whereas guides made by conventional procedure had an excellent accuracy, the fitting accuracy of those produced by DICOM datasets was not sufficient. Deviations ranged between 2.0 and 3.5 mm.

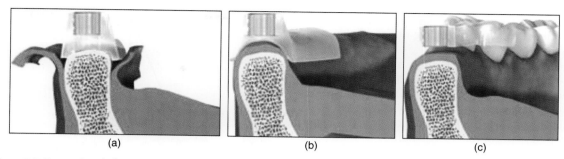

(a)   (b)   (c)

Figure 7.7 Types of guided surgery templates. (a) Bone-supported. (b) Mucosa-supported. (c) Teeth-supported.

Surgical guide fixation methods

There are three types of surgical guides: bone-, mucosa-, and tooth-supported (Figure 7.7). A recent review article has focused on the accuracy of computer-assisted template-guided implant placement in studies published between 2002 and 2009 (Schneider *et al.*, 2009). Overall, eight of them were included, resulting in one model, four cadaver and three clinical studies. The results showed average deviations of 1.1–1.5 mm with particularly considerable maximum deviations failing to justify flapless implantation. Moreover, no significant differences could be identified between bone-, tooth-, and mucosa-supported guides. In a comparative study of Ozan *et al.* (2009) with stereolithographically designed guides, significantly lower deviation values were determined with tooth-supported versus bone- and mucosa-supported guides, especially with regard to the angular deviations and the deviations observed at the implant apex level. Ersoy *et al.* (2008) also found significantly lower deviations with purely tooth-supported guides than with mixed supported or purely mucosa-supported guides. Similarly, Van Assche *et al.* (2007) reported significantly higher deviations with guides with mixed support (especially at terminal gaps) versus purely tooth-supported guides on the mesiodistal deviation. He indicated mucosal resilience as well as distortion of the guide as possible explanations. Therefore, it has been suggested that to use purely or partially mucosa-supported guides should make the accurate intraoperative repositioning of the guide more difficult and thus affect implantation precision. This might be due to alterations in the local mucosal environment and

increased resilience. This is a very important point to take consider, since, as maximum implantation precision is required for mucosa-borne guides allowing no direct control of the implants inserted, especially if a flapless approach is performed (Vercruyssen *et al.*, 2008). The use of flapless implant placement needs to be critically evaluated in clinical studies (Van Assche *et al.*, 2007; Dreiseidler *et al.*, 2009), although template-guided minimally invasive implantology has already become a commonly used treatment concept. It has been claimed that tooth-supported SLA surgical guides were more accurate than bone- or mucosa-supported guides (Pettersson *et al.*, 2010), but these findings need to be interpreted with caution as the implants were placed *in vitro* under ideal, identical conditions.

Effectiveness of computer-guided surgery

Accuracy

During the last decade, special attention has been given to a "prosthesis-driven" implant placement. Three-dimensional imaging (showing the alveolar bone in relation to the ideal tooth position), obtainable with relative CBCT low-radiation dosages (Loubele *et al.*, 2009; Pauwels *et al.*, 2012) and planning software, opened the possibility for preoperative planning and proper communication between the patient, the surgeon, and the prosthodontist. During the last few years, different strategies have been developed to transfer the digitally planned implant to its clinical position in the patient's mouth. The most commonly used system is the implant placement guided by customized surgical guides. However, many doubts have arisen regarding their usefulness and especially their accuracy.

The template-guided surgery involves several steps that result in deviations between the planned and the clinically placed implant positions. The overall accuracy of the implant placement is the sum of all errors that arise during the whole treatment procedure. Although it is difficult to detect deviations that possibly occur in each step, it is essential for clinicians to learn to what extent the deviations occur between the virtually planned and the actual final implant position in order to avoid surgical as well as prosthetic complications. Accuracy is also a great concern in case the clinician opts for the immediate delivery of a prefabricated prosthesis.

To assess the accuracy of the various implant systems, most of the studies available in the literature (Jung *et al.*, 2009; Schneider *et al.*, 2009; Van Assche *et al.*, 2012), evaluated the following parameters or outcome variables.

Outcome variables (Figure 7.8)

- Figure 7.8 Deviation at the entry point of the implant or cavity.
- Deviation at the apex of the implant or cavity.
- Deviation of the axis of the cavity or implant.
- Deviation in height/depth.

The accuracy of static computer-guided surgery was overall evaluated in a recent review, which is an update of two previous studies published by the same group of researchers. A total of 1688 implants, 1326 *in vivo*, 104 *in vitro*, and 218 *ex vivo* were planned on a CBCT scan and actually placed. A second CBCT scan was taken postoperatively and a comparison was made between the preoperative and the postoperative position (Jung *et al.*, 2009; Schneider *et al.*, 2009; Van Assche *et al.*, 2012)

The overall mean deviation at the entry point was 0.99 mm (SE 0.12 mm, 95% CI 0.75–1.22), ranging from 0 to 6.5 mm. The corresponding data at the apex was 1.24 mm (SE 0.13 mm, 95% CI 1.01–1.56), ranging from 0 to 6.9 mm. The overall mean angulation was 3.81° (SE 0.32°, 95% CI 3.18–4.43), ranging from 0.00° to 24.9°. The overall mean vertical deviation (based on five studies)

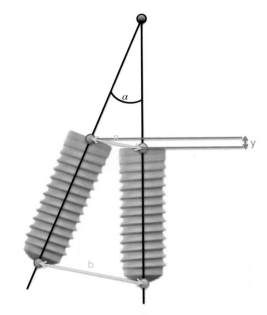

Figure 7.8 Outcome variables. (a) Deviation at the entry point of the implant or cavity. (b) Deviation at the apex of the implant or cavity; (α) Deviation of the axis of the cavity or implant; (y) Deviation in height/depth. Blue: planned/red: performed.

was 0.46 mm (SE 0.14, 95% CI 0.20–0.72), ranging from −2.33 to 4.2 mm.

Influencing factors

Several factors have been claimed to affect the aforementioned outcomes, and we can classify them into guide-, software-, operator-, and patient-related.

Guide-related factors

Guides can be bone-, mucosa-, and tooth-supported. Although it has been pointed out that the difference between them is insignificant (Ersoy *et al.*, 2008), a recent clinical study that compares in the same cohort of patients different type of guides suggests that tooth-supported guides are more accurate (Ozan *et al.*, 2009).

Another variable to consider is the number of guides that are used during the surgery. Some systems rely on different guides for each single surgical drill that is used for the implant osteotomy, while others employ a single guide that fits multiple drills. The evidence is inconclusive. Some authors did not report any difference between the two methods (Arisan *et al.*, 2010), while others stated that bone- and mucosa-supported single guide systems are more reliable (Cassetta *et al.*, 2011). Moreover, multiple fixation pins can be used in order to stabilize bone- and mucosa-supported guides, and it seems that the more pins are used, the less inaccuracy will result. Finally, it has been stated that the accuracy, in terms of apical and angular deviation, is significantly lower for laboratory-produced guides. However, only one clinical study has been conducted, examining 52 partially edentulous patients rehabilitated with 132 dental implants (Behneke *et al.*, 2011). On average linear deviations at the implant neck and apex were 0.27 mm (range 0.01–0.97 mm) and 0.46 mm (range 0.03–1.38 mm), respectively. The angular deviation was instead 1.84°, with a range of 0.07–6.26°.

Software-related factors

Software planning, in other words CBCT conversion, volume rendering, visualization detail accuracy, and referential marker registration, is a possible additional factor influencing the precision in the planning stage. Horwitz *et al.* were able to compute the inaccuracy that derives exclusively from the CT image processing and the presurgical planning phase of the software Med3D (Heidelberg, Germany) in an *in vitro* study. They stated that it results in a mean linear deviation of 0.31 ± 0.15 mm at the level of the implant shoulder, a linear deviation of 0.4 ± 0.1 mm at the apex and an angular deviation of $1.33 \pm 0.69°$ (Horwitz *et al.*, 2009). The same software was evaluated in an *in vivo* study (Behneke *et al.*, 2011). The mean angular and linear deviations were 2.11 and 0.32 mm at the implant shoulder and 0.49 mm at the implant tip, respectively. If we focus on the linear deviation at the implant shoulder, in the first study the inaccuracy was 0.31 ± 0.15 mm and, in the second, 0.32. So the software Med3D (Heidelberg, Germany) has the same performance in a clinical as well as in an experimental environment, suggesting that its inaccuracy derives from the presurgical phase of the treatment rather than from the surgical one. To draw a definitive conclusion about the influence

of the presurgical phase on the performance of guided surgery, it is necessary to compare different systems. In an *in vitro* study, Abboud *et al.* (2013) used exactly the same radiographic and planning protocol, implant system, instrumentation, and drilling protocol to place two implants (implant 1 and 2) in 18 models. They compared two groups. In the first, they used the coDiagnostiX system (Institut Straumann AG, Basel, Switzerland) that relies on cylindrical shape fiducial markers, while in the second they used the Med3D system that is characterized by rectangular brick-shaped ones. The horizontal deviation of the final implant placement was higher for coDiagnostiX (0.65 mm for implant 1 and 1.13 for implant 2) compared to Med3D (0.33 mm for implant 1 and 2). A possible explanation of the first group inaccuracy is the inability of the software to detect precisely the metal reference markers present in the radiological guide. Information regarding the ability of CBCT scan devices to detect different shaped objects has been already discussed in Section 1.3.1. To sum up, the type of system can play a key role in the final outcome, but further studies are needed to confirm these preliminary results.

Another important variable is the type of implant placement that the software allows. Some systems allow a full guided surgery from the very first drill to the final implant placement, while others support the clinician during osteotomy, but leave the implant placement as freehand. In order to understand the real advantages of both a partially and fully guided implant placement, it is important to keep in mind that the freehand implant placement technique, in conjunction with digital planning, results in deviation of 1.5 mm and a maximum of 1.8 mm at the entry point and a mean of 2.1 mm and a maximum of 3.7 at the apex of the implant (Sarment, 2003). If we consider data from single tooth implant placement, the accuracy is slightly better: 1.35 mm with a maximum of 2.16 mm at the entrance and 1.62 with a maximum of 2.68 mm at the apex (Sarment, 2003). Those are *in-vitro* data. In other words, the conditions for the implant placement are ideal. Instead most of the studies that evaluate the accuracy of partially and fully guided implant placement are *ex vivo* or clinical studies.

There are three studies that compared the accuracy of guided with not guided implant

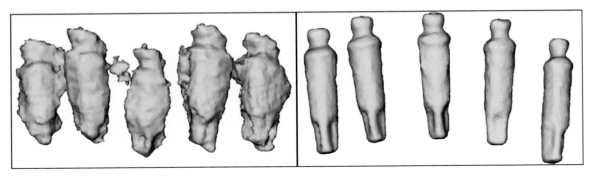

Figure 7.9 Pettersson *et al.*, (2010). (Figure 4, page 533. Reproduced with permission of John Wiley & Sons, Inc.)

surgery. Unfortunately, the two groups differed also for other variables, such as type of support and guiding system (Arisan *et al.*, 2010; Behneke *et al.*, 2011; Cassetta *et al.*, 2011). The mean deviation at the entry point *in vivo* was 0.87 mm (SE 0.11, max 3) when the implant placement was fully guided and 1.34 mm (SE 0.06, max 6.5) when it was not. The mean deviation at the apex was respectively 1.15 mm (SE 0.12, max 4.2) and 1.69 mm (SE 0.08, max 6.9). The mean deviation in angulation was 3.06° (SE 0.27, max 15.25) and 5.6° (SE 0.4, max 24.9). To sum up, all the deviation parameters were significantly lower for implants placed with a fully guided technique. Those data were, however, not confirmed by other studies where the accuracy of the horizontal coronal position of the implants was comparable between those placed with conventional guides and those placed with CAD/CAM guides. In addition, CAD/CAM-guided implants showed more consistency in accuracy than conventional guided ones (Farley *et al.*, 2013).

Operator-related factors, experience

The question whether the guided surgery technique could compensate for the lack of operator experience raises a big interest. Hinckfuss in 2012 stated that surgeon's experience had minimal effect on the accuracy of implant placement, if the implants are digitally planned and placed with a guided system. However, although minimal, an angular displacement in the buccolingual dimension was less likely to occur in the group of experienced clinicians and this difference could yield to less esthetic and functional problems.

The maximum deviation error produced by experienced, intermediate, and novice surgeons were respectively 6.68°, 9.08°, and 9.78°. An effort was made to simulate the clinical environment as much as possible, but invariably the laboratory environment is more controlled and those values could be underestimated.

Patient-related factors

Pettersson *et al.* (2010) published an interesting study, which evaluated the differences between virtually planned and inserted implants in both maxilla and mandible. During the matching procedure, it was apparent that in some cases the segmented implants from the 1-year follow-up CT scan were not cylindrical in shape as the original implant shape (Figure 7.9). The authors attributed this finding to patient movement during CT scanning. One radiologist reviewed all the CT images obtained from the patients' preoperative and postoperative scans. Double contours, implying that the patient had moved during the scans, were found from both the preoperative and postoperative CT data.

Of all the 139 inserted implants, 90 implants were placed in patients, who did not move during the preoperative and postoperative scan. Movement was noted in preoperative CT images for 21 implants and for 43 implants in postoperative images. Fifteen implants were from three patients, who moved during both the preoperative and postoperative CT scans. Comparing the results, statistical significance was found when combining

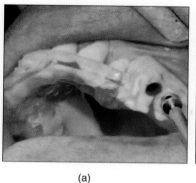
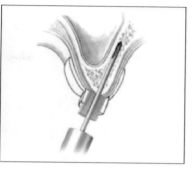
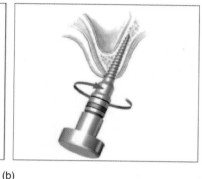

(a)   (b)

Figure 7.10 Technique described by Fortin (2006). (a) Implants are placed using guided surgery to avoid a sinus elevation procedure. (b) A bone recipient site close to and parallel to the sinus wall is prepared to avoid bone augmentation.

the movement of the preoperative and the postoperative scans with the results of the deviation at the level of the hex and apex of the implants.

In conclusion, the accuracy of image-guided systems for oral implant surgery depends on guide-, software-, operator-, and patient-based factors. A safety distance of at least the equivalent of the maximum deviation of the individual system is necessary. Similar accuracy data has been reported for bur tracking and image-guided guide production. Both methods allow precise positioning of oral implants. Compared to freehand dental implant surgery, the computer-aided approach requires a substantially greater effort in time, but seems to be superior on the account of its potential to reduce error and systematize reproducible treatments success. It also enables the protection of critical anatomic structures and the esthetic and functional advantages of prosthodontics-driven implant positioning.

Reduction of surgery time, flapless approach

Owing to the recent development of diagnostic tools for precise evaluation of potential implant sites such as CT and 3D implant planning software, application of the flapless technique has become feasible and fairly common. It has been reported that minimally invasive flapless implant placement significantly reduced postoperative discomfort, especially compared to the conventional open-flap surgery. (Fortin *et al.*, 2006; Nkenke *et al.*, 2007; Cannizzaro *et al.*, 2008). Moreover, the

flapless technique is faster. It takes 24 minutes, on average for a flapless guided surgery, while it takes 61 minutes for an open-flap guided surgery and 69 minutes for a conventional freehand implant surgery (Arisan *et al.*, 2010). Nevertheless, the flapless guided surgery procedure is technically demanding and suitable only for selected patients. As implant therapy is conceived as a long-standing treatment modality, the reduction of surgery time and postoperative morbidity in the immediate days following flapless implant surgery may not be sufficient to support this approach on a routine basis. In summary, by using computer generated guides, not only is the time required for incision and flap exposure eliminated, but also postoperative patient morbidity and discomfort may be reduced due to the noninvasive nature of the procedure. As a result, when indicated and if adequately planned, implant placement surgery may become "easier" and "faster."

Reduced need for bone regeneration

It is a common belief that computer aided surgery can be a tool for avoiding major bone regenerative procedures. However, the evidence available in the literature is very limited. Only one study has reported on guided implant placement as an alternative to bone augmentation (Fortin *et al.*, 2006). Implants were planned upright at all locations, where the CT scan demonstrated sufficient bone volume (Figure 7.10). Otherwise, the practitioner attempted to find a bone recipient site close to and parallel to the anterior or posterior sinus wall, in the palatal curvature or a septum, to avoid bone augmentation. It is important to mention that the practitioner had to adjust the axis of the eventually tilted implant in a manner that intersected the planned tooth crown, which resulted in a both bone- and prosthesis-driven, rather than merely bone-driven implant placement.

Following this procedure, implant axes resulted frequently in a tilted position, which did not seem to represent a prosthetic drawback and succeeded in avoiding guided bone regeneration. Preliminary studies of fixed prostheses supported by a combination of upright and tilted implants have confirmed high implant survival rates (Krekmanov et al., 2000; Calandriello and Tomatis, 2005). By means of guided surgery, bone augmentation may be avoided in specific situations. This can reduce overall treatment duration by decreasing surgery times and eliminating the need for bone grafting, which usually requires longer healing periods. Moreover, the cost of treatment, patient discomfort, and morbidity may be lower. Nevertheless, long-term studies will have to provide evidence that such approaches can be recommended for broader use.

Surgical and prosthetic complications

The concept of computer-guided surgery and immediate loading are usually presented in combination as a surgical and prosthetic treatment that is easy, safe, and predictable. Unfortunately, this is not true, as several complications both during the surgical procedure and during the prosthesis connection can occur. According to the literature, surgical complications are more likely to happen. Hultin et al. (2012) indicated that the surgical complications are almost 70% and that the fracture of the surgical guide is the most common one. Instead, the most common complication associated with the immediate connection of the prosthesis, which represents the 39% of the total, is its misfit. Implant and prosthesis failures are late complications.

Implant survival after 1 year ranged between 89% and 100% (mean 97%) and the corresponding prosthesis survival between 62% and 100% (study mean 95%). It sounds interesting to compare implant and prosthesis survival of implants placed with a conventional technique and those installed in conjunction with guided surgery. There is no difference in implant survival (Nkenke et al., 2007; Danza et al., 2009; Berdougo et al., 2009), as well as in prosthesis survival (Nkenke et al., 2007). In addition, no obvious difference in implant survival rate can be expected for implants restored with an immediate protocol, although data regarding prosthesis survival is not reported.

In conclusion, the most common complications are fracture of the surgical guide and misfit of the prosthesis. When conventional implant surgical techniques are used, however, these kinds of events are not referred to as complications. Therefore, direct comparison of complication rate between conventional and guided surgeries is not possible. It is instead important to recognize the fact that several unexpected adverse events can occur during guided implant treatment, indicating that the clinical demands on the surgeon are not less during guided implant placement than during the conventional one.

Computer guided implant surgery workflow

The actual workflow for producing surgical guides is quite complex, because several patient appointments and waiting periods are necessary to prepare the prosthetic setup, do the radiological examination, produce the surgical guide and finally place the implant. This is not only time consuming for the patient, but it is also work intensive and generates cost (Vercruyssen et al., 2008). Various options are being developed to optimize this workflow. Digital technology has tremendously improved conventional laboratory work in recent years (Nelson et al., 2008). Digital impression techniques have been available for more than 20 years as single-shot impressions (Fuster-Torres et al., 2009; Pieper, 2009) and are now also offered with video capturing (Pieper, 2009). To optimize precision, the most accurate techniques should be used, such as the high-frequency blue-light technique in conjunction with digital impression (Birnbaum and Aaronson, 2008). The high-frequency light features high-precision transfer without noise,

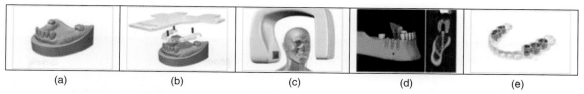

Figure 7.11 Single-scan systems. (a) Step 1. The master cast represents the patient situation and is the basis for the production of the scan and surgical guide. (b) Step 2. The scan guide contains information about the desired prosthetic outcome in the form of radiopaque teeth (visible in CT/CBCT scan). The scan guide is connected to a plate containing reference landmarks (in this particular example three pins) in order to ensure the link between digital implant planning and surgical guide fabrication. (c) Step 3. The patient is scanned wearing the scan guide with a commercially available 3D CT/CBCT scanner. (d) Step 4. The user can import the 3D dataset (DICOM) directly into the planning software. The implant is positioned with respect to the patient's anatomy and the desired prosthetic outcome. After completion of the implant planning, the software provides the plan for surgical guide production (Laboratory-based, milled or printed) and the surgical plan for the guided surgery kit (explaining step by step the drilling sequence). (e) Step 5. The surgical guide is produced according to the guide plan provided by the planning software. The surgical guide contains the surgical sleeves that guide the surgical instruments and the implant.

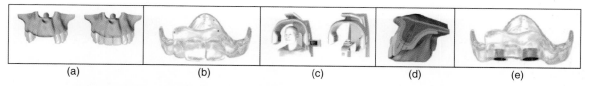

Figure 7.12 Double-scan systems. (a) Step 1. Clinical diagnostics by examination of the patient and impression making for study casts. Fabrication and clinical validation of diagnostic tooth setup. (b) Step 2. Transformation of tooth setup into a radiographic guide – the prosthetic reference during planning. (c) Step 3. Digitization of patient and radiographic guide using a (CB)CT scanner, following the double-scan protocol. (d) Step 4. 3D diagnostics and treatment planning in the software, defining implant position(s) from a clinical, anatomical, and prosthetic perspective, by combining tooth setup with patient anatomy. (e) Step 5. Guided insertion of implants through a custom-manufactured surgical guide based on the treatment plan.

because there is no need for summarizing multiple frames. This allows a digital waxup for planning after the radiological scan instead of the cost-intensive preparation of barium sulfate teeth as the scan reference in a laboratory environment (Figures 7.11–7.13). With this technique, at least one step could be eliminated (Ritter *et al.*, 2009).

Presurgical study phase

Implant installation in partially edentulous cases with a flapless approach requires surgical guides with 5 mm high metallic sleeves due to anatomical factors. Through the sleeve, the drills are inserted for the implant osteotomy, but the drills need to be stabilized with a corresponding drill handle. Usually the company that produces the software provides written instructions with the sequence of the drills with the matching drill handles. If the

implant is placed with the help of specific guiding devices, the surgery is full-guided. If instead the implant is installed just utilizing the surgical guide, as shown in the case below, the placement is partially guided (Figure 7.13).

Clinical applications of computer-guided surgery – case reports

Flapless placement and immediate restoration of single implant

A 25-year-old male has a congenitally missing lateral incisor. After a 2-year-long orthodontic treatment, the patient is ready for the implant placement. Clinical and radiographic examination showed a 7 mm mesiodistal and 6.5 mm buccolingual dimension, which was judged adequate for the placement of a Narrow Crossfit (NC) 10 mm

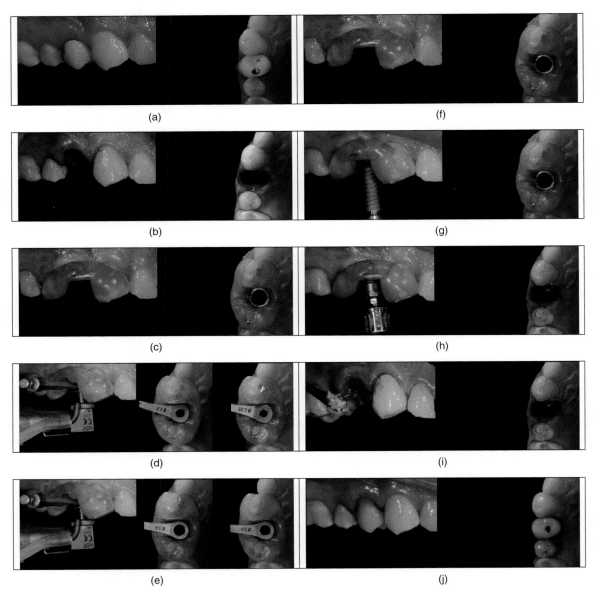

Figure 7.13 Surgical procedure. (a) Clinical and radiographic examination precedes every implant treatment procedure. (b) In this particular case, an atraumatic extraction with simultaneous implant placement is performed. (c) The surgical guide, fabricated with the help of the software Sicat, is inserted. (d) For the osteotomy, the company provides the sequence of drills that needs to be used. (e) Each drill is inserted through the hole of a drill handle that has a matching diameter. (f) After the drilling process, the surgical guide is kept in place. (g) A partially guided implant placement, without a handle, is performed. (h) The implant is placed in the prosthetically desired position. (i) The gap between the buccal bone and the implant surface is filled with a xenograft. (j) A provisional crown fabricated before implant placement is delivered immediately after surgery.

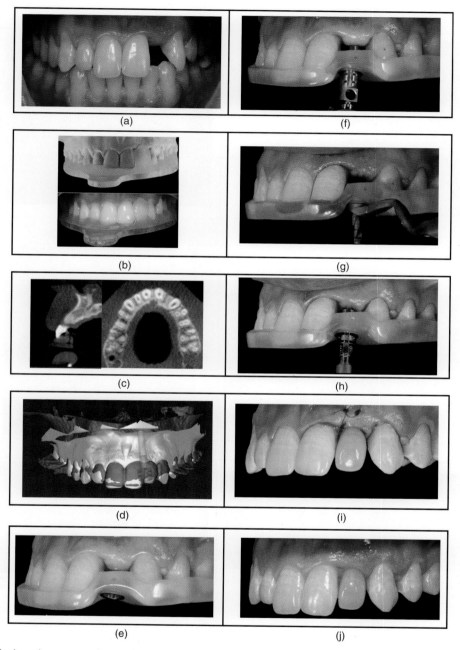

Figure 7.14 Flapless placement and immediate restoration of a single implant. (a) Patient presents with a congenitally missing left lateral incisor. (b) A laboratory-based radiographic guide with 3 reference pins in the plate is used (templiX™). (c) Bone volume is assessed. A 3.3 x 12 mm bone level implant is selected. (d) By using a computer-aided surgery software, the implant is digitally placed in reference to the position of the final restoration and the crestal bone. (e) A laboratory-made surgical guide is used to drive implant placement. (f) A flapless approach is selected and a soft tissue pouch removed with a specific instrument present in the Straumann® guided surgery cassette. (g) An osteotomy is created by drilling through the drill handles and the metallic sleeves present in the surgical guide. (h) The implant placement is fully guided by using a special transfer piece with reference lines. (i) The final crown is delivered the same day of the implant placement. A connective tissue graft is sutured in place to compensate the horizontal defect at the level of the lateral. (j) Healing after 4 weeks shows adequate papilla fill in the interproximal areas.

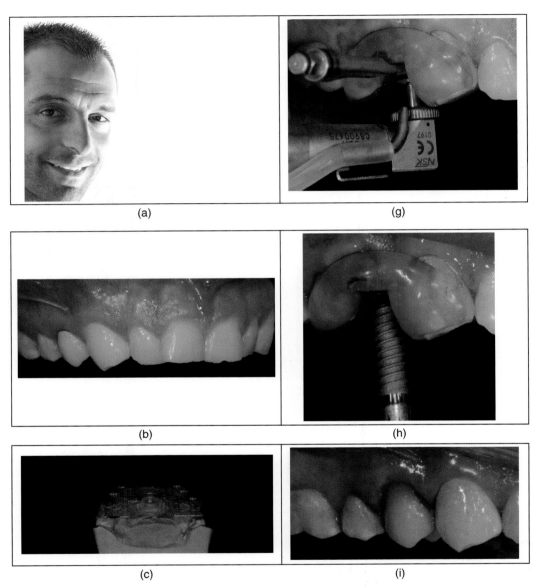

Figure 7.15 Immediate placement and restoration of single implant. (a) Patient presents with chief complaint: "I want a solution for the infection that I have in my tooth, and I don't want to have a hole". His esthetic expectations are high. (b) The right first premolar needs to be extracted for restorative reasons. (c) A special plate with radiopaque landmarks is used for the radiographic guide. (d) 3D reconstruction of the patient's maxillary bone and implant. (e) SICAT surgical software planning is used for virtual implant placement. (f) Presurgical intraoral view. (g) After an atraumatic extraction, the buccal bone integrity is verified and an immediate implant placement performed with guided surgery. (h) A 4.1 × 12 mm implant (Klockner®) is fully guided through the 5 mm sleeve. (i) After implant placement, a prefabricated provisional crown is delivered. (j) Final restoration at the 2-year follow-up. (k) The soft tissue and the color of the crown are in excellent harmony with the natural dentition. (l) A 2-year postoperative CBCT shows maintenance of the buccal bone.

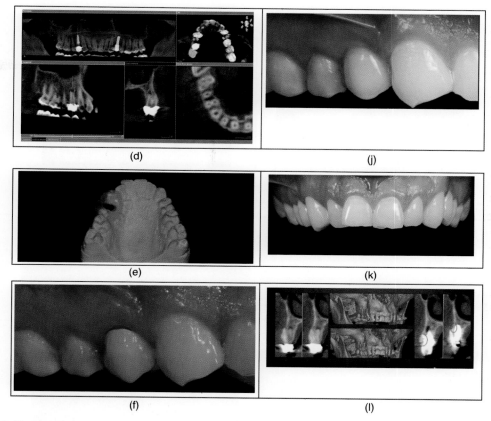

(d)

(j)

(e)

(k)

(f)

(l)

Figure 7.15 (*Continued*)

Straumann® bone level implant (Straumann, Switzerland). Owing to the high esthetic demand of the patient and in order to do a minimally invasive procedure, it was opted for a flapless guided surgery in conjunction with a connective tissue flap to compensate for the horizontal ridge deficiency. The diagnostic cast with a validated waxup was scanned and the soft tissue profile combined with the digital data obtained from the CBCT scan. The digital planning was carried out with the coDiagnostiX software and implant position was planned according to the bone available and the position of the implant-supported restoration. A laboratory-derived guide was fabricated according to the manufacturer's instructions and used preoperatively with the diagnostic cast in order to place the implant analog and create an IPS e.max® Press crown that would be the final implant restoration. No temporarization

was performed (IPS e.max Press crown fabricated by dental technician Daniel del Solar) (see Figure 7.14).

Immediate placement and restoration of single implant

A 32-year-old male needed to have his right first premolar removed due to untreatable root caries. The tooth was previously treated endodontically, and the radiographic evaluation showed a periapical radiolucency. As the CBCT confirmed the integrity of the buccal bone on the crestal aspect of the tooth, an immediate implant placement was planned. The software Sicat™ (Sirona®, Germany) was used to digitally place the implant. A laboratory-based guide was fabricated and used preoperatively in the master model to obtain a

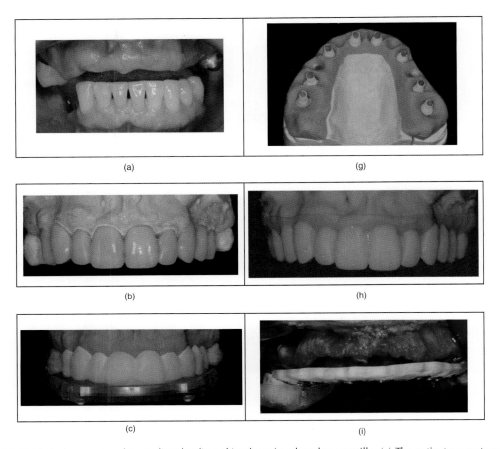

(a)   (g)

(b)   (h)

(c)   (i)

Figure 7.16 Guided placement and immediate loading of implants in edentulous maxilla. (a) The patient presents wearing an acrylic RPD. She wants a fixed restoration. (b) The future implant position is planned in the diagnostic and treatment planning phase. (c) The validated initial setup is used as a guide for the fabrication of the radiographic guide. A bite plate with fiducial markers is bonded to the barium sulfate teeth. (d) After CBCTs were obtained, SICAT Planning Software was used for implant virtual placement. (e) Surgical guide fabricated by the manufacturer (SICAT GmbH & Co. KG Brunnenalle, Bonn, Germany). (f) Before surgery, the diagnostic cast is modified. Using the surgical guide, for the placement of implant analogs. (g) Eight provisional abutments were placed on top of the analogs. (h) Self-polymerizing (New Outline®, anaxdent GmbH, Stuttgart, Germany) was used for the fabrication of a provisional full-mouth restoration. (i) Due to the limited bone availability, a full-thickness flap needed to be reflected. (j) Eight implants were placed in the maxilla and five in the mandible in the same surgery, using the computer-aided surgery guide. (k) After some adjustments, the full-mouth provisional restoration is screwed on top of the eight implants. (l) Postsurgical panoramic radiograph taken after delivery of the temporary prosthesis. Note the small implant/abutment misfit. This expected prosthetic complication was corrected by means of postoperative adjustments to the temporary provisional.

screw-retained temporary crown. After the atraumatic extraction of the premolar, the integrity of the buccal bone was verified and a tissue level implant (Klockner®, Spain) was placed with the help of the guide. Immediately afterward, the provisional crown was inserted. After 2 years of follow-up, the clinical and radiographic examination revealed that the buccal bone was maintained, as well as a scalloped soft tissue architecture (see Figure 7.15).

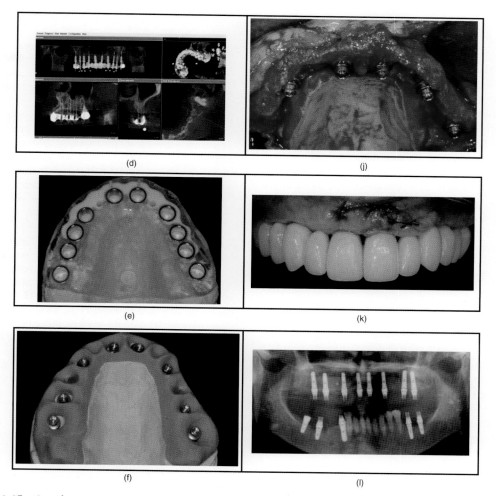

(d) (j)

(e) (k)

(f) (l)

Figure 7.16 *(Continued)*

Guided placement and immediate loading of implants in edentulous maxilla

A 62-year partially edentulous patient with a history of recurrent caries and improper follow-up expressed the desire to have a fixed restoration. The patient was wearing an acrylic resin removable partial denture for a long time and requested an immediate restoration. A full maxillary implant-supported reconstruction with immediate loading and 5 posterior mandibular implants were digitally planned. Then a tooth-supported guide was fabricated. At the time of the surgery, the guide was placed and the first implant positioned at the central incisor to increase the stability of the guide. The remaining implants were installed. Since adequate primary stability was obtained, all the implants were immediately loaded. Due to the great number of implants placed and the complexity of the case, some implant-prostheses mismatch was expected and occurred, but was resolved with intraoperative adjustments. In these cases, a team approach (surgeon, prosthodontist, dental technician) is preferable (Figure 7.16).

Summary

The use of computer-guided surgery allows for the placement of dental implants with high clinical accuracy. According to Nickenig *et al.* (2012), an average positional precision of ≤ 1 mm and within 5 degrees of deviation in inclination can be achieved. Their study documented that the axis and implant position is significantly more precise when using a three-dimensional surgical guide compared to freehand placement. The three-dimensional assessment of the restorative plan via radiopaque duplication of the dental mock-up in the scanning guide allows for highly accurate virtual planning of implants. This enables the clinician to optimally position the implants through the guided surgery guide during implant surgery. Three-dimensional diagnostics are recommended primarily in advanced and complex cases. If they indicated, it is important to assure from the outset that the CBCT data can be used as planning data for a guided surgery guide. The successful application of guided surgery requires comprehensive knowledge and experience. While guided surgery protocols in optimal scenarios are very precise, inaccuracies, and uncertainties still exist. Thus, it is recommended that minimum safety distances to vital structures adjacent to the planned implants be maintained.

Acknowledgments

The authors thank *Mr. Daniel del Solar, CDT*, Badajoz, Spain, for the dental laboratory work presented in the three cases. They also acknowledge the contributions made by Dr. Pedro Lázaro, Periodontics, Madrid, Spain, in some of the cases where he worked with Dr. Cano.

References

Abboud, M., Guirado, J.L.C., Orentlicher, G., & Wahl, G. (2013) Comparison of the accuracy of cone beam computed tomography and medical computed tomography: implications for clinical diagnostics with guided surgery. *International Journal of Oral and Maxillofacial Implants*, **28**, 536–42.

Andersson, M., Carlsson, L., Persson, M., & Bergman, B. (1996) Accuracy of machine milling and spark erosion with a CAD/CAM system. *Journal of Prosthetic Dentistry*, **76**, 187–93.

Arısan, V., Karabuda, Z.C., & Özdemir, T. (2010) Accuracy of two stereolithographic guide systems for computer-aided implant placement: a computed tomography-based clinical comparative study. *Journal of Periodontology*, **81**, 43–51.

Azari, A. & Nikzad, S. (2008) Computer-assisted implantology: historical background and potential outcomes-a review. *International Journal of Medical Robotics*, **4**(2), 95–104.

Behneke, A., Burwinkel, M., Knierim, K., & Behneke, N. (2011) Accuracy assessment of cone beam computed tomography-derived laboratory-based surgical templates on partially edentulous patients. *Clinical Oral Implants Research*, **23**, 137–43.

Berdougo, M., Fortin, T., Blanchet, E., Isidori, M., & Bosson, J.L. (2009) Flapless implant surgery using an image-guided system. A 1- to 4-year retrospective multicenter comparative clinical study. *Clinical Implant Dentistry and Related Research*, **12**, 142–52.

Birnbaum, N.S. & Aaronson, H.B. (2008) Dental impressions using 3D digital scanners: virtual becomes reality. *Compendium of Continuing Education in Dentistry*, **29**(8494, 496), 498–505.

Blanchet, E., Lucchini, J.P., Jenny, R., et al. (2004) An image-guided system based on custom templates: case reports. *Clinical Implant Dentistry and Related Research*, **1**, 40–47.

Brief, J., Edinger, D., Hassfeld, S., & Eggers, G. (2005) Accuracy of image-guided implantology. *Clinical Oral Implants Research*, **16**, 495–501.

Calandriello, R. & Tomatis, M. (2005) Simplified treatment of the atrophic posterior maxilla via immediate/early function and tilted implants: a prospective 1-year clinical study. *Clinical Implant Dentistry and Related Research*, **7**(suppl1), S1–S12.

Cannizzaro, G., Leone, M., Consolo, U., Ferri, V., & Esposito, M. (2008) Immediate functional loading of implants placed with flapless surgery versus conventional implants in partially edentulous patients: a 3-year randomized controlled clinical trial. *International Journal of Oral and Maxillofacial Implants*, **23**, 867–75.

Cassetta, M., Giansanti, M., Di Mambro, A., Calasso, S., & Barbato, E. (2011) Accuracy of two stereolithographic surgical templates: a retrospective study. *Clinical Implant Dentistry and Related Research*, **15**, 448–459.

Danforth, R.A., Peck, J., & Hall, P. (2003) Cone beam volume tomography: an imaging option for diagnosis of complex mandibular third molar anatomical relationships. *Journal of the California Dental Association*, **31**, 847–852.

Danza, M., Zollino, I., & Carinci, F. (2009) Comparison between implants inserted with and without computer planning and custom model coordination. *Journal of Craniofacial Surgery*, **20**, 1086–92.

D'haese, J., van de Velde, T., Komiyama, A., Hultin, M., & De Bruyn, H. (2010) Accuracy and complications using computer-designed stereolithographic surgical guides for oral rehabilitation by means of dental implants: a review of the literature. *Clinical Implant Dentistry and Related Research*, **14**, 321–35.

Dreiseidler, T., Neugebauer, J., Ritter, L., *et al.* (2009) Accuracy of a newly developed integrated system for dental implant planning. *Clinical Oral Implants Research*, **20**, 1191–9.

Duret, F. & Preston, J.D. (1991) CAD/CAM imaging in dentistry. *Current Opinion in Dentistry*, **1**, 150–4.

Eggers, G., Muhling, J., & Marmulla, R. (2006) Image-to-patient registration techniques in head surgery. *International Journal of Oral and Maxillofacial Surgery*, **35**, 1081–1095.

Ersoy, A.E., Turkyilmaz, I., Ozan, O., & McGlumphy, E.A. (2008) Reliability of implant placement with stereolithographic surgical guides generated from computed tomography: clinical data from 94 implants. *Journal of Periodontology*, **79**, 1339–45.

Farley, N.E., Kennedy, K., McGlumphy, E.A., & Clelland, N.L. (2013) Split-mouth comparison of the accuracy of computer-generated and conventional surgical guides. *International Journal of Oral and Maxillofacial Implants*, **28**, 563–72.

Finkle, D.R., Ringler, S.L., Luttenton, C.R., Beernink, J.H., Peterson, N.T., & Dean, R.E. (1985) Comparison of the diagnostic methods used in maxillofacial trauma. *Plastic and Reconstructive Surgery*, **75**, 32–41.

Fortin, T., Bosson, J.L., Isidori, M., & Blanchet, E. (2006) Effect of flapless surgery on pain experienced in implant placement using an image-guided system. *International Journal of Oral and Maxillofacial Implants*, **21**, 298–304.

Fuster-Torres, M.A., Albalat-Estela, S., Alcaniz-Raya, M., *et al.* (2009) CAD/CAM dental systems in implant. Dentistry: update. *Medicina Oral, Patología Oral y Cirugía Bucal*, **3**, E141–E145.

Hämmerle, C.H.F., Stone, P., Jung, R.E., Kapos, T., & Brodala, N. (2009) Consensus statements and recommended clinical procedures regarding computer-assisted implant dentistry. *International Journal of Oral and Maxillofacial Implants*, **24**(Suppl), 126–31.

Hashimoto, K., Kawashima, S., Araki, M., *et al.* (2006) Comparison of image performance between cone-beam computed tomography for dental use and four-row multidetector helical CT. *Journal of Oral Sciences*, **48**, 27–34.

Heiland, M., Schulze, D., Blake, F., *et al.* (2005) Intraoperative imaging of zygomaticomaxillary complex fractures using a 3D C-arm system. *International Journal of Oral and Maxillofacial Surgery*, **34**, 369–375.

Hinckfuss, S., Conrad, H.J., Lin, L., Lunos, S., & Seong, W.-J. (2012) Effect of surgical guide design and surgeon's experience on the accuracy of implant placement. *Journal of Oral Implantology*, **38**, 311–23.

Honda, K., Larheim, T.A., Maruhashi, K., *et al.* (2006) Osseous abnormalities of the mandibular condyle: diagnostic reliability of cone beam computed tomography compared with helical computed tomography based on an autopsy material. *Dento Maxillo Facial Radiology*, **35**, 152–157.

Horwitz, J., Zuabi, O., & Machtei, E.E., (2009) Accuracy of a computerized tomography-guided template-assisted implant placement system: an in vitro study. *Clinical Oral Implants Research*. **20**, 1156–62.

Hounsfield, G.N. (1973) Computerized transverse axial scanning (tomography). 1. Description of system. *British Journal of Radiology*, **46**, 1016–22.

Hultin, M., Svensson, K.G., & Trulsson, M. (2012) Clinical advantages of computer-guided implant placement: a systematic review. *Clinical Oral Implants Research*, **23**, 124–35.

Jabero, M. & Sarment, D.P. (2006) Advanced surgical guidance technology: a review. *Implant Dentistry*, **2**, 135–142.

Jung, R.E., Schneider, D., Ganeles, J., *et al.* (2009) Computer technology applications in surgical implant dentistry: a systematic review. *International Journal of Oral and Maxillofacial Implants*, **24**(Suppl), 92–109.

Kapos, T., *et al.* (2009) Computer-aided design computer-assisted manufacturing in prosthetic dentistry. *International Journal of Oral & Maxillofacial Implants*, **8**, 1–8.

Krekmanov, L., Kahn, M., Rangert, B., & Lindström, H. (2000) Tilting of posterior mandibular and maxillary implants for improved prosthesis support. *International Journal of Oral and Maxillofacial Implants*, **15**, 405–14.

Loubele, M., Bogaerts, R., Van Dijck, E., *et al.* (2009) Comparison between effective radiation dose of CBCT and MSCT scanners for dentomaxillofacial applications. *European Journal of Radiology*, **71**, 461–468.

Mah, J.K., Danforth, R.A., Bumann, A., *et al.* (2003) Radiation absorbed in maxillofacial imaging with a new dental computed tomography device. *Oral Surgery, Oral Medicine, Oral Pathology, Oral Radiology & Endodontics*, **96**, 508–513.

Mischkowski, R.A., Zinser, M.J., Neugebauer, J., *et al.* (2006) Comparison of static and dynamic computer-assisted guidance methods in implantology. *International Journal of Computerized Dentistry*, **9**, 23–35.

Miyazaki, T., Hotta, Y., Kunii, J., Kuriyama, S., & Tamaki, Y. (2009) A review of dental CAD/CAM: current status and future perspectives from 20 years of experience. *Dental Materials Journal*, **28**, 44–56.

Mörmann, W.H., Brandestini, M., Lutz, F., & Barbakow, F. (1989) Chairside computer-aided direct ceramic inlays. *Quintessence International*, **20**, 329–39.

Nelson, K., Hildebrand, D., & Mehrhof, J. (2008) Fabrication of a fixed retrievable implant-supported prosthesis based on electroforming: a technical report. *Journal of Prosthodontics*, **7**, 591–595.

Neugebauer, J., Stachulla, G., Ritter, L., *et al.* (2010) Computer-aided manufacturing technologies for guided implant placement. *Expert Review of Medical Devices*, **7**, 113–29.

Nickenig, H.J., Eitner, S., Rothamel, D., Wichmann, M., & Zöller, J.E. (2012) Possibilities and limitations of implant placement by virtual planning data and surgical guide templates. *International Journal of Computerized Dentistry*, **15**, 9–21.

Nkenke, E., Eitner, S., Radespiel-Tröger, M., Vairaktaris, E., Neukam, F.-W., & Fenner, M. (2007) Patient-centred outcomes comparing transmucosal implant placement with an open approach in the maxilla: a prospective, non-randomized pilot study. *Clinical Oral Implants Research*, **18**, 197–203.

Oh, S., Kim, S., & Suh, T.S. (2007a) How image quality affects determination of target displacement when using kilovoltage cone-beam computed tomography. *Journal of Applied Clinical Medical Physics*, **8**, 101–107.

Oh, T.J., Shotwell, J., Billy, E., *et al.* (2007b) Flapless implant surgery in the esthetic region: advantages and precautions. *International Journal of Periodontics & Restorative Dentistry*, **1**, 27–33.

Ozan, O., Turkyilmaz, I., Ersoy, A.E., McGlumphy, E.A., & Rosenstiel, S.F. (2009) Clinical accuracy of 3 different types of computed tomography-derived stereolithographic surgical guides in implant placement. *Journal of Oral and Maxillofacial Surgery*, **67**, 394–401.

Pauwels, R., Beinsberger, J., Collaert, B., *et al.* (2012) Effective dose range for dental cone beam computed tomography scanners. *European Journal of Radiology*, **81**, 267–271.

Pettersson, A., Komiyama, A., Hultin, M., Nässtrom, K., & Klinge, B. (2010) Accuracy of virtually planned and template guided implant surgery on edentate patients. *Clinical Implant Dentistry and Related Research*, **14**, 527–37.

Pieper, R. (2009) Digital impressions – easier than ever. *International Journal of Computerized Dentistry*, **1**, 47–52.

Priest, G. (2005) Virtual-Designed and Computer-Milled Implant Abutments. *Journal of Oral and Maxillofacial Surgery*, **63**, 22–32.

Ritter, L., Neugebauer, J., Dreiseidler, T., *et al.* (2009) 3D x-ray meets CAD/CAM dentistry: a novel procedure for virtual dental implant planning. *International Journal of Computerized Dentistry*, **1**, 29–40.

Rosenfeld, A. & Mandelaris, G. (2006) Prosthetically directed implant placement using computer software to ensure precise placement and predictable prosthetic outcomes. *International Journal of Periodontics & Restorative Dentistry*, **26**, 215–21.

Sarment, D.P. (2003) Accuracy of Implant Placement with a Stereolithographic Surgical Guide. *International Journal of Oral & Maxillofacial Implants*, **24**, 1–7.

Schneider, D., Marquardt, P., Zwahlen, M., & Jung, R.E. (2009) A systematic review on the accuracy and the clinical outcome of computer-guided template-based implant dentistry. *Clinical Oral Implants Research*, **20**, 73–86.

Sharpe, M.B., Moseley, D.J., Purdie, T.G., Islam, M., Siewerdsen, J.H., & Jaffray, D.A. (2006) The stability of mechanical calibration for a kV cone beam computed tomography system integrated with linear accelerator. *Medical Physics*, **33**, 136–144.

Stein, W., Hassfeld, S., Brief, J., *et al.* (1998) CT-based 3D-planning for dental implantology. *Studies in Health Technology and Informatics*, **50**, 137–143.

Stopp, S., Wolff, T., Irlinger, F., & Lueth, T. (2008) A new method for printer calibration and contour accuracy manufacturing with 3D- print technology. *Rapid Prototyping Journal*, **14**, 167–172.

Stopp, S., Deppe, H., & Lueth, T. (2007) Manufacturing drill templates for dental implantology using a 3D printer. *Rapid Prototyping Journal*, **14**, 167–172.

Stratemann, S.A., Huang, J.C., Maki, K., Miller, A.J., & Hatcher, D.C. (2008) Comparison of cone beam computed tomography imaging with physical measures. *Dento Maxillo Facial Radiology*, **37**, 80–93.

Sukovic, P. (2003) Cone beam computed tomography in craniofacial imaging. *Orthodontics and Craniofacial Research*, **6**(Suppl. 1), 31–36.179–182

Van Assche, N., van Steenberghe, D., Guerrero, M.E., *et al.* (2007) Accuracy of implant placement based on pre-surgical planning of three-dimensional cone-beam images: a pilot study. *Journal of Clinical Periodontology*, **34**, 816–21.

Van Assche, N., van Steenberghe, D., Quirynen, M., & Jacobs, R. (2010) Accuracy assessment of computer-assisted flapless implant placement in partial edentulism. *Journal of Clinical Periodontology*, **37**, 398–403.

Van Assche, N., Vercruyssen, M., Coucke, W., Teughels, W., Jacobs, R., & Quirynen, M. (2012) Accuracy of computer-aided implant placement. *Clinical Oral Implants Research*, **23**, 112–23.

Van Steenberghe, D., Glauser, R., Blomback, U., *et al.* (2005) A computed tomographic scan-derived customized surgical template and fixed prosthesis for flapless surgery and immediate loading of implants in fully edentulous maxillae: a prospective multicenter study. *Clinical Implant Dentistry and Related Research,* 7(Suppl. 1), S111–20.

Vannier, M.W. (2003) Craniofacial computed tomography scanning technology, applications and future trends. Section 2: Multi-dimensional imaging. *Orthodontics and Craniofacial Research,* 1, 23–30.

Varvara, G., Esposito, P., Franchini, F., *et al.* (2003) A positioning device for computed tomography: a clinical report. *Journal of Prosthetic Dentistry,* 2, 123–126.

Vercruyssen, M., Jacobs, R., Van Assche, N., & van Steenberghe, D. (2008) The use of CT scan based planning for oral rehabilitation by means of implants and its transfer to the surgical field: a critical review on accuracy. *Journal of Oral Rehabilitation,* 35, 454–74.

Weitz, J., Deppe, H., Stopp, S., Lueth, T., Mueller, S., & Hohlweg-Majert, B. (2010) Accuracy of templates for navigated implantation made by rapid prototyping with DICOM datasets of cone beam computer tomography (CBCT). *Clinical Oral Investigations,* 15, 1001–6.

Widmann, G. & Bale, R.J. (2006) Accuracy in computer-aided implant surgery–a review. *International journal of Oral and Maxillofacial Implants,* 21, 305–313.

Widmann, G., Widmann, R., Widmann, E., *et al.* (2007) Use of a surgical navigation system for CT-guided template production. *International Journal of Oral and Maxillofacial Implants,* 1, 72–78.

Winter, A.A., Pollack, A.S., Frommer, H.H., *et al.* (2005) Cone beam volumetric tomography vs. medical CT scanners. *New York State Dental Journal,* 71, 28–33.

Wittwer, G., Adeyemo, W.L., Schicho, K., Birkfellner, W., & Enislidis, G. (2007) Prospective randomized clinical comparison of 2 dental implant navigation systems. *International Journal of Oral and Maxillofacial Implants,* 22, 785–90.

8 Digital Design and Manufacture of Implant Abutments

Radi Masri, Joanna Kempler, and Carl F. Driscoll

Introduction

Since their introduction more than three decades ago, endosseous implants have transformed prosthetic dentistry. Removable prosthodontics ceased to be the only option for completely edentulous patients, and the functional and esthetic outcomes of restorations were greatly improved to achieve unprecedented patient satisfaction.

The restoration of dental implants follows similar principles to those described for the restoration of natural teeth. An accurate rendition of implant position in the dental arch (impression) is necessary to design and fabricate a foundation for the restoration – an implant abutment. An implant-retained restoration, whether cement- or screw-retained, can then be fabricated on top of the implant abutment.

Implant abutments

Implant abutments can be generally classified into two types: (i) prefabricated implant abutments and (ii) custom-made implant abutments.

Prefabricated abutments

Prefabricated abutments are manufactured using subtractive manufacturing technology described in detail in Chapter 3. The seating surface of these abutments is precision milled to passively fit the head of the implant with very low machining tolerance (Malaguti *et al.*, 2011; Ma *et al.*, 1997). The height of the abutment, location and width of the finish line, and the axial walls can be modified manually by the technician or the dentist to accommodate a full coverage restoration. Like any item used in dentistry, these abutments are manufactured from biocompatible materials, typically a titanium alloy or ceramic, that do not promote plaque accumulation and can withstand masticatory forces. An example of a prefabricated abutment is shown in Figure 8.1.

Prefabricated abutments are readily available, economical, and can be easily modified; thus, they are widely used. However, their contours are rarely anatomic and do not support the surrounding soft tissues making managing the emergence profile of an implant restoration difficult. They

Clinical Applications of Digital Dental Technology, First Edition. Edited by Radi Masri and Carl F. Driscoll.
© 2015 John Wiley & Sons, Inc. Published 2015 by John Wiley & Sons, Inc.

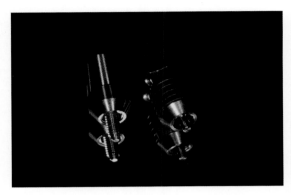

Figure 8.1 A titanium prefabricated abutment designed for an implant with an external connection. Note the gold abutment screw that is used to retain the abutment and the impression coping used to make an impression from the head of the implant.

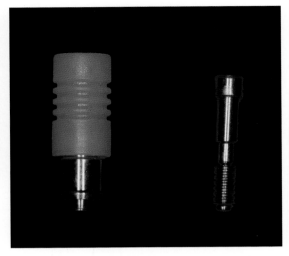

Figure 8.2 A Gold Adapt (NobelBiocare) custom abutment and retaining screw, before fabrication.

are also difficult to use in patients where there is excessive implant angulation. To circumvent these caveats, custom abutments are indicated.

Custom abutments

Custom abutments were first described in 1988 (Lewis *et al.*, 1988; Lewis *et al.*, 1989). Traditionally, these abutments consisted of a plastic sleeve or a gold cylinder that could be waxed to specification and cast in metal alloy to fabricate an abutment that sits on dental implants. These abutments are prepared, finished, and polished like any traditional casting and can be designed for cement- or screw-retained restorations. In Figure 8.2, a custom abutment is shown before fabrication.

With the continued evolution of dental technology, abutments can now be designed digitally and fabricated using milling technology for each individual patient. Thus, by definition these CAD/CAM abutments are classified as custom abutments.

There is no longer a need to wax and cast abutments, and dentists and technicians can design and fabricate custom abutments from the comfort of their seats. CAD/CAM custom abutments are economical to fabricate and provide optimum contours for the restoration resulting in better esthetics and function.

CAD/CAM abutment design

Similar to CAD/CAM crown fabrication, there are two digital workflows to fabricate a custom abutment (see Boxes 4.1 and 4.2; Chapter 4). In the first workflow, a conventional impression is made of the head of the implant to fabricate a master cast in which implant position and angulation relative to other structures in the dental arch is registered. This master cast is then verified for accuracy and scanned using a desktop scanner (Persson *et al.*, 2008; Persson *et al.*, 2009), to fabricate a digital master cast. Custom abutments can be digitally created and designed with optimum anatomical contours to provide adequate resistance and retention form, esthetic emergence profile, and optimum hygiene. Abutment margin type, width and location, and restorative space can be manipulated to produce an abutment that can accommodate a full coverage restoration. The majority of custom abutments fabricated these days utilize this workflow.

In the second workflow, a digital impression is made using impression copings specifically designed for digital impressions, and they are referred to as scan bodies (Figure 8.3). A scan body is used to index the implant position and used to obtain a digital master cast. The digital master cast can then be used to virtually design a custom abutment, which can be later milled

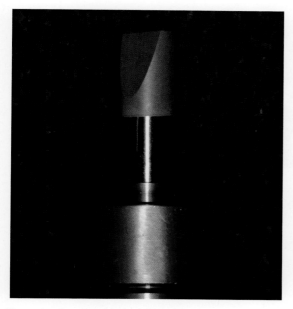

Figure 8.3 An example of a Nobel Biocare Scan Body.

shape resulting in abutments with anatomical contours that provide for excellent function and esthetics (Garg, 2002). ATLANTIS abutments are made from Grade 5 titanium alloy (Titanium-6 Alumninum-4Vanadium; Ti-6Al-4V), which can be shaded with titanium nitride (TiN) to give a gold hue, or from zirconia (yttria-stabilized tetragonal zirconia polycrystals; Y-TZP) in four different shades. ATLANTIS abutments are compatible with all major implant companies including but not limited to Nobel Biocare, Straumann, DENTSPLY, and Biomet 3I implants. Although Atlantis abutments fit implants with excellent precision (Kerstein and Radke, 2008), the connecting surface of ATLANTIS abutments differ from that of the original abutments for these implants and therefore, higher rotational misfit is expected (Gigandet *et al.*, 2014).

and sent to the clinician. The use of this workflow will obviate the need for elastomeric impression material, produce more accurate restorations, and streamline dental treatment. Almost all intraoral scanners (iTero, 3D Shape, 3M TrueDefinition, and Cerec OmniCam, see Chapter 2) have the capability to make impressions of implant scan bodies to design and fabricate a custom abutment just like that described for the fabrication of crowns (Chapter 4).

If an intraoral scanner is not available in the clinic, there are several digital solutions for the fabrication of custom abutments (Kapos and Evans, 2014; Priest, 2005). These include ATLANTIS abutments (DENTSPLY Implants) (Garg, 2002), NobelProcera (Nobel Biocare), and Bella Tek Encode Impression System (Biomet 3I) (Mahn and Prestipino, 2013).

ATLANTIS abutments

ATLANTIS abutments are individually designed to fabricate cement- or screw-retained abutments. Patented software, Virtual Abutment Design (ATLANTIS VAD, DENTSPLY Implants), is used to design the abutments from the final tooth

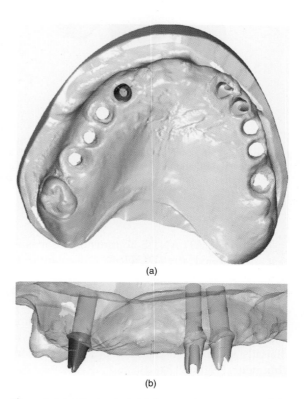

(a)

(b)

Figure 8.4 (a) Occlusal view of scanned master cast and the design of CAD/CAM custom abutments. White color represents the location of implants and abutments are in green. (b) Frontal view of scanned master cast and abutments design.

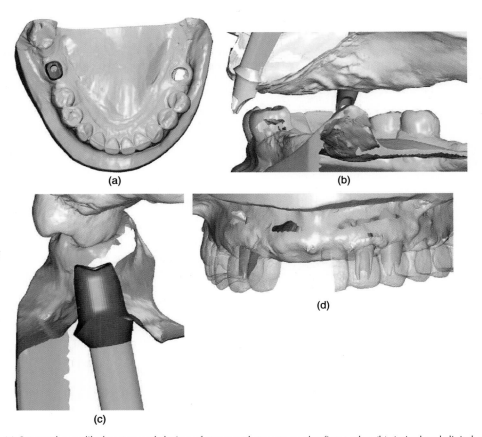

(a)

(b)

(c)

(d)

Figure 8.5 (a) Scanned mandibular cast and design of custom abutment on the first molar. (b) Articulated digital casts with a superimposed scan of the provisional restoration. This will allow for the design of a custom abutment within the confines of the provisional restoration and the available space. In this figure, maxillary anterior custom abutments are shown. (c) Designed mandibular custom abutment is shown. (d) Frontal view of designed abutments with a superimposed scan of the provisional restoration.

To fabricate ATLANTIS abutments, the master cast is scanned (by DENTSPLY Implants) to fabricate a digital master cast with accurate representation of soft tissues, remaining teeth and implant (Figure 8.4a, b). The opposing cast is also scanned along with the occlusal registration and the provisional restoration or (waxup) to digitally articulate the casts and design the custom abutments (Figure 8.5a–d).

Once the abutments are designed, a link is sent to the dentist or laboratory technicians to review the abutment design and edit it using ATLANTIS 3D Editor software. ATLANTIS 3D Editor software is an online, easy to use, graphic supported communication tool for the dental laboratories and dentists. Using this software, the dentist/laboratory technician can evaluate articulated casts and edit the abutment design. A superimposed view of the provisional restoration can be used to investigate the available restorative space, margin type, width, and location relative to soft tissues and emergence profile of the designed custom abutment. The occlusal and frontal views can also be used to evaluate the path of insertion of the restoration. Once the design of custom abutments is finalized and approved, the abutments are fabricated (by DENTSPLY Implants) (Figure 8.6a, b) and returned to the dentist to try in

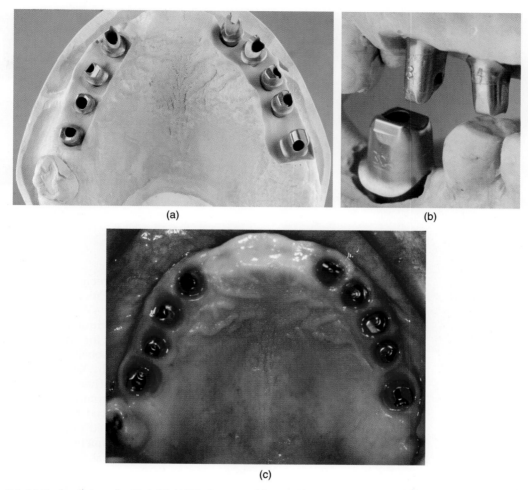

(a)

(b)

(c)

Figure 8.6 (a) Occlusal view of milled ATLANTIS abutments fabricated by DENTSPLY Implants. The abutments are coated with TiN to give gold shading. (b) Lateral view of ATLANTIS custom abutments. (c) Try-in of abutments in the mouth.

the mouth (Figure 8.6c) and to fabricate the final restoration (Figure 8.7a, b).

Having designed the abutments digitally, the clinician, or the technician can easily fabricate identical functional duplicates of the original abutments. These abutments can be used as a master die to evaluate the final restoration or as a temporary means to retain a provisional restoration while the final restoration is fabricated. The final restorations (crowns or fixed dental prostheses) can be fabricated using conventional methods or using digital technology as described earlier in Chapter 5.

NobelProcera abutments

NobelProcera abutments are fabricated in a process similar to that described for ATALANTIS abutments. The master cast is scanned using an automated desktop scanner (2G scanner, Nobel Biocare). This scanner is a 3D noncontact laser scanner for surface data acquisition. It uses a unique technology known as conoscopic holography. Conoscopic holography is a technology based on polarized light interference whereby dimensions and surface details are derived from solid angle measurement (cone of light) rather than

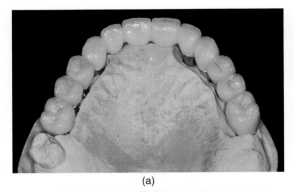

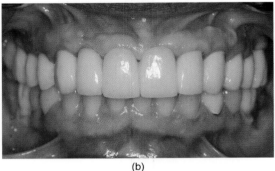

Figure 8.7 (a) Occlusal view of metal ceramic-restorations fabricated on the master cast. (b) Frontal view of restorations inserted in the mouth.

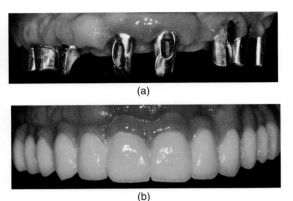

Figure 8.8 (a) Custom abutments designed using NobelProcera system. (b) Final prosthesis cemented on NobelProcera abutments.

from a single ray as performed previously using traditional laser scanners (Burgner *et al.*, 2013). This makes conoscopic holography more precise, stable, and robust than laser triangulation-based methods (Burgner *et al.*, 2013), especially in complex cases with multiple implants and severe angulation (Holst *et al.*, 2012).

Scanning of the master cast can be performed in the laboratory rather than sending it to a central location (as described above for ATLANTIS abutments). Scan bodies or abutment position locators (Nobel Biocare) are used to index the implant position and scanned. The NobelProcera software can then be used to virtually design abutments, fixed dental prostheses, bars, and crowns. Virtual design of the abutment is performed in the laboratory and similar to ATLANTIS abutments, the technician or dentist can design and edit the abutment design according to their specifications. An example of custom abutments fabricated

using NobelProcera abutment system is shown in Figure 8.8a, b. NobelProcera abutments can be fabricated from Ti-6Al-4V, zirconia, alumina, base metal alloy (cobalt chromium), IPS e.max, and acrylic (Telio CAD) for the fabrication of provisional restorations. NobelProcera abutments are also compatible with 3D Shape intraoral scanners (see Chapter 2). Therefore, an abutment can be designed directly from an intraoral digital impression without the need to obtain and scan a master cast. The finalized design can be sent online to order milled abutments.

In addition to the fabrication of custom abutments, NobelProcera software can be used to fabricate milled bars. Several implant bar systems are supported, these include Dolder, Hader, Round, Paris, and free form milled bars. Screw-retained attachments and clips can also be provided. NobelProcera bars are compatible with Ball attachments (Bredent), Dalbo attachments (Zest), and Anchor Bar Locators (Zest). In Figure 8.9a, a free form milled bar (substructure made from Ti-6Al-4V) that was fabricated using the NobelProcera system is shown (Figure 8.9b).

To fabricate an implant-retained bar, the master cast is scanned and the digital file is opened using the NobelProcera software (Figure 8.10a). The waxup, or the provisional restoration, is also scanned to be used as a reference to fabricate the bar (Figure 8.10b). Virtual design of the bar is accomplished by installing digital abutments on

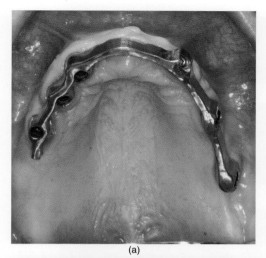

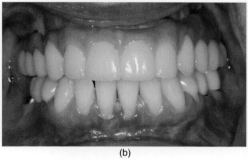

(a)

(b)

Figure 8.9 (a) Occlusal view of free form milled bar fabricated using NobelProcera system. (b) Frontal view of the final prosthesis retained on the substructure using lateral retaining screws.

the digital master cast and allowing the software to connect these abutments with a bar, using preset bar designs programmed into the software. Bar dimensions, location, distance from soft tissue can be intuitively and easily edited according to the specifications provided by the dentist. In Figure 8.10a–i, steps of designing a virtual bar are shown. The virtual design can be sent to Nobel Biocare, online, to mill the bar.

Abutments and bars fabricated using the NobelProcera System exhibit clinically acceptable fit. In a study comparing the fit of CAD/CAM implant abutments fabricated using NobelProcera, Hamilton et al. found that, for most implant systems, the difference of fit between CAD/CAM abutments and prefabricated abutments was less than 4 μm. However, the difference in fit was more in abutments fabricated for Straumann implants (bone level), using ProceraNobel software. The difference was approximately 15 μm (Hamilton et al., 2013).

BellaTek encode system

In this system, a custom-designed coded healing abutment (Encode abutment) is used to convey implant position in the dental arch. The abutment is engraved with specific occlusal surface coding (Figure 8.11) and can be used instead of an impression coping or a scan body. As such, there is no need for an implant level impression, there is less tissue trauma because there is no need to remove the healing abutment and there is reduction of chair time needed. The use of this technology is simple and as described earlier, the digital master cast can be made either directly using an intraoral digital impression system of the coded healing abutment or indirectly by scanning a cast made from a conventional impression. However, the accuracy of this system is not fully characterized.

A study by Al-Abdullah et al. revealed that definitive casts fabricated from coded abutment impressions are less accurate than those fabricated from conventional impression techniques (Al-Abdullah et al., 2013). Two other studies reached the same conclusions (Eliasson and Ortorp, 2012; Howell et al., 2013). However, in all of these studies, a master cast containing implant analogs was fabricated from the coded abutment impression and none of these studies evaluated the accuracy of a digital master cast obtained using this system. Therefore, more studies are needed to evaluate the accuracy and the potential of this system.

Similarly, there are very few studies in the literature investigating the accuracy of fit of CAD/CAM abutments fabricated using intraoral digital scanners. While their accuracy is expected to be high for single implant restorations, their accuracy in situations where multiple implants are being restored remains to be examined.

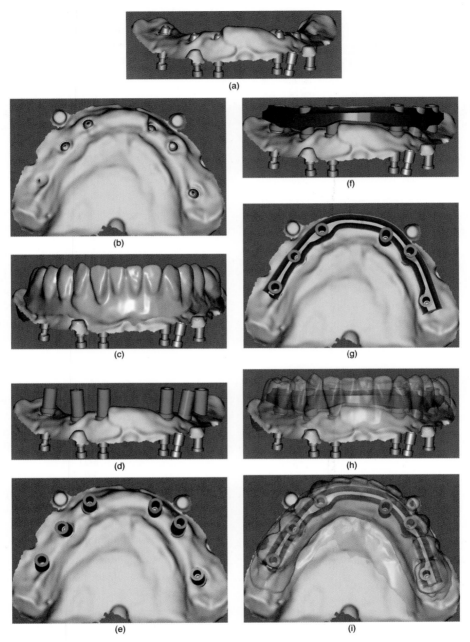

Figure 8.10 (a) Frontal view of master cast that is scanned into NobelProcera software to design an implant-retained bar. (b) Occlusal view of master cast that is scanned into NobelProcera software to design an implant-retained bar. (c) Waxup of final prosthesis is scanned into NobelProcera software (frontal view). (d) Virtual abutments are placed on the virtual master cast (frontal view). (e) Virtual abutments are placed on the virtual master cast (occlusal view). (f) Virtual bar is designed (frontal view). (g) Virtual bar is designed (occlusal view). (h) Waxup is superimposed on top of the designed bar to evaluate space available for restorative material (frontal view). (i) Waxup is superimposed on top of the designed bar to evaluate space available for restorative material (occlusal view).

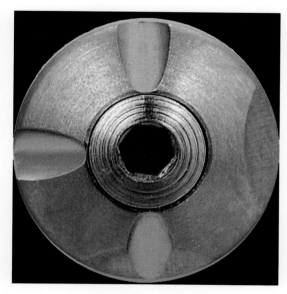

Figure 8.11 The Encode healing abutment (Biomet 3I).

Summary

A description of three commercially available systems for the fabrication of CAD/CAM abutments was included in this chapter. Common to all these systems is the need to "digitize" implant position, location, and angulation relative to other structures (teeth or implants) in the dental arch. The digital master cast is then used to design abutments that can precisely fit the implants. The virtual design is translated into a plan that can be transmitted to a milling machine to produce the abutments. In addition to the systems described here, several other systems exist. However, they all follow the same principles. Before choosing a system, it is imperative that the clinician evaluates the available evidence supporting its use. Data that describe tolerance, fit, and longevity of restorations must be considered.

References

Al-Abdullah, K., Zandparsa, R., & Finkelman, M., et al. (2013) An in vitro comparison of the accuracy of implant impressions with coded healing abutments and different implant angulations. *The Journal of Prosthetic Dentistry*, **110**, 90–100.

Burgner, J., Simpson, A.l., & Fitzpatrick, J.M., et al. (2013) A study on the theoretical and practical accuracy of conoscopic holography-based surface measurements: toward image registration in minimally invasive surgery. *International Journal of Medical Robotics and Computer Assisted Surgery*, **9**, 190–203.

Eliasson, A. & Ortorp, A. (2012) The accuracy of an implant impression technique using digitally coded healing abutments. *Clinical Implant Dentistry and Related Research*, **14**(Suppl 1), e30–e38.

Garg, A.K. (2002) The Atlantis Components Abutment: simplifying the tooth implant procedure. *Dental Implantology Update*, **13**, 65–70.

Gigandet, M., Bigolin, G., & Faoro, F., et al. (2014) Implants with Original and Non-Original Abutment Connections. *Clinical Implant Dentistry and Related Research*, **16**(2), 303–311.

Hamilton, A., Judge, R.B., & Palamara, J.E., et al. (2013) Evaluation of the fit of CAD/CAM abutments. *The International Journal of Prosthodontics*, **26**, 370–380.

Holst, S., Persson, A., & Wichmann, M., et al. (2012) Digitizing implant position locators on master casts: comparison of a noncontact scanner and a contact-probe scanner. *The International Journal of Oral & Maxillofacial Implants*, **27**, 29–35.

Howell, K.J., McGlumphy, E.A., & Drago, C., et al. (2013) Comparison of the accuracy of Biomet 3i Encode Robocast Technology and conventional implant impression techniques. *The International Journal of Oral & Maxillofacial Implants*, **28**, 228–240.

Kapos, T. & Evans, C. (2014) CAD/CAM technology for implant abutments, crowns, and superstructures. *The International Journal of Oral & Maxillofacial Implants*, **29**(Suppl), 117–136.

Kerstein, R.B. & Radke, J. (2008) A comparison of fabrication precision and mechanical reliability of 2 zirconia implant abutments. *The International Journal of Oral & Maxillofacial Implants*, **23**, 1029–1036.

Lewis, S., Beumer, J. 3rd., & Hornburg, W., et al. (1988) The "UCLA" abutment. *The International Journal of Oral & Maxillofacial Implants*, **3**, 183–189.

Lewis, S., Avera, S., & Engleman, M., et al. (1989) The restoration of improperly inclined osseointegrated implants. *The International Journal of Oral & Maxillofacial Implants*, **4**, 147–152.

Ma, T., Nicholls, J.I., & Rubenstein, J.E. (1997) Tolerance measurements of various implant components. *The International Journal of Oral & Maxillofacial Implants*, **12**, 371–375.

Mahn, D.H. & Prestipino, T. (2013) CAD/CAM implant abutments using coded healing abutments: a detailed description of the restorative process. *The Compendium of Continuing Education in Dentistry*, **34**, 612–615.

Malaguti, G., Denti, L., & Bassoli, E., et al. (2011) Dimensional tolerances and assembly accuracy of dental implants and machined versus cast-on abutments. *Clinical Implant Dentistry and Related Research*, **13**, 134–140.

Persson, A.S., Andersson, M., & Oden, A., *et al.* (2008) Computer aided analysis of digitized dental stone replicas by dental CAD/CAM technology. *Dental Materials*, **24**, 1123–1130.

Persson, A.S., Oden, A., & Andersson, M., *et al.* (2009) Digitization of simulated clinical dental impressions: virtual three-dimensional analysis of exactness. *Dental Materials*, **25**, 929–936.

Priest, G. (2005) Virtual-designed and computer-milled implant abutments. *Journal of Oral and Maxillofacial Surgery*, **63**, 22–32.

9 Digital Applications in Endodontics

Ashraf F. Fouad

Introduction

Endodontics is a specialty that fundamentally deals with diagnosis and treatment of diseases of the dental pulp and periapical tissues. These tissues are unique among oral tissues in many ways. They are invisible to the clinician even with magnification. The pulp space is very small with complex anatomy and physiology. Moreover, the pulp is frequently rendered devoid of vital tissues and host responses by irreversible disease. The periapical tissues respond to pulpal disease and its treatment but are not directly manipulated clinically, except during surgical procedures.

Endodontic disease is an infectious process that is secondary to caries, trauma, advanced periodontal disease, congenital anomalies of teeth, and severe abrasion or attrition. Therefore, the treatment of endodontic pathosis focuses on prevention or elimination of infection of the root canal space. The instrumentation of the canal space is intended to provide adequate cleaning of this space but also provides a convenient way to obturate it. The obturation is frequently done in a way that allows retreatment or revision of initial therapy, as the conditions of the coronal restoration, tooth function, and future disease risk change.

This chapter will describe digital technologies that support the basic goals of diagnosis and treatment as well as provide some information on their efficacy and effectiveness where appropriate. In describing these technologies, it is essential to remember that the most important objective of these technologies is to improve diagnostic acumen and treatment outcomes. Naturally, other goals include efficiency and convenience for the practitioner; however, these additional goals would only be justified if they do not interfere with the first objective and provide safety and cost-effectiveness for the patient.

Diagnostic technologies

Conventional pulp testing

One of the most fundamental processes for endodontic diagnosis is pulp testing. This basic procedure, which has been available for several decades, allows the clinician to determine whether the pulp is vital or necrotic. Contemporary techniques allow the determination of pulp sensitivity, also known as sensibility, rather than vitality. The assumption is that the vital pulp contains actively

Clinical Applications of Digital Dental Technology, First Edition. Edited by Radi Masri and Carl F. Driscoll.
© 2015 John Wiley & Sons, Inc. Published 2015 by John Wiley & Sons, Inc.

conducting neurons that can be easily stimulated by thermal or electrical stimuli. The limitations of available technologies are that the clinician frequently wishes to determine reversible from irreversible pulpitis. This is important because this distinction is essential in determining whether endodontic therapy is necessary. If so, this should be performed before a costly restoration is fabricated. In addition, pulpal sensitivity may be lost when the pulp still has intact vascularity, such as following traumatic injuries. Finally, restorations, caries, and difficulty in moisture control and mineralization within the pulp – dentin complex frequently modify the response of the patient yielding limited test reliability.

Because of these limitations, pulp sensitivity testing has to be conducted with care to achieve the most reliable results. The teeth involved need to be adequately isolated with cotton rolls and dried. Control teeth need to be tested first, to assure baseline response and educate the patient on test expectations. The probe of the electrical pulp tester (EPT) or cotton pellet in a cold test should be applied with light pressure to assure contact, but not to stimulate periapical responses, particularly in cases with severe periapical pain.

The principal goal for conventional pulp sensitivity testing is to determine whether the pulp is vital or necrotic. Contemporary data show that the EPT has high specificity (ability to determine that the disease is absent when the pulp is truly vital) and that cold in the form of Endo Ice or CO_2 snow has high sensitivity (ability to determine if the pulp is necrotic, when it is truly necrotic) (Weisleder et al., 2009). Therefore, both tests complement one another, and provide a reasonably good accuracy in measuring pulp vitality. One study has shown that cold testing has a high false negative response in patients older than age 50, presumably due to dentin sclerosis (Peters et al., 1994). While cold testing is a good test for reproducing and localizing a symptom of thermal hyperalgesia, there is no universal agreement on how long the pain from the cold stimulus needs to persist, in order to determine if the pulp is reversibly or irreversibly inflamed. Heat testing generally has low accuracy and is used only to reproduce a symptom of heat sensitivity.

Other pulp vitality testing technologies

Other technologies have been used to measure pulp vitality, by attempting to detect an intact vascular supply in the pulp. Laser Doppler flowmetry is the oldest of these technologies. Laser Doppler has been to be able to detect resumption of vitality of a traumatized tooth long before the EPT can register a response (Mesaros and Trope, 1997; Gazelius et al., 1988). However, this technology has not gained widespread adoption because the probe needs to be stabilized with respect to the tooth to avoid erroneous measurement, may detect gingival blood flow and requires that the pulp chamber extend into or close to the crown of the tooth to allow direct reflection of the Doppler signal (Polat et al., 2004). Moreover, the size of the pulp chamber and the presence of restorations have been shown to significantly affect the pulpal blood flow, as measured by laser Doppler flowmetry (Chandler et al., 2010). Recent work has shown that with tooth isolation, significant changes in the pulpal blood flow, such as with the use of local anesthesia with a vasoconstrictor, can be reliably measured (Setzer et al., 2013).

Pulse oximetry was introduced for the measurement of pulp vitality over 20 years ago (Schnettler and Wallace, 1991; Noblett et al., 1996; Kahan et al., 1996). This method relies on measurement of oxygen saturation with pulpal blood, as a method of assessing pulp vitality. One study showed that a custom made pulse oximeter had a sensitivity of 1.00, compared with 0.81 for cold test, and 0.71 for the electrical test (Gopikrishna et al., 2007). More recently, it was shown that the mean oxygen saturation levels were as follows: normal pulp: 92.2%, reversible pulpitis: 87.4%, irreversible pulpitis: 83.1%, pulp necrosis: 74.6%, and endodontically-treated tooth: 0% (Setzer et al., 2012a). The differences between the groups in that study were statistically significant, indicating promise for the use of this technology in pulp testing.

Allodynia measuring device

Dentists commonly percuss teeth as part of endodontic diagnosis. However, they rely on the patient's subjective response in assessing the results of this test. Patients are frequently not sure if the percussion caused sensitivity, or was just different in sensation from a neighboring normal tooth. Moreover, there are factors related to percussion that may lead to differences in response such as the magnitude of the force, the location on the tooth of percussion and the direction of percussion (occlusal or buccal). Percussion sensitivity is referred to as allodynia (or mechanical allodynia), as under normal circumstances teeth do not hurt with percussion. It is useful in identifying periapical inflammation, periodontal abscess, cracked teeth and occlusal trauma. One device was proposed to measure the degree of occlusal force that is exerted by the patient as an objective measure of mechanical allodynia (Khan *et al.*, 2007a, b). A follow-up study using this device showed that mechanical allodynia is associated with 57% of cases with irreversible pulpitis (Owatz *et al.*, 2007). The diagnosis of mechanical allodynia in conjunction with symptomatic irreversible pulpitis is of clinical importance, because it necessitates that the emergency visit to relieve the symptoms include working length determination and total pulpal debridement, rather than just a pulpotomy, if allodynia is absent (Hasselgren and Reit, 1989).

Optical coherence tomography (OCT)

OCT is an imaging technology that analyzes the scattered reflections of light close to the infra-red region, to determine the structure of a biological tissue. An advantage of OCT is that it is not biologically hazardous and is not invasive. However, technologies that employ OCT in dentistry are still in their infancy. In endodontics, OCT has been used to characterize enamel cracks (Imai *et al.*, 2012) and to detect coronal cracks (Nakajima *et al.*, 2012) and vertical root fractures (Shemesh *et al.*, 2008; Yoshioka *et al.*, 2013). However, all these efforts have been used on extracted teeth, and no clinical devices are currently available for this purpose. This is an important clinical area as these clinical conditions are frequently difficult to diagnose without removal of restorations or surgical exploration.

Digital radiography and cone beam computed tomography (CBCT)

In the past two decades, digital radiography has replaced film radiography as the primary imaging modality in dentistry. The advantages to digital radiography are numerous, but include reduced exposure to ionizing radiation, speedy processing of the image, image enhancement to facilitate diagnosis, adequate archival and exchange of images and elimination of hazardous chemicals and the need for a dark room (see Chapter 1). However, studies have generally shown that direct digital and film radiography have equivalent clinical accuracy in detecting periapical lesions and estimation of working length measurements (Kullendorff *et al.*, 1996; Almenar Garcia *et al.*, 1997).

As detailed in Chapter 1, the true innovation in radiographic imaging in recent years has been the advent of CBCT. This technology allows observation of the tooth and its surrounding structures in the coronal, sagittal and axial planes, which have many advantages in clinical endodontics (Cotton *et al.*, 2007) (Figure 9.1).

CBCT was shown to have higher accuracy compared to traditional radiography in detecting periapical lesions (de Paula-Silva *et al.*, 2009; Estrela *et al.*, 2008), assessment of healing following treatment (Patel *et al.*, 2012; Christiansen *et al.*, 2009) identification of root fractures (Kamburoglu *et al.*, 2009; Edlund *et al.*, 2011) and detection of root resorption (Durack *et al.*, 2011). The resolution of images varies widely among different CBCT machines. Studies have shown that the higher the resolution the more accurate the ability to detect aspects of endodontic interest, such as root resorption (Liedke *et al.*, 2009). CBCT scans that yield image stack with voxel sizes of 76–100 μm and reduced edge streak artifacts provide the best use for endodontic applications.

Magnetic resonance imaging (MRI)

MRI represents a noninvasive imaging technology that does not use ionizing radiation, and so does not have health hazards. It relies on the use of a strong magnetic field that excites hydrogen atoms within tissues. The resonant frequencies of

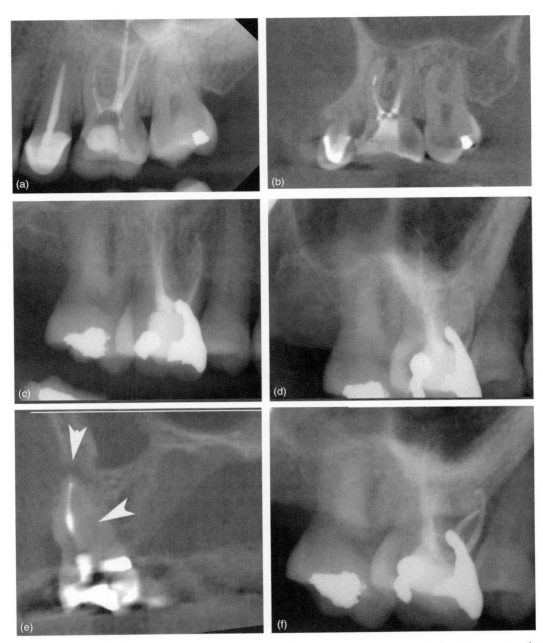

Figure 9.1 Traditional (a) and CBCT (b) radiographs of maxillary left first molar with previous endodontic treatment and a separated instrument in the MB canal. Note that the CBCT image showed a large periapical lesion that the periapical radiograph did not show. Root end surgery confirmed that there was a thick cortical plate of bone and a lesion present in the medullary bone. (c) and (d): Show two angles using periapical radiography that suggest a missed MB2 canal and a periapical lesion. (e) CBCT confirms that a missed canal and a lesion existed and shows their location and extent (arrows). (f) Completed retreatment of MB1 and MB2.

the atoms are detected as they return to equilibrium state. Attempts have been made to image teeth with MRI for a long time (Lockhart *et al.*, 1992). However, it was not until the advent of newer modifications of the technology, such as SWIFT-MRI, that image details potentially useful in endodontic applications could be shown (Idiyatullin *et al.*, 2011) (Figure 9.2).

Ultrasound real-time imaging of periapical lesions

Another noninvasive imaging technology that does not utilize ionizing radiation is ultrasound imaging combined with color power Doppler. This technology was introduced about a decade ago, with evidence of being able to not only detect the presence of periapical lesions but also differentiate granulomas from cysts (Cotti *et al.*, 2003, 2002). The ability of this technology to differentiate cysts and granulomas was confirmed in a more recent trial (Aggarwal *et al.*, 2008). Some have even used it to monitor healing of periapical lesions following nonsurgical treatment, showing that ultrasound can detect healing earlier than radiography (Rajendran and Sundaresan, 2007; Maity *et al.*, 2011). However, it is still generally recognized that radiographic techniques are more accurate than ultrasound, and the differentiation of granuloma and cyst does not yield any differences in treatment planning at this time.

There is growing interest in the use of ultrasound to aid in healing of dental lesions because of its anti-inflammatory and disease suppressing capabilities, however, this area has not been sufficiently studies in dentistry (Scheven *et al.*, 2009a, b).

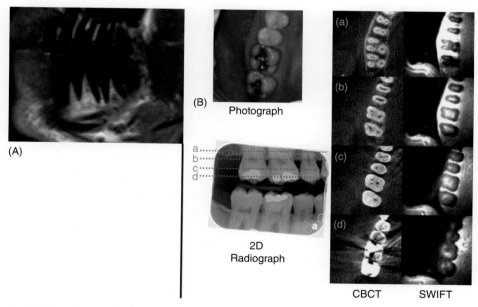

Figure 9.2 (a) Typical MRI image of posterior teeth and surrounding tissues, showing contrast for different tissues but low resolution to discern dentin and pulp detail. (b) SWIFT-MRI shown in comparison with traditional radiography and CBCT. The photograph depicts the maxillary teeth that are also imaged with a traditional two-dimensional radiograph used to detect interproximal caries. The dotted lines, represented by a, b, c, and d, correlate with the cross-sectional CBCT and SWIFT images at those levels, from more superior closer to the root tip moving inferiorly to the crown of the teeth. Note the higher resolution for SWIFT-MRI (FOV diameter of 110 mm and an isotropic voxel size of 430) and the lack of streaking artifacts associated with metallic restoration that are present in CBCT. (Image reproduced with permission from Idiyatullin *et al.*, 2011.)r

Electronic technologies in local anesthesia

Effective local anesthesia is clearly of great importance for endodontic treatment. Historically, two electronic technologies that showed a lot of promise in this area were electronic dental anesthesia (EDA) (Gerschman and Giebartowski, 1991), and iontophoresis of local anesthetic agents (Gangarosa, 1981). However, effective anesthesia using these technologies could never be achieved, especially for endodontic treatment.

More recently, The Wand (Aseptico) (also known as Computer-Controlled Local Anesthetic Delivery (C-CLAD™) system, or CompuDent®) was introduced to minimize pain during anesthetic process (Fukayama et al., 2003). The Wand consists of a foot pedal-operated pump delivery system, which delivers a constant slow rate of anesthesia, and does not utilize a traditional syringe. In addition to reducing pain from the pressure of anesthesia, particularly in painful injections such as palatal infiltration and incisive blocks, the lack of a traditional syringe is purported to reduce apprehension of patients, particularly children, who may be scared by the sight of a dental syringe, and elevation of pulse with some injections such as periodontal ligament or intraosseous injections. Studies have shown that The Wand may be beneficial in reducing the pain of palatal anesthesia in children (Gibson et al., 2000), but no real advantage in adults (Saloum et al., 2000). The Wand was comparable to *slow* intraosseous injection in maintaining normal patient's pulse, compared with a fast intraosseous injection that elevated the pulse (Susi et al., 2008).

Another electronic device that is claimed to reduce the pain of anesthetic injection is the DentalVibe (DentalVibe Inc.). This is a two-pronged fork that is applied to soft tissues around the area of needle injection, and activated to deliver soft vibrations that minimize the sensation of the needle penetration of the tissues. Objective evaluation of this device's efficacy has not been reported.

Electronic technologies in endodontic treatment

Magnification technologies: microscopes and endoscopes

The use of magnification technologies in endodontics has gained considerable popularity in the past two decades. While magnifying loupes, especially those with adjunctive lighting sources, have become standard among numerous dentists, endodontic applications call for a higher level of magnification and illumination, which can only be accomplished by surgical operating microscopes and endoscopes (American Academy of Endodontics, 2012). One study showed that dental students significantly enhanced their accuracy in cutting endodontic access preparations and identifying canals if they used the operating microscope (Rampado et al., 2004). Another study showed no differences among endodontists between those who used microscopes and those who used dental loupes in the incidence of locating MB2 canals in maxillary molars, but that both technologies allowed the a detection rate to be almost three fold that of no magnification (Buhrley et al., 2002).

Studies have shown that the use of the microsurgical technique in endodontic surgery has been associated with a dramatic improvement of the prognosis of endodontic surgery in recent years (Azarpazhooh, 2010; Setzer et al., 2012b). It should be noted, however, the microsurgical technique involves reduced resection angle of the root, ultrasonic root end preparation (which reduces the size of the osteotomy) and filling with mineral trioxide aggregate (MTA) which is much more biocompatible than older materials. Randomized analysis of the effect of endoscopes vs. dental loupes on outcomes of surgery did not show significant differences (Taschieri et al., 2006). However, it was shown that endoscopy at 64× magnification was more accurate in diagnosing root end cracks than microscopy at 16× and 24× magnification (von Arx et al., 2010).

In addition to these objective demonstrations for the importance of magnification in endodontics, endodontic practitioners have found magnification to be useful in identifying calcified and bifurcating canals, and removal of obstructions such as pulp stones, posts, and separated instruments. It is also important in assessing and negotiating complex canal anatomy, removal of gross debris and a multitude of other tasks performed in endodontics.

Sonic and ultrasonic technologies

Sonic and ultrasonic devices have been utilized extensively in endodontic practice in the past two decades. Initially, active root canal instrumentation was undertaken with files that were activated by sonic or ultrasonic devices. However, these devices were shown to not be more effective than regular instrumentation, and in some cases were more aggressive than traditional hand instrumentation. Currently, sonic and ultrasonic devices are most commonly used in endodontic access preparation and identification of root canals, root end preparation during surgeries, passive sonic or ultrasonic irrigation and needle activation during sonic or ultrasonic irrigation.

Using an ultrasonic tip, which is typically diamond coated during access preparation, is very useful. Tips that vary in sizes are used to identify canals, negotiate obstructions, removal of posts or separated instruments and breaking through a paste/cement fill during retreatment (Figure 9.3).

The advantages of ultrasonic tips include that they are narrow allowing precise cutting and permitting visualization under the microscope without interference by the handpiece head. Ultrasonic drivers are usually set to an intensity that ranges from 1 to 10. The higher the intensity the more energy is given. This is necessary for activating the tip on the left in Figure 9.3(a) vertically, over a post to loosen it. Other tips may be used at reduced intensity to carve out a space around the post to isolate it, remove the composite in the pulp chamber without gouging and/or negotiate intracanal obstruction at lower intensities.

Passive sonic or ultrasonic instrumentation allows the file or a plastic tip to vibrate freely inside a root canal that is filled with antimicrobial irrigant. While several *in vitro* studies have shown advantages for these devices in antimicrobial activity or removal of smear layer, randomized

clinical trials have thus far not shown the effectiveness of the these devices compared with traditional irrigation (Paiva *et al.*, 2013; Huffaker *et al.*, 2010). One study showed that passive ultrasonic irrigation results in deeper penetration in the canal if a size 10 file is first introduced 1 mm beyond the foramen to maintain patency (Vera *et al.*, 2011). This suggests that these devices may also push irrigants beyond the apical foramen.

Ultrasonic (and recently sonic) irrigation is a different technology that relies on vibrating the irrigating needle itself, thus enhancing the flushing and permeation of the root canal system. Initial studies showed remarkable advantages in cleaning and disinfecting the canal system (Burleson *et al.*, 2007; Carver *et al.*, 2007). However, recent independent evaluation could not confirm these findings, nor show differences in short-term healing with passive ultrasonic irrigation (Beus *et al.*, 2012; Liang *et al.*, 2013).

Ultrasonic root end cavity preparation has revolutionized endodontic surgery. The reason for this is that it has allowed root end cavity preparation with minimal size osteotomy, compared with previously used micro handpieces, and with a high degree of precision and control. The ultrasonic tip is bent at 3 mm (the optimal depth of the preparation), and has different shank angulations for teeth in different sites in the oral cavity. Initial concerns about the induction of microcracks with these tips have been attributed to the drying of teeth specimens for processing for imaging with scanning electron microscopy rather than the ultrasonic cavity preparation. Currently, longer tips (up to 9 mm bend) are available for preparing poorly prepared root canals from a root end direction, if space allows. Careful monitoring of the intensity of ultrasonic energy is needed to avoid fracture of the tips in the surgery site.

Electronic working length determination (electronic apex locators)

Electronic apex locators (EALs) have been around for several decades. The most significant innovation in the technologies of EALs was the introduction of units that emit two or more currents that have different frequencies (Fouad *et al.*, 1993; Shabahang *et al.*, 1996). The impedance of

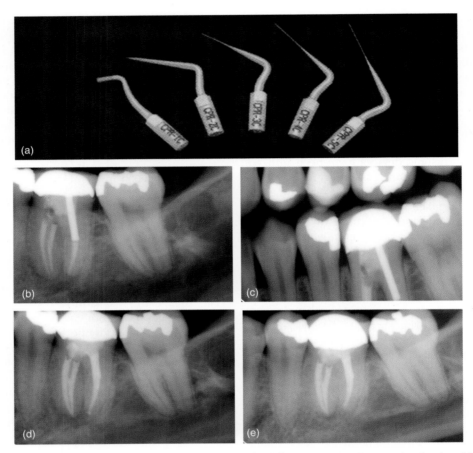

Figure 9.3 (a) Ultrasonic instruments of varying types and sizes for different purposes. Preoperative (b, c) and Postoperative radiographs (d) of a retreatment case that required the used of several of these ultrasonic tips in removing the composite and the post through the existing crown, without disrupting the crown. (e) Six month recall shows healing.

these different current signals, which these units measures, changes as the unit approaches the apical constriction, thus indicating the position of the apical foramen (Meredith and Gulabivala, 1997). This innovation allowed these units to work despite the presence of conductive fluids in the root canal such as irrigants, blood, or tissue fluid. Current models provide a smaller size with a more user-friendly interface, but no significant differences in efficacy from earlier multi-frequency current models (Comin Chiaramonti et al., 2012).

EALs provide reasonably accurate estimate of the working length compared with preoperative radiographs (Fouad and Reid, 2000). However,

working radiographs (with files or gutta percha cones) are still necessary to assure accuracy of technique. Metallic restorations, retreatments, apical root resorption, and immature apex continue to be limitations for the use of these instruments.

Root canal instrumentation

Rotary and reciprocating files

The advent of nickel titanium rotary root canal instruments almost two decades ago was quite revolutionary. It provided significant efficiency in the process of instrumenting most root canals, while maintaining the shape of the canal. The flexibility of the metal allowed the fabrication of files with higher taper that could prepare the canal more efficiently in a "crown-down" manner, thus minimizing the preparation time and the amount of periapical debris extrusion (Reddy and Hicks, 1998).

Today there are dozens of different types of rotary files available for the dentist. Earlier file designs included radial lands in the cross section that allowed cleaving of the dentinal wall without sharp edges that could bind and potentially separate under torsional forces. Instruments such as the Profile (Tulsa, Dentsply), Quantec, or K3 (SybronEndo) are examples of these so called "landed" instruments. This was followed about a decade ago by "nonlanded" instruments (such as Endosequence (Brasseler) and Protaper (Tulsa, Dentsply), which had sharp edges in the cross section to allow more efficient cutting of dentin, at higher rotational speeds. The Protaper relied on the novel idea of variable taper within the same instrument, to minimize the number of needed instruments and facilitate the overall preparation. The nonlanded instruments, while very popular among practitioners, appeared to have more instrument separation (Wolcott *et al.*, 2006; Herold *et al.*, 2007).

More recently, innovations in the metallurgical properties of the nickel titanium instruments by proprietary work hardening methods led to the production of instruments with more superior mechanical properties such as the M-wire (Vortex and Vortex Blue; Tulsa Dentsply), R-phase (Twisted Files, SybronEndo), and controlled memory (Hyflex, Coltène/Whaledent Inc.). Efficiency and effectiveness of these newer instruments compared with traditional files in clinical trials have not been reported.

In the last two years, a technology that relies on reciprocation of NiTi files has been introduced (Wave One, Tulsa Dentsply; and Reciproc, VDW). The technology utilizes different motors with a more expansive array of rotation and reciprocation. The latter is claimed to utilize one disposable instrument (of three available sizes) for preparing the root canal (Figure 9.4), based on a principle that was published in 2008 (Yared, 2008).

Again, this technology appears to be quite popular among clinicians, although verification of

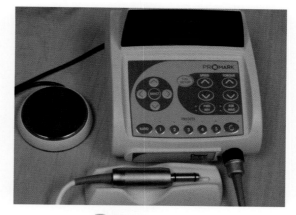

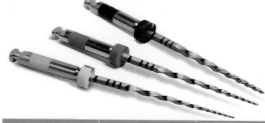

Files	Size	Taper
Small	21	o6
Primary	25	o8
Large	40	o8

Figure 9.4 Wave One reciprocating motor and instruments.

its effectiveness in clinical practice has not been reported. Of particular concern is the ability of the one instrument used to perform adequate apical preparation to disrupt and disperse microbial biofilms that may be adherent to canal walls in the apical third of the root canal.

It is noteworthy that most of the newer root canal instruments have a shorter shank than previous instruments. These instruments were designed this way to fit handpieces with a smaller head than traditional handpieces (Figure 9.5).

This reduction in shank and handpiece lengths allows the practitioner to more easily negotiate root canals in posterior teeth, particularly second and third molars in patients with limited mouth opening. When files with shorter shanks are used in traditional handpieces, their available usable length is reduced by 2–3 mm.

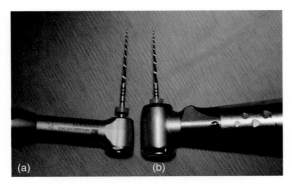

Figure 9.5 Comparison of traditional (b) and small head (a) handpieces holding 25 mm Vortex files of the same size that have a small shank. Only 22.5 mm of the file on the right is available for use.

instrument and the canal walls while irrigating is intended to assure effective debridement. Small canals need to be prepared to at least a size 25/0.04 to allow the instrument to access the entire working length.

Several studies have shown the superiority of the SAF in preparation and antibacterial action of the SAF system particularly in oval or irregular shaped canals (Siqueira *et al.*, 2010; Paque and Peters, 2011; Peters and Paque, 2011; Neves *et al.*, 2014). However, other research has shown limitation of the system in performing effective apical preparation and irrigation (Paranjpe *et al.*, 2012), or comparable results to other contemporary systems (Siqueira *et al.*, 2013).

Self-adjusting file (SAF)

The SAF (Re Dent-Nova) (Figure 9.6) represents a different concept in root canal preparation (Metzger *et al.*, 2010a; Metzger *et al.*, 2010b). The instrument is composed of compressible leaflets that expand inside the root canal to adapt to the shape of the canal, and oscillate in a vertical manner to prepare the canal. Irrigation is achieved at the same time as instrumentation, via an attached tube. Continuous mechanical friction between the

Root canal obturation

The obturation of root canal with gutta percha and sealer has been the same for a very long time. The use of heat has served to mold the gutta percha mass to better fit the intricacies of the root canal system, but it has long been recognized that it is ultimately the sealer that seals the root canal system, not the gutta percha. Studies have shown that different obturation techniques, whether or not they utilize heat, do not seem to affect

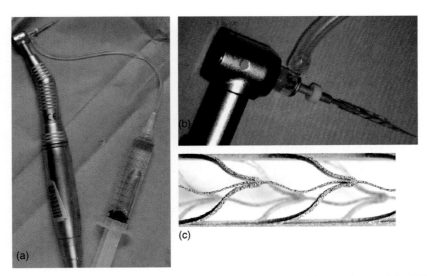

Figure 9.6 (a) Set up of the SAF instrument with the irrigation syringe. (b) Close-up of the attachment of the SAF to the handpiece and the irrigation tube. (c) The SAF lattice structure.

the prognosis (Ng *et al.*, 2008). However, recent analysis of healing of periapical lesions following endodontic treatment with CBCT showed that the density of root filling is a predictor of healing (Liang *et al.*, 2011). The following are the three main technologies utilized in thermoplasticized gutta percha to aid in the efficiency and improved density of the root canal filling material:

Down pack technologies

Heating devices such as Touch and Heat and System B (SybronEndo) have been available for over a decade. These devices utilize autoclavable tips of various sizes that allow the operator to perform vertical compaction of gutta percha, after coating it and the canal wall with adequate amounts of sealer. It is generally recognized that for the continuous wave technique of obturation to be effective in compacting gutta percha master cone in the apical third, the hot plugger tip needs to be advanced to a depth that is 4–5 mm from the working length, at a temperature of about 200 °C. The tip is then cooled while maintaining constant pressure and then heated and withdrawn followed by condensation with an appropriately sized cold plugger.

Recent wireless devices such as DownPak (EI, Hu-Friedy, Chicago, IL) or the Endotec II (Medidenta International Inc; Woodside, NY) are battery operated and allow convenience during the technique. The DownPak utilizes heat and vibration for vertical and lateral condensation. This minimizes the need for high temperatures during obturation.

Thermoplasticized gutta percha

Following down packing of the master cone, a space is created in the coronal two thirds of the root canal. At this time more sealer is added, and then molten gutta percha can be injected into the empty space using one of the available devices. The Obtura 3 (Obtura), Calamus (Tulsa, Dentsply), Ultrafil 3D (Hygienic-Coltene-Whaledent, Akron, OH) or Elements Obturation unit (Sybron Endo) are the most commonly used devices for this purpose. The effective technique necessitates that this be done incrementally, with vertical compaction performed between the increments, to assure better compaction of gutta percha.

Carrier-based technologies

Thermafil (Tulsa, Dentsply), Successfil (Hygienic-Coltene-Whaledent, Akron, OH), and SimpliFill (Discus Dental, Culver City, CA) are examples of carrier-based gutta percha systems. Again, all of these systems are used with sealer, and utilize a carrier made of metal, plastic or more recently harder gutta percha (GuttaCore, Tulsa Dentsply). The prepared root canal is sized using a sizing instrument. A carrier coated with gutta percha that is slightly larger in size than the sizing instrument is placed in an oven until the gutta percha is sufficiently soft. It is then inserted with sealer to the working length and the excess material removed. These carrier-based systems are popular among practitioners because of the simplicity and ease of use. However, they are usually more difficult to remove for post preparation or during retreatment than other root canal obturation methods.

As noted before, outcome studies have not shown differences among root canal obturation techniques. Clearly, there are many other variables, including the complexity of the root canal anatomy, the type of sealer used, the residual microbial irritants in the canal and the promptness and effectiveness of restoration that would play a significant role in the ultimate outcome of the case.

Summary

Advanced instrumentation and digital technology continue to improve the techniques used in endodontic diagnosis and treatment. With proper use, the application of new technology is bound to reduce patient treatment time, reduce pain, expedite healing and improve the overall outcome of endodontic treatment.

References

AAE Position Statement (2012) Use of microscopes and other magnification techniques. *Journal of Endodontics*, **38**, 1153–1155.

Aggarwal, V., Logani, A., & Shah, N. (2008) The evaluation of computed tomography scans and ultrasounds in the differential diagnosis of periapical lesions. *Journal of Endodontics*, **34**, 1312–1315.

Almenar Garcia, A., Forner Navarro, L., Ubet Castello, V., & Minana Laliga, R. (1997) Evaluation of a digital radiography to estimate working length. *Journal of Endodontics*, **23**, 363–365.

Azarpazhooh, A. (2010) Surgical endodontic treatment under magnification has high success rates. *Evidence Based Dentistry*, **11**, 71–72.

Beus, C., Safavi, K., Stratton, J., & Kaufman, B. (2012) Comparison of the effect of two endodontic irrigation protocols on the elimination of bacteria from root canal system: a prospective, randomized clinical trial. *Journal of Endodontics*, **38**, 1479–1483.

Buhrley, L.J., Barrows, M.J., Begole, E.A., & Wenckus, C.S. (2002) Effect of magnification on locating the MB2 canal in maxillary molars. *Journal of Endodontics*, **28**, 324–327.

Burleson, A., Nusstein, J., Reader, A., & Beck, M. (2007) The in vivo evaluation of hand/rotary/ultrasound instrumentation in necrotic, human mandibular molars. *Journal of Endodontics*, **33**, 782–787.

Carver, K., Nusstein, J., Reader, A., & Beck, M. (2007) In vivo antibacterial efficacy of ultrasound after hand and rotary instrumentation in human mandibular molars. *Journal of Endodontics*, **33**, 1038–1043.

Chandler, N.P., Pitt Ford, T.R., & Monteith, B.D. (2010) Effect of restorations on pulpal blood flow in molars measured by laser Doppler flowmetry. *International Endodontic Journal*, **43**, 41–46.

Christiansen, R., Kirkevang, L.L., Gotfredsen, E., & Wenzel, A. (2009) Periapical radiography and cone beam computed tomography for assessment of the periapical bone defect 1 week and 12 months after root-end resection. *Dentomaxillofacial Radiology*, **38**, 531–536.

Comin Chiaramonti, L., Menini, M., & Cavalleri, G. (2012) A comparison between two fourth generation apex locators. *Minerva Stomatologica*, **61**, 183–196.

Cotti, E., Campisi, G., Garau, V., & Puddu, G. (2002) A new technique for the study of periapical bone lesions: ultrasound real time imaging. *International Endodontic Journal*, **35**, 148–152.

Cotti, E., Campisi, G., Ambu, R., & Dettori, C. (2003) Ultrasound real-time imaging in the differential diagnosis of periapical lesions. *International Endodontic Journal*, **36**, 556–563.

Cotton, T.P., Geisler, T.M., Holden, D.T., Schwartz, S.A., & Schindler, W.G. (2007) Endodontic applications of cone-beam volumetric tomography. *Journal of Endodontics*, **33**, 1121–1132.

De Paula-Silva, F.W., Wu, M.K., Leonardo, M.R., Da Silva, L.A., & Wesselink, P.R. (2009) Accuracy of periapical radiography and cone-beam computed tomography scans in diagnosing apical periodontitis using histopathological findings as a gold standard. *Journal of Endodontics*, **35**, 1009–1012.

Durack, C., Patel, S., Davies, J., Wilson, R., & Mannocci, F. (2011) Diagnostic accuracy of small volume cone beam computed tomography and intraoral periapical radiography for the detection of simulated external inflammatory root resorption. *International Endodontic Journal*, **44**, 136–147.

Edlund, M., Nair, M.K., & Nair, U.P. (2011) Detection of vertical root fractures by using cone-beam computed tomography: a clinical study. *Journal of Endodontics*, **37**, 768–772.

Estrela, C., Bueno, M.R., Leles, C.R., Azevedo, B., & Azevedo, J.R. (2008) Accuracy of cone beam computed tomography and panoramic and periapical radiography for detection of apical periodontitis. *Journal of Endodontics*, **34**, 273–279.

Fouad, A.F. & Reid, L.C. (2000) Effect of using electronic apex locators on selected endodontic treatment parameters. *Journal of Endodontics*, **26**, 364–367.

Fouad, A.F., Rivera, E.M., & Krell, K.V. (1993) Accuracy of the Endex with variations in canal irrigants and foramen size. *Journal of Endodontics*, **19**, 63–67.

Fukayama, H., Yoshikawa, F., Kohase, H., Umino, M., & Suzuki, N. (2003) Efficacy of anterior and middle superior alveolar (AMSA) anesthesia using a new injection system: the Wand. *Quintessence International*, **34**, 537–541.

Gangarosa, L.P., Sr, (1981) Newer local anesthetics and techniques for administration. *Journal of Dental Research*, **60**, 1471–1480.

Gazelius, B., Olgart, L., & Edwall, B. (1988) Restored vitality in luxated teeth assessed by laser Doppler flowmeter. *Endodontics and Dental Traumatology*, **4**, 265–268.

Gerschman, J.A. & Giebartowski, J. (1991) Effect of electronic dental anesthesia on pain threshold and pain tolerance levels of human teeth subjected to stimulation with an electric pulp tester. *Anesthesia Progress*, **38**, 45–49.

Gibson, R.S., Allen, K., Hutfless, S., & Beiraghi, S. (2000) The Wand vs. traditional injection: a comparison of pain related behaviors. *Pediatric Dentistry*, **22**, 458–462.

Gopikrishna, V., Tinagupta, K., & Kandaswamy, D. (2007) Evaluation of efficacy of a new custom-made pulse oximeter dental probe in comparison with the electrical and thermal tests for assessing pulp vitality. *Journal of Endodontics*, **33**, 411–414.

Hasselgren, G. & Reit, C. (1989) Emergency pulpotomy: pain relieving effect with and without the use of sedative dressings. *Journal of Endodontics*, **15**, 254–256.

Herold, K.S., Johnson, B.R., & Wenckus, C.S. (2007) A scanning electron microscopy evaluation of microfractures, deformation and separation in EndoSequence and Profile nickel-titanium rotary files using an extracted molar tooth model. *Journal of Endodontics*, **33**, 712–714.

Huffaker, S.K., Safavi, K., Spangberg, L.S., & Kaufman, B. (2010) Influence of a passive sonic irrigation system on the elimination of bacteria from root canal systems: a clinical study. *Journal of Endodontics*, **36**, 1315–1318.

Idiyatullin, D., Corum, C., Moeller, S., Prasad, H.S., Garwood, M., & Nixdorf, D.R. (2011) Dental magnetic resonance imaging: making the invisible visible. *Journal of Endodontics*, **37**, 745–752.

Imai, K., Shimada, Y., Sadr, A., Sumi, Y., & Tagami, J. (2012) Noninvasive cross-sectional visualization of enamel cracks by optical coherence tomography in vitro. *Journal of Endodontics*, **38**, 1269–1274.

Kahan, R.S., Gulabivala, K., Snook, M., & Setchell, D.J. (1996) Evaluation of a pulse oximeter and customized probe for pulp vitality testing. *Journal of Endodontics*, **22**, 105–109.

Kamburoglu, K., Ilker Cebeci, A.R., & Grondahl, H.G. (2009) Effectiveness of limited cone-beam computed tomography in the detection of horizontal root fracture. *Dental Traumatology*, **25**, 256–261.

Khan, A.A., Mccreary, B., Owatz, C.B., *et al.* (2007a) The development of a diagnostic instrument for the measurement of mechanical allodynia. *Journal of Endodontics*, **33**, 663–666.

Khan, A.A., Owatz, C.B., Schindler, W.G., Schwartz, S.A., Keiser, K., & Hargreaves, K.M. (2007b) Measurement of mechanical allodynia and local anesthetic efficacy in patients with irreversible pulpitis and acute periradicular periodontitis. *Journal of Endodontics*, **33**, 796–799.

Kullendorff, B., Nilsson, M., & Rohlin, M. (1996) Diagnostic accuracy of direct digital dental radiography for the detection of periapical bone lesions: overall comparison between conventional and direct digital radiography. *Oral Surgery, Oral Medicine, Oral Pathology, Oral Radiology and Endodontics*, **82**, 344–350.

Liang, Y.H., Li, G., Wesselink, P.R., & Wu, M.K. (2011) Endodontic outcome predictors identified with periapical radiographs and cone-beam computed tomography scans. *Journal of Endodontics*, **37**, 326–331.

Liang, Y.H., Jiang, L.M., Jiang, L., *et al.* (2013) Radiographic healing after a root canal treatment performed in single-rooted teeth with and without ultrasonic activation of the irrigant: a randomized controlled trial. *Journal of Endodontics*, **39**, 1218–1225.

Liedke, G.S., Da Silveira, H.E., Da Silveira, H.L., Dutra, V., & De Figueiredo, J.A. (2009) Influence of voxel size in the diagnostic ability of cone beam tomography to evaluate simulated external root resorption. *Journal of Endodontics*, **35**, 233–235.

Lockhart, P.B., Kim, S., & Lund, N.L. (1992) Magnetic resonance imaging of human teeth. *Journal of Endodontics*, **18**, 237–244.

Maity, I., Kumari, A., Shukla, A.K., Usha, H., & Naveen, D. (2011) Monitoring of healing by ultrasound with color power doppler after root canal treatment of maxillary anterior teeth with periapical lesions. *Journal of Conservative Dentistry*, **14**, 252–257.

Meredith, N. & Gulabivala, K. (1997) Electrical impedance measurements of root canal length. *Endodontics and Dental Traumatology*, **13**, 126–131.

Mesaros, S.V. & Trope, M. (1997) Revascularization of traumatized teeth assessed by laser Doppler flowmetry: case report. *Endodontics and Dental Traumatology*, **13**, 24–30.

Metzger, Z., Teperovich, E., Zary, R., Cohen, R., & Hof, R. (2010a) The self-adjusting file (SAF). Part 1: respecting the root canal anatomy--a new concept of endodontic files and its implementation. *Journal of Endodontics*, **36**, 679–690.

Metzger, Z., Zary, R., Cohen, R., Teperovich, E., & Paque, F. (2010b) The quality of root canal preparation and root canal obturation in canals treated with rotary versus self-adjusting files: a three-dimensional micro-computed tomographic study. *Journal of Endodontics*, **36**, 1569–1573.

Nakajima, Y., Shimada, Y., Miyashin, M., Takagi, Y., Tagami, J., & Sumi, Y. (2012) Noninvasive cross-sectional imaging of incomplete crown fractures (cracks) using swept-source optical coherence tomography. *International Endodontic Journal*, **45**, 933–941.

Neves, M.A., Rocas, I.N., & Siqueira, J.F., Jr, (2014) Clinical antibacterial effectiveness of the self-adjusting file system. *International Endodontic Journal.*, **7**, 356–365.

Ng, Y.L., Mann, V., Rahbaran, S., Lewsey, J., & Gulabivala, K. (2008) Outcome of primary root canal treatment: systematic review of the literature – Part 2. Influence of clinical factors. *International Endodontic Journal*, **41**, 6–31.

Noblett, W.C., Wilcox, L.R., Scamman, F., Johnson, W.T., & Diaz-Arnold, A. (1996) Detection of pulpal circulation in vitro by pulse oximetry. *Journal of Endodontics*, **22**, 1–5.

Owatz, C.B., Khan, A.A., Schindler, W.G., Schwartz, S.A., Keiser, K., & Hargreaves, K.M. (2007) The incidence of mechanical allodynia in patients with irreversible pulpitis. *Journal of Endodontics*, **33**, 552–556.

Paiva, S.S., Siqueira, J.F., Jr,, Rocas, I.N., *et al.* (2013) Molecular microbiological evaluation of passive ultrasonic activation as a supplementary disinfecting step: a clinical study. *Journal of Endodontics*, **39**, 190–194.

Paque, F. & Peters, O.A. (2011) Micro-computed tomography evaluation of the preparation of long oval root canals in mandibular molars with the self-adjusting file. *Journal of Endodontics*, **37**, 517–521.

Paranjpe, A., De Gregorio, C., Gonzalez, A.M., *et al.* (2012) Efficacy of the self-adjusting file system on cleaning and shaping oval canals: a microbiological and microscopic evaluation. *Journal of Endodontics*, **38**, 226–231.

Patel, S., Wilson, R., Dawood, A., Foschi, F., & Mannocci, F. (2012) The detection of periapical pathosis using digital periapical radiography and cone beam computed tomography – part 2: a 1-year post-treatment follow-up. *International Endodontic Journal*, **45**, 711–723.

Peters, O.A. & Paque, F. (2011) Root canal preparation of maxillary molars with the self-adjusting file: a micro-computed tomography study. *Journal of Endodontics*, **37**, 53–57.

Peters, D.D., Baumgartner, J.C., & Lorton, L. (1994) Adult pulpal diagnosis. I. Evaluation of the positive and negative responses to cold and electrical pulp tests. *Journal of Endodontics*, **20**, 506–511.

Polat, S., Er, K., Akpinar, K.E., & Polat, N.T. (2004) The sources of laser Doppler blood-flow signals recorded from vital and root canal treated teeth. *Archives of Oral Biology*, **49**, 53–57.

Rajendran, N. & Sundaresan, B. (2007) Efficacy of ultrasound and color power Doppler as a monitoring tool in the healing of endodontic periapical lesions. *Journal of Endodontics*, **33**, 181–186.

Rampado, M.E., Tjaderhane, L., Friedman, S., & Hamstra, S.J. (2004) The benefit of the operating microscope for access cavity preparation by undergraduate students. *Journal of Endodontics*, **30**, 863–867.

Reddy, S.A. & Hicks, M.L. (1998) Apical extrusion of debris using two hand and two rotary instrumentation techniques. *Journal of Endodontics*, **24**, 180–183.

Saloum, F.S., Baumgartner, J.C., Marshall, G., & Tinkle, J. (2000) A clinical comparison of pain perception to the Wand and a traditional syringe. *Oral Surgery, Oral Medicing, Oral Pathology, Oral Radiology and Endodontics*, **89**, 691–695.

Scheven, B.A., Man, J., Millard, J.L., *et al.* (2009a) VEGF and odontoblast-like cells: stimulation by low frequency ultrasound. *Archives of Oral Biology*, **54**, 185–191.

Scheven, B.A., Shelton, R.M., Cooper, P.R., Walmsley, A.D., & Smith, A.J. (2009b) Therapeutic ultrasound for dental tissue repair. *Medical Hypotheses*, **73**, 591–593.

Schnettler, J.M. & Wallace, J.A. (1991) Pulse oximetry as a diagnostic tool of pulpal vitality. *Journal of Endodontics*, **17**, 488–490.

Setzer, F.C., Kataoka, S.H., Natrielli, F., Gondim-Junior, E., & Caldeira, C.L. (2012a) Clinical diagnosis of pulp inflammation based on pulp oxygenation rates measured by pulse oximetry. *Journal of Endodontics*, **38**, 880–883.

Setzer, F.C., Kohli, M.R., Shah, S.B., Karabucak, B., & Kim, S. (2012b) Outcome of endodontic surgery: a meta-analysis of the literature--Part 2: Comparison of endodontic microsurgical techniques with and without the use of higher magnification. *Journal of Endodontics*, **38**, 1–10.

Setzer, F.C., Challagulla, P., Kataoka, S.H., & Trope, M. (2013) Effect of tooth isolation on laser Doppler readings. *International Endodontic Journal*, **46**, 517–522.

Shabahang, S., Goon, W.W., & Gluskin, A.H. (1996) An in vivo evaluation of Root ZX electronic apex locator. *Journal of Endodontics*, **22**, 616–618.

Shemesh, H., Van Soest, G., Wu, M.K., & Wesselink, P.R. (2008) Diagnosis of vertical root fractures with optical coherence tomography. *Journal of Endodontics*, **34**, 739–742.

Siqueira, J.F., Jr,, Alves, F.R., Almeida, B.M., De Oliveira, J.C., & Rocas, I.N. (2010) Ability of chemomechanical preparation with either rotary instruments or self-adjusting file to disinfect oval-shaped root canals. *Journal of Endodontics*, **36**, 1860–1865.

Siqueira, J.F., Jr,, Alves, F.R., Versiani, M.A., *et al.* (2013) Correlative bacteriologic and micro-computed tomographic analysis of mandibular molar mesial canals prepared by self-adjusting file, reciproc, and twisted file systems. *Journal of Endodontics*, **39**, 1044–1050.

Susi, L., Reader, A., Nusstein, J., Beck, M., Weaver, J., & Drum, M. (2008) Heart rate effects of intraosseous injections using slow and fast rates of anesthetic solution deposition. *Anesthesia Progress*, **55**, 9–15.

Taschieri, S., Del Fabbro, M., Testori, T., Francetti, L., & Weinstein, R. (2006) Endodontic surgery using 2 different magnification devices: preliminary results of a randomized controlled study. *Journal of Oral and Maxillofacial Surgery*, **64**, 235–242.

Vera, J., Arias, A., & Romero, M. (2011) Effect of maintaining apical patency on irrigant penetration into the apical third of root canals when using passive ultrasonic irrigation: an in vivo study. *Journal of Endodontics*, **37**, 1276–1278.

Von Arx, T., Kunz, R., Schneider, A.C., Burgin, W., & Lussi, A. (2010) Detection of dentinal cracks after root-end resection: an ex vivo study comparing microscopy and endoscopy with scanning electron microscopy. *Journal of Endodontics*, **36**, 1563–1568.

Weisleder, R., Yamauchi, S., Caplan, D.J., Trope, M., & Teixeira, F.B. (2009) The validity of pulp testing: a clinical study. *Journal of American Dental Association*, **140**, 1013–1017.

Wolcott, S., Wolcott, J., Ishley, D., *et al.* (2006) Separation incidence of protaper rotary instruments: a large cohort clinical evaluation. *Journal of Endodontics*, **32**, 1139–1141.

Yared, G. (2008) Canal preparation using only one Ni-Ti rotary instrument: preliminary observations. *International Endodontic Journal*, **41**, 339–344.

Yoshioka, T., Sakaue, H., Ishimura, H., Ebihara, A., Suda, H., & Sumi, Y. (2013) Detection of root surface fractures with swept-source optical coherence tomography (SS-OCT). *Photomedicine and Laser Surgery*, **31**, 23–27.

From Traditional to Contemporary: Imaging Techniques for Orthodontic Diagnosis, Treatment Planning, and Outcome Assessment

10

Georgios Kanavakis and Carroll Ann Trotman

Introduction

Orthodontic diagnosis and treatment planning requires an extensive clinical evaluation that includes a detailed analysis of radiographic images. According to the American Association of Orthodontists (AAO), the current standard of care for initial orthodontic diagnosis requires that all patients have a panoramic and/or periapical radiograph(s) as well as a cephalometric radiograph of the craniofacial region. Computer tomography (CT) imaging, specifically, three-dimensional (3D) images recorded with contemporary *cone-beam* computer tomography (CBCT) may be used as an alternative to cephalometrics. More recently, with the advent of newer technologies, the focus in orthodontics has shifted toward analyses of the facial soft tissues both under static conditions (at rest) and during 4D dynamic functional movements, to detect soft tissue functional impairments in patients. This chapter will review traditional and contemporary hard and soft tissue imaging techniques used in orthodontic practice.

Traditional cephalometrics

Radiographic cephalometry was introduced in 1931 by Broadbent in the United States (Broadbent, 1931) and Hofrath in Germany (Hofrath, 1931). Both clinicians developed the technique independently and around the same time. Today, cephalometric radiographs remain a mainstay for orthodontic diagnostic purposes, treatment planning, and outcome assessment. Several cephalometric analyses (Figure 10.1) using linear and angular measurements have been developed by orthodontists over the years to identify normal facial morphology and dysmorphology (Steiner, 1953; Tweed, 1954; Kim and Vietas, 1978; Jacobson, 1975).

For many years, orthodontists made measurements on radiographs manually, using an illuminated viewbox, lead pencils and acetate paper. Subsequently, with the development of digital radiography, the image quality and accuracy improved (Liu *et al.*, 2000; Chen *et al.*, 2000). Nonetheless, shortcomings that can significantly affect the diagnostic value of cephalometric

Clinical Applications of Digital Dental Technology, First Edition. Edited by Radi Masri and Carl F. Driscoll.
© 2015 John Wiley & Sons, Inc. Published 2015 by John Wiley & Sons, Inc.

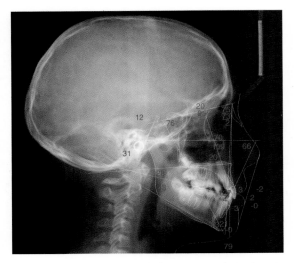

Figure 10.1 Traditional cephalometric analysis in two dimensions.

radiographs remain. These include imaging errors created when a 3D structure such as the craniofacial bony skeleton is projected as a 2D image and can lead to errors associated with magnification, landmark obscuration due to structural superimpositions, and distortions of angular and linear measurements (Harrell *et al.*, 2002; Tsao *et al.*, 1983). Operator errors also occur, such as when the orthodontist does not accurately identify specific cephalometric landmarks (Houston, 1983; Baumrind and Frantz, 1971).

CT scanning and cone-beam computed tomography (CBCT)

Several of the limitations of cephalometric radiographs can be overcome with the use of high-resolution medical CT scans that provide very detailed and accurate images of the hard tissues of the craniofacial complex (see Chapter 1). However, the radiation dose required as well as the associated costs continue to be prohibitive factors for routine use of this particular imaging modality as a standard of care in orthodontic practice (Silva *et al.*, 2008; Halazonetis, 2005). More recently – in the late 1990s – CBCT was introduced in orthodontics as an alternative to CT scans (Arai *et al.*, 1999; Mozzo *et al.*, 1998), and since then,

there has been increasing interest in this technology. CBCT, also known as volumetric CT (VCT), uses a cone-shaped tube instead of a collimated fan beam with spiral CT scanners. The resulting cone-shaped X-ray beam performs a 360° rotation, synchronously with an area detector, around the object being scanned while its angulation remains constant throughout the entire scanning period. This movement allows an entire region, such as the craniofacial region, to be captured in a single rotation of the radiation source instead of "multiple slices" that are being generated by conventional CT units (Mozzo *et al.*, 1998). Moreover, the CBCT X-ray beams are almost parallel and close to the sensor, therefore, providing an orthogonal beam projection that minimizes image distortion (Haney *et al.*, 2010).

During the scanning, raw data are produced as voxels, which are cuboid structures representing a certain degree of beam absorption. The final image is a 3D reconstruction of the region performed by sophisticated computer software using specific algorithms. The main advantage of CBCT, compared to traditional imaging modalities, is the high quality of the images it provides. This advantage becomes particularly helpful when evaluating hard tissue structures. In orthodontics, 3D reconstructed CBCTs are primarily used to determine accurate tooth structure and position, assess alveolar bone dimensions, diagnose skeletal

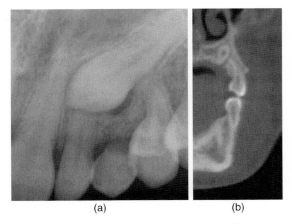

(a)   (b)

Figure 10.2 (a) On the periapical radiograph, the first premolar appears to have a malformed root. (b) The CBCT image (coronal slice) reveals that the premolar has a significant palatal angulation.

dysmorphology, and evaluate and assess the airway in the craniofacial complex. These particular applications are discussed in greater detail in the following sections.

Tooth structure and position

CBCT reconstructions provide a more accurate representation of mesiodistal root angulations than periapical radiographs (White and Pharoah, 2008). In addition, buccolingual root angulations can be identified (Figure 10.2).

These features become especially important in cases of impacted teeth where an exact determination of 3D root position is essential in order to formulate an appropriate treatment plan (Becker et al., 2010; Botticelli et al., 2011; Haney et al., 2010; Katheria et al., 2010). In particular, for patients with impacted canines, CBCTs allow the orthodontist to accurately locate teeth (Nakajima et al., 2005), assess root proximity to surrounding anatomical structures, and diagnose possible root resorption on teeth adjacent to the canine (Alqerban et al., 2011) (Figure 10.3).

The orthodontist is able to provide more efficient planning in terms of treatment mechanics to correct the impacted tooth, thus avoiding "blind" manipulation that may result in damage to adjacent teeth. Moreover, when exposure of an impacted tooth is deemed necessary, the surgeon

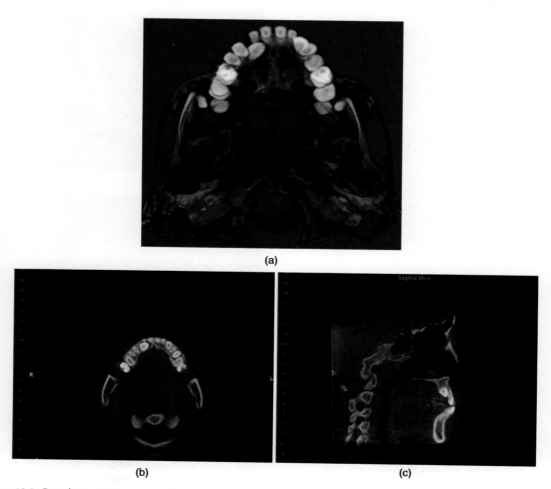

(a)

(b)   (c)

Figure 10.3 Cone-beam CT image of a palatally impacted canine. (a) Maxillary reconstruction. (b) Axial view. (c) Sagittal view.

is able to visualize the 3D surgical field from reconstructed images prior to the actual surgery resulting in more efficient surgical treatment with the potential for minimal trauma (Becker *et al.*, 1983) and improved periodontal outcomes for the exposed tooth (Kohavi *et al.*, 1984).

Crown and root morphology

Abnormal dental crown and root morphology can pose a challenge for the orthodontist when planning an appropriate treatment strategy that results in ideal tooth relationships posttreatment. Examples of dental crown abnormalities include fusion of teeth, gemination, macrodontia, and/or other conditions that influence the normal shape and size of teeth. CBCT provides an opportunity to accurately measure enamel thickness and visualize the dental pulp. This information can be very helpful when the orthodontist needs to determine the amount of enamel reduction that has to be performed in order to achieve good tooth alignment and proper interarch relationships.

Furthermore, the entire dentition can be reconstructed to allow intra- and inter-arch measurements (Baumgaertel *et al.*, 2009), calculation of tooth size-arch length discrepancies, and an evaluation of occlusal relationships.

A more common problem for the orthodontist is root resorption in patients during treatment. Although mild root resorption is generally uneventful (Lupi *et al.*, 1996), there are a limited number of cases where patients suffer severe root resorption during active orthodontic treatment (Harris *et al.*, 1997; Sameshima and Sinclair, 2001). Early diagnosis and management of such occurrences is key for good prognosis. CBCT imaging is much more efficient in facilitating early detection of root resorption compared with traditional 2D radiographs (Alqerban *et al.*, 2011), and therefore serves as an important diagnostic tool in such cases (Figure 10.4).

Alveolar bone assessment

Alveolar bone is clearly depicted on CBCT 3D reconstructions (Figure 10.5). Specific regions with limited bone in the dentoalveolar process, as well as regions with greater likelihood of developing bone loss during orthodontic tooth movement can be easily identified. (Baysal *et al.*, 2013).

Moreover, it is possible to visualize the amount of bone available for molar distalization in the posterior maxilla distal to the erupted molars and the amount of bone lateral to the buccal maxillary segments (Müssig *et al.*, 2005). Lateral alveolar bone thickness becomes very important in patients

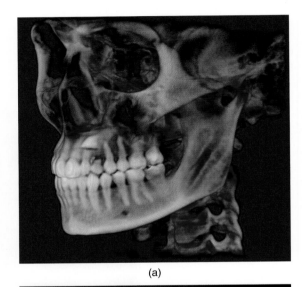

(a)

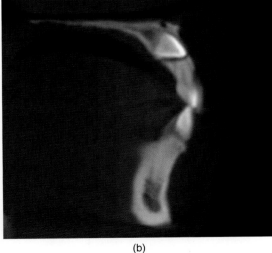

(b)

Figure 10.4 CBCT image revealing resorption of the lateral incisor root, caused by the erupting permanent canine. (a) Facial reconstruction. (b) Sagittal view of the affected area.

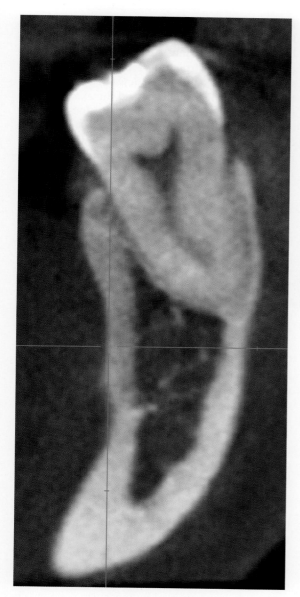

Figure 10.5 Cortical bone thickness measurements at different areas. (Image is courtesy of Dr. Björn Ludwig, Traben-Trarbach, Germany.)

that require expansion of the maxilla by means of rapid palatal expansion (RPE). Studies on the skeletal and periodontal effects of RPE (Garrett *et al.*, 2008) have demonstrated that maxillary expansion is accompanied by a degree of buccal tipping of the posterior maxillary dentition along with splitting of the maxillary midpalatal suture.

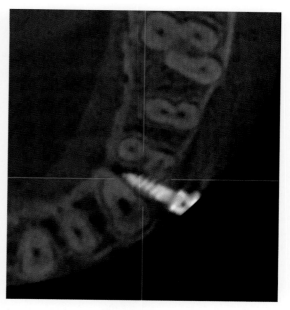

Figure 10.6 Interproximal placement of a temporary anchorage device (TAD). (Image is courtesy of Dr. Björn Ludwig, Traben-Trarbach, Germany.)

As a result of the buccal tipping, there is a decrease in buccal bone thickness and marginal bone height in patients post-expansion (Rungcharassaeng *et al.*, 2007). Using the CBCT images, the orthodontist can evaluate the extent of the marginal bone height and plan treatment mechanics in order to avoid irreversible damage to the periodontal tissues.

Furthermore, with the introduction of temporary skeletal anchorage devices (TADs) and bone plates- that are fixed to the bone and act as absolute anchors for tooth movement-, there has been an increased interest among clinicians and researchers regarding the most appropriate bony regions for the placement of these devices. Studies using CBCT technology have provided specific guidelines for clinicians (Baumgaertel and Hans, 2009; Baumgaertel, 2011; Ludwig *et al.*, 2011) and have significantly improved our ability to successfully utilize skeletal anchorage in daily orthodontic practice (Figure 10.6).

Skeletal dysmorphology

A major indication for a CBCT image in clinical orthodontics is the diagnosis of skeletal

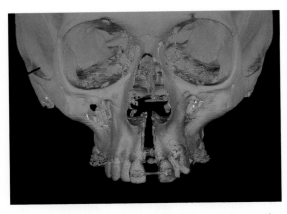

Figure 10.7 Superimposition of CBCT images in a patient undergoing orthopedic palatal expansion. (Image is courtesy of Dr. Björn Ludwig, Traben-Trarbach, Germany.)

discrepancies. Because CBCTs provide high-quality reconstructions of the whole craniofacial complex including the temporomandibular joints, these reconstructions allow for 3D evaluation of maxillomandibular relationships, specific abnormalities associated with patients who have craniofacial anomalies, and skeletal asymmetries (De Vos *et al.*, 2009; Hodges *et al.*, 2013). Physiologic changes due to craniofacial growth are also more easily visualized using 3D superimpositions on the anterior cranial base (Cevidanes *et al.*, 2006) (Figure 10.7).

For orthognathic surgery patients, 3D surgical treatment planning provides valuable anatomical insight for the surgeon (Jayaratne *et al.*, 2010; Tucker *et al.*, 2010). This is particularly the case for patients with craniofacial anomalies who may require cranial vault reconstruction and/or placement of distraction osteogenesis devices. For the latter situation, the reconstructed images can be used to build an accurate acrylic model of the craniofacial region, and the distraction devices fabricated to fit the model prior to surgery, thus saving on the actual length of the surgery (Quereshy *et al.*, 2012) (Figure 10.8).

When the dysmorphology involves the temporomandibular joint (TMJ), a comprehensive radiologic examination would include an MRI and a CT scan of the joint(s). Although both techniques are extremely helpful from a diagnostic standpoint, they are expensive, time consuming, and in the case of CT scans, involve exposing patients to a high-radiation doses. CBCTs can provide a localized image with high diagnostic quality in less time and using lower radiation than conventional CT scans (Mah *et al.*, 2003). Manipulation of the 3D reconstruction of the TMJs allows for sagittal, coronal, and axial views of the joints and the surrounding structures, and the exact location of the condyle in the mandibular fossa can be detected (Tsiklakis *et al.*, 2004). Degenerative changes on the occlusal surface of the condylar head are clearly outlined and asymmetries can be measured with accuracy (Figure 10.9).

Airway visualization and measurement

Diagnostic evaluations and investigational projects on the airway were conducted with the use of 2D cephalometric radiographs (Poole *et al.*, 1980). As mentioned earlier in this chapter, the use of these radiographs was associated with significant inaccuracies especially with the higher morphological variability of the airway that cannot be depicted accurately on a 2D image. CBCT images and 3D reconstructions of the head and neck complex have increased our ability to inspect and identify diffuse narrowing (narrowing disturbed over a large distance) or focal narrowing (encroachments) of the airway (Hatcher, 2012). The images clearly delineate the soft tissue contour of the airway (Mah *et al.*, 2010), allow for a complete volumetric analysis (Osorio *et al.*, 2008), and provide information from cross-sectional areas (Tso *et al.*, 2009) (Figure 10.10).

This type of information has empowered health-care professionals in the field of sleep medicine and dentistry to improve their services to patients with sleep disorders such as obstructive sleep apnea. Areas of obstruction can be detected easier prior to treatment, and posttreatment outcomes can be quantified by measuring changes in airway dimensions.

One caveat that should be mentioned is that despite the undeniable superiority of CBCT imaging in providing high-quality reconstructions of the facial structures, there has been controversy surrounding the applicability of this technology for routine orthodontic practice. In 2010, an article published in the New York Times raised concerns of unnecessary radiation exposure to orthodontic patients with the use of CBCTs (Bogdanich and

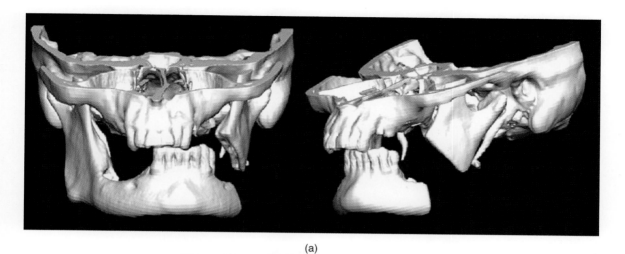

(a)

(b)

Figure 10.8 (a) CBCT image of a patient requiring mandibular reconstruction surgery. (b) Virtual design and fabrication of acrylic model. (Image is courtesy of Dr. Constantinos Laskarides, Boston MA.)

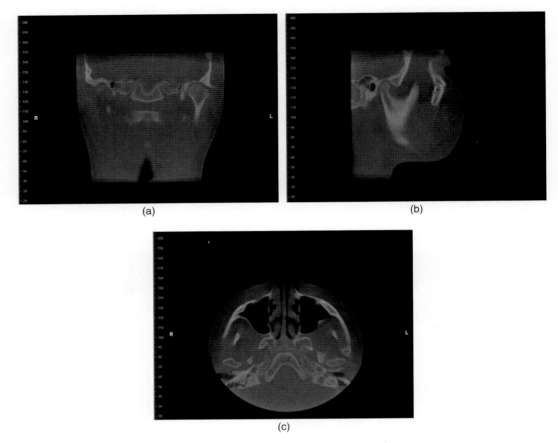

Figure 10.9 CBCT image of a normal TMJ. (a) Coronal view. (b) Sagittal view. (c) Axial view.

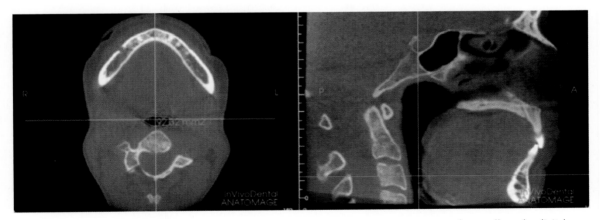

Figure 10.10 Axial and sagittal view of the airway created from a CBCT image. Contemporary software allows for digital measurements of the airway dimensions.

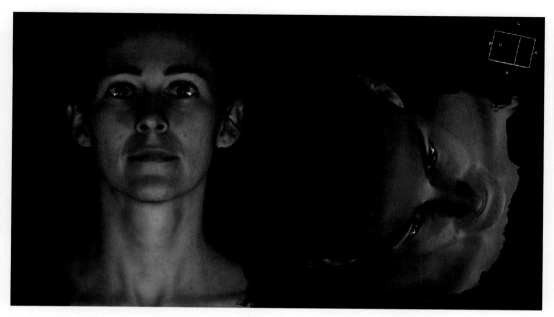

Figure 10.11 3D facial image of a subject. The image can be rotated in different direction (right image) and measures recorded. (Virginie Sirianna.)

Craven, 2010). Subsequently, and in large part because of public awareness, the American Association of Orthodontists (AAO) issued a resolution stating *"while there may be clinical situations where a CBCT radiograph may be of value, the use of such technology is not routinely required for orthodontic radiography."* Several studies have demonstrated that acquiring a CBCT image at the beginning of orthodontic treatment does not significantly impact treatment decisions (Kapila *et al.*, 2011). Moreover, there is no clear evidence that obtaining detailed information regarding the specific location of impacted canines (Halazonetis, 2012) or the exact position of the condyle in the mandibular fossa (Petersson, 2010; Rinchuse and Kandasamy, 2012) alters orthodontic mechanotherapy or treatment modalities – this is an inferred conclusion. The radiation exposure of CBCTs compared with the more traditional imaging technique of a lateral cephalometric radiograph is high enough to exclude routine use of CBCTs for orthodontic purposes (Grunheid *et al.*, 2012; Ludlow *et al.*, 2003; Ludlow *et al.*, 2006; Roberts *et al.*, 2009).

Limiting scanning time and increasing voxel size can reduce the radiation exposure using CBCTs; however, these adjustments significantly compromise the diagnostic quality of the images. An additional complication for the immediate future is that most, if not all, the analyses used for the purpose of orthodontic diagnosis have been established using 2D cephalometrics. With the advent of 3D CBCT reconstructions, most orthodontists use specific software to reconstruct 2D images from the 3D reconstructions in order to be able to perform the traditional analyses (Grauer *et al.*, 2010; van Vlijmen *et al.*, 2009; Zamora *et al.*, 2011). In short, with the use of this approach, orthodontists do not utilize the entire 3D information for diagnosis and treatment planning, questioning the routine need for the 3D data/information. Thus, CBCT imaging should not be used routinely for all orthodontic patients, but only in cases where it can provide information that could significantly impact treatment. These cases refer to patients with severe root resorption, root resorption due to impacted adjacent teeth, obstructive sleep apnea, craniofacial anomalies, impacted teeth, and skeletal asymmetries.

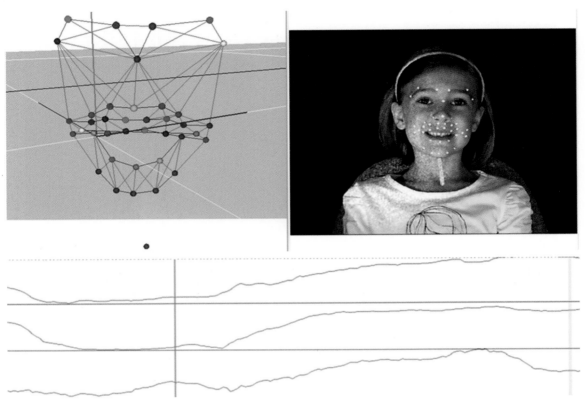

Figure 10.12 Markers are secured to specific facial landmarks. Subjects are instructed to perform different facial movements (animations). The landmarks are tracked in real time and x, y, and z data are captured over time (lower panel). (Penelope Sirianna by Virginie Sirianna.)

Imaging the facial soft tissues

Novel technologies exist for imaging the facial soft tissues. These technologies range from laser scanning to 3D photographic imaging devices. The latter is the least invasive of these and uses cameras that simultaneously capture images of the static face from different directions. The images then are reconstructed using proprietary software to produce a highly accurate 3D facial soft tissue image that can be rotated in different directions, and allow for landmark identification and recording of various measurements (e.g., linear, angular, volume, e.g., 3dMDface™ by 3dMD). Alternatively, more sophisticated surface analyses can be computed and comparisons can be made between normative data and data from patients with different craniofacial malformations. These types of comparisons are most useful for the assessment of surgical outcomes (Figure 10.11).

Dynamic functional movements of the facial soft tissues can also be captured during different facial animations (Faraway and Trotman, 2011; Trotman et al., 2010; Trotman, 2011). This approach to functional soft tissue imaging is important for the assessment of facial soft tissue motor movements in patients who require rehabilitative surgery, for example, patients born with cleft lip and palate (Faraway and Trotman, 2011; Trotman et al., 2010; Trotman, 2011). These patients require an initial (primary) lip repair surgery, and later in life, may need subsequent (revision) surgeries of the lip. The extent of the circumoral (lip) soft tissue functional impairment can be assessed before surgery, as well as the degree of normalization of the soft tissue function postsurgery. The method involves capturing the 3D movements of small diameter markers secured to specific landmarks on the face from cameras located around the face

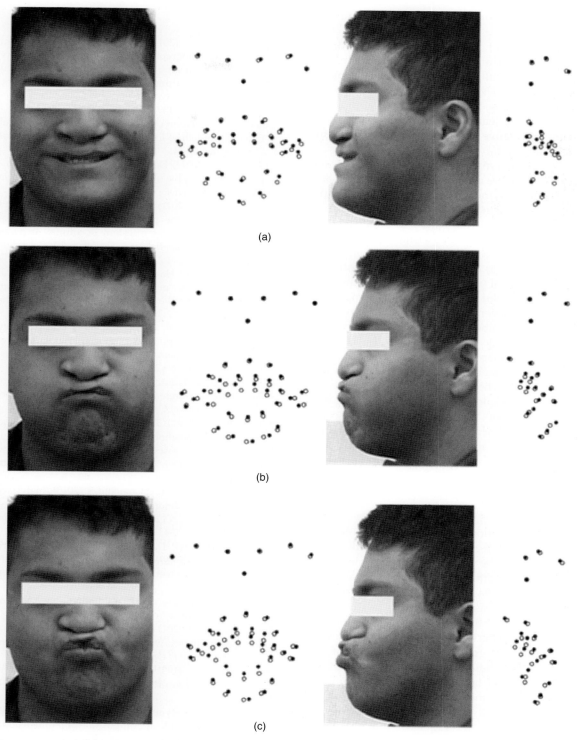

Figure 10.13 A cleft lip patient performing three maximum facial movements: (a) smile, (b) cheek puff, and (c) lip purse. The average/mean smile of the patient is superimposed on the average smile for control patients.

(e.g., Motion Analysis, Santa Rosa, California) (Figure 10.12).

The x, y, and z coordinates of the landmarks are captured during each animation (smile, lip purse, cheek puff, grimace, and mouth opening) at a rate of 60 Hz and for 4 seconds. These data then are processed offline. Using this approach, an individual patient's movement can be compared to the normative movement for each animation (Trotman *et al.*, 2013a). The comparisons can be modeled dynamically; in Figure 10.13 static captures of these dynamic comparisons are shown to demonstrate the approach and patient's impairment. The patient has a repaired cleft of the lip and it is important for the reader to understand that these comparisons can be visualized as the facial movement is occurring (Trotman *et al.*, 2013b). For example, (a) during the smile animation, the mean of several (maximum) smile movements for the patient (solid black dots) is superimposed on the mean of several (maximum) smile movements for a large number of noncleft "normal" subjects (open dots). Clear differences at the maximum of the movement can be visualized. The same comparisons can be made for the other animations shown in (b) cheek puff and (c) lip purse. This statistical modeling provides a quantitative visual comparison of surgical outcomes associated with surgery for the upper lip in these patients. Obviously, this approach can be applied to other patients who have facial soft tissue impairments.

Summary

Digital applications have significantly enhanced diagnosis and treatment planning in orthodontics. Treatment can be performed more efficiently with fewer complications. In addition to using bony landmarks as basis for treatment planning and as a way to measure progress in treatment, new advances allow the orthodontist to evaluate and predict the effect of changes in dentoalveolar structures and growth on the position of facial soft tissues. These technologies remain in early stages and can be improved upon significantly. However, with the rate at which new technology is introduced, it will not be long before new advanced digital techniques become a practical reality in orthodontics.

References

Alqerban, A., et al. (2011) Comparison of 6 cone-beam computed tomography systems for image quality and detection of simulated canine impaction-induced external root resorption in maxillary lateral incisors. *American Journal of Orthodontics and Dentofacial Orthopedics*, **140**, e129–e139.

American Association of Orthodontists (2008) Clinical Practice Guidelines for Orthodontics and Dentofacial Orthopedics. 1–34.

Arai, Y., et al. (1999) Development of a compact computed tomographic apparatus for dental use. *Dento Maxillo Facial Radiology*, **28**, 245–248.

Baumgaertel, S. (2011) Cortical bone thickness and bone depth of the posterior palatal alveolar process for mini-implant insertion in adults. *American Journal of Orthodontics and Dentofacial Orthopedics*, **140**, 806–811.

Baumgaertel, S. & Hans, M.G. (2009) Buccal cortical bone thickness for mini-implant placement. *American Journal of Orthodontics and Dentofacial Orthopedics*, **136**, 230–235.

Baumgaertel, S., et al. (2009) Reliability and accuracy of cone-beam computed tomography dental measurements. *American Journal of Orthodontics and Dentofacial Orthopedics*, **136**, 19–25.Discussion 25.

Baumrind, S. & Frantz, R.C. (1971) The reliability of head film measurements. 1. Landmark identification. *American Journal of Orthodontics*, **60**, 111–127.

Baysal, A., et al. (2013) Alveolar bone thickness and lower incisor position in skeletal Class I and Class II malocclusions assessed with cone-beam computed tomography. *Korean Journal of Orthodontics*, **43**, 134–140.

Becker, A., Chaushu, G., & Chaushu, S. (2010) Analysis of failure in the treatment of impacted maxillary canines. *American Journal of Orthodontics and Dentofacial Orthopedics*, **137**, 743–754.

Becker, A., Kohavi, D., & Zilberman, Y. (1983) Periodontal status following the alignment of palatally impacted canine teeth. *American Journal of Orthodontics*, **84**, 332–336.

Bogdanich, W. & Craven, J. (2010) Radiation worries for children in dentists' chairs. New York Times, 1–11.

Botticelli, S., et al. (2011) Two- versus three-dimensional imaging in subjects with unerupted maxillary canines. *European Journal of Orthodontics*, **33**, 344–349.

Broadbent, B.H. (1931) A new x-ray technique and its application to orthodontia. *Angle Orthodontist*, **1**, 45–66.

Cevidanes, L.H., Styner, M.A., & Proffit, W.R. (2006) Image analysis and superimposition of 3-dimensional cone-beam computed tomography models. *American*

Journal of Orthodontics and Dentofacial Orthopedics, **129**, 611–618.

Chen, Y.J., *et al.* (2000) Comparison of landmark identification in traditional versus computer-aided digital cephalometry. *Angle Orthodontist*, **70**, 387–392.

De Vos, W., Casselman, J., & Swennen, G.R. (2009) Cone-beam computerized tomography (CBCT) imaging of the oral and maxillofacial region: a systematic review of the literature. *International Journal of Oral and Maxillofacial Surgery*, **38**, 609–625.

Faraway, J.J. & Trotman, C.A. (2011) Shape change along geodesics with application to cleft lip surgery. *Journal of the Royal Statistical Society: Series C: Applied Statistics*, **60**, 743–755.

Garrett, B.J., *et al.* (2008) Skeletal effects to the maxilla after rapid maxillary expansion assessed with cone-beam computed tomography. *American Journal of Orthodontics and Dentofacial Orthopedics*, **134**, 8–9.

Grauer, D., *et al.* (2010) Accuracy and landmark error calculation using cone-beam computed tomography-generated cephalograms. *Angle Orthodontist*, **80**, 286–294.

Grunheid, T., *et al.* (2012) Dosimetry of a cone-beam computed tomography machine compared with a digital x-ray machine in orthodontic imaging. *American Journal of Orthodontics and Dentofacial Orthopedics*, **141**, 436–443.

Halazonetis, D.J. (2005) From 2-dimensional cephalograms to 3-dimensional computed tomography scans. *American Journal of Orthodontics and Dentofacial Orthopedics*, **127**, 627–637.

Halazonetis, D.J. (2012) Cone-beam computed tomography is not the imaging technique of choice for comprehensive orthodontic assessment. *American Journal of Orthodontics and Dentofacial Orthopedics*, **141**, 403–411.

Haney, E., *et al.* (2010) Comparative analysis of traditional radiographs and cone-beam computed tomography volumetric images in the diagnosis and treatment planning of maxillary impacted canines. *American Journal of Orthodontics and Dentofacial Orthopedics*, **137**, 590–597.

Harrell, W.E.J., Hatcher, D.C., & Bolt, R.L. (2002) In search of anatomic truth: 3-dimensional digital modeling and the future of orthodontics. *American Journal of Orthodontics and Dentofacial Orthopedics*, **122**, 325–330.

Harris, E.F., Kineret, S.E., & Tolley, E.A. (1997) A heritable component for external apical root resorption in patients treated orthodontically. *American Journal of Orthodontics and Dentofacial Orthopedics*, **111**, 301–309.

Hatcher, D.C. (2012) Cone beam computed tomography: craniofacial and airway analysis. *Dental Clinics of North America*, **56**, 343–357.

Hodges, R.J., Atchison, K.A., & White, S.C. (2013) Impact of cone-beam computed tomography on orthodontic diagnosis and treatment planning. *American Journal of Orthodontics and Dentofacial Orthopedics*, **143**, 665–674.

Hofrath, H. (1931) Die bedeutung der röntgenfern-und abstandsaufnahme für die diagnostik der kieferanomalien. *Fortschritte der Orthodontik in Theorie und Praxis*, **1**, 232–258.

Houston, W.J. (1983) The analysis of errors in orthodontic measurements. *American Journal of Orthodontics*, **83**, 382–390.

Jacobson, A. (1975) The "Wits" appraisal of jaw disharmony. *American Journal of Orthodontics*, **67**, 125–138.

Jayaratne, Y.S., *et al.* (2010) Computer-aided maxillofacial surgery: an update. *Surgical Innovation*, **17**, 217–225.

Kapila, S., Conley, R.S., & Harrell, W.E.J. (2011) The current status of cone beam computed tomography imaging in orthodontics. *Dento Maxillo Facial Radiology*, **40**, 24–34.

Katheria, B.C., *et al.* (2010) Effectiveness of impacted and supernumerary tooth diagnosis from traditional radiography versus cone beam computed tomography. *Pediatric Dentistry*, **32**, 304–309.

Kim, Y.H. & Vietas, J.J. (1978) Anteroposterior dysplasia indicator: an adjunct to cephalometric differential diagnosis. *American Journal of Orthodontics*, **73**, 619–633.

Kohavi, D., Becker, A., & Zilberman, Y. (1984) Surgical exposure, orthodontic movement, and final tooth position as factors in periodontal breakdown of treated palatally impacted canines. *American Journal of Orthodontics*, **85**, 72–77.

Liu, J.K., Chen, Y.T., & Cheng, K.S. (2000) Accuracy of computerized automatic identification of cephalometric landmarks. *American Journal of Orthodontics and Dentofacial Orthopedics*, **118**, 535–540.

Ludlow, J.B., Davies-Ludlow, L.E., & Brooks, S.L. (2003) Dosimetry of two extraoral direct digital imaging devices: NewTom cone beam CT and Orthophos Plus DS panoramic unit. *Dento Maxillo Facial Radiology*, **32**, 229–234.

Ludlow, J.B., *et al.* (2006) Dosimetry of 3 CBCT devices for oral and maxillofacial radiology: CB Mercuray, NewTom 3G and i-CAT. *Dento Maxillo Facial Radiology*, **35**, 219–226.

Ludwig, B., *et al.* (2011) Anatomical guidelines for miniscrew insertion: vestibular interradicular sites. *Journal of Clinical Orthodontics*, **45**, 165–173.

Lupi, J.E., Handelman, C.S., & Sadowsky, C. (1996) Prevalence and severity of apical root resorption and alveolar bone loss in orthodontically treated adults. *American Journal of Orthodontics and Dentofacial Orthopedics*, **109**, 28–37.

Mah, J.K., et al. (2003) Radiation absorbed in maxillofacial imaging with a new dental computed tomography device. Oral Surgery, Oral Medicine, Oral Pathology, Oral Radiology & Endodontics, 96, 508–513.

Mah, J.K., Huang, J.C., & Choo, H. (2010) Practical applications of cone-beam computed tomography in orthodontics. Journal of the American Dental Association, 141(Suppl. 3), 7S–13S.

Mozzo, P., et al. (1998) A new volumetric CT machine for dental imaging based on the cone-beam technique: preliminary results. European Radiology, 8, 1558–1564.

Müssig, E., Wörtche, R., & Lux, C.J. (2005) Einsatzmöglichkeiten der digitalen Volumentomographie in der kieferorthopädischen Diagnostik. Journal of Orofacial Orthopedics, 66, 241–249.

Nakajima, A., et al. (2005) Two- and three-dimensional orthodontic imaging using limited cone beam-computed tomography. Angle Orthodontist, 75, 895–903.

Osorio, F., et al. (2008) Cone beam computed tomography: an innovative tool for airway assessment. Anesthesia and Analgesia, 106, 1803–1807.

Petersson, A. (2010) What you can and cannot see in TMJ imaging–an overview related to the RDC/TMD diagnostic system. Journal of Oral Rehabilitation, 37, 771–778.

Poole, M.N., Engel, G.A., & Chaconas, S.J. (1980) Nasopharyngeal cephalometrics. Oral Surgery, Oral Medicine, and Oral Pathology, 49, 266–271.

Quereshy, F.A., et al. (2012) Use of cone beam computed tomography to volumetrically assess alveolar cleft defects–preliminary results. Journal of Oral and Maxillofacial Surgery, 70, 188–191.

Rinchuse, D.J. & Kandasamy, S. (2012) Orthodontic dental casts: the case against routine articulator mounting. American Journal of Orthodontics and Dentofacial Orthopedics, 141, 9–16.

Roberts, J.A., et al. (2009) Effective dose from cone beam CT examinations in dentistry. British Journal of Radiology, 82, 35–40.

Rungcharassaeng, K., et al. (2007) Factors affecting buccal bone changes of maxillary posterior teeth after rapid maxillary expansion. American Journal of Orthodontics and Dentofacial Orthopedics, 132, 428.e1–428.e8.

Sameshima, G.T. & Sinclair, P.M. (2001) Predicting and preventing root resorption: Part I. Diagnostic factors. American Journal of Orthodontics and Dentofacial Orthopedics, 119, 505–510.

Silva, M.A., et al. (2008) Cone-beam computed tomography for routine orthodontic treatment planning: a radiation dose evaluation. American Journal of Orthodontics and Dentofacial Orthopedics, 133, 640.e1–640.e5.

Steiner, C.C. (1953) Cephalometrics for you and me. American Journal of Orthodontics, 39, 729–755.

Trotman, C.A. (2011) Faces in 4 dimensions: why do we care, and why the fourth dimension? American Journal of Orthodontics and Dentofacial Orthopedics, 140, 895–899.

Trotman, C.A., et al. (2013a) Facial soft tissue dynamics before and after primary lip repair. Cleft Palate-Craniofacial Journal, 50, 315–322.

Trotman, C.A., et al. (2010) Effects of lip revision surgery in cleft lip/palate patients. Journal of Dental Research, 89, 728–732.

Trotman, C.A., et al. (2013b) Influence of objective three-dimensional measures and movement images on surgeon treatment planning for lip revision surgery. Cleft Palate-Craniofacial Journal, 50, 684–695.

Tsao, D.H., Kazanoglu, A., & McCasland, J.P. (1983) Measurability of radiographic images. American Journal of Orthodontics, 84, 212–216.

Tsiklakis, K., Syriopoulos, K., & Stamatakis, H.C. (2004) Radiographic examination of the temporomandibular joint using cone beam computed tomography. Dento Maxillo Facial Radiology, 33, 196–201.

Tso, H.H., et al. (2009) Evaluation of the human airway using cone-beam computerized tomography. Oral Surgery, Oral Medicine, Oral Pathology, Oral Radiology & Endodontics, 108, 768–776.

Tucker, S., et al. (2010) Comparison of actual surgical outcomes and 3-dimensional surgical simulations. Journal of Oral and Maxillofacial Surgery, 68, 2412–2421.

Tweed, C.H. (1954) The Frankfort-Mandibular incisor angle (FMIA) in orthodontic diagnosis, treatment planning and prognosis. American Journal of Orthodontics, 32, 121–169.

van Vlijmen, O.J., et al. (2009) Comparison of cephalometric radiographs obtained from cone-beam computed tomography scans and conventional radiographs. Journal of Oral and Maxillofacial Surgery, 67, 92–97.

White, S.C. & Pharoah, M.J. (2008) Oral Radiology: Principles and Interpretation. Elsevier Health Sciences.

Zamora, N., et al. (2011) Cephalometric measurements from 3D reconstructed images compared with conventional 2D images. Angle Orthodontist, 81, 856–864.

11 Clinical Applications of Digital Dental Technology in Oral and Maxillofacial Surgery

Jason Jamali, Antonia Kolokythas, and Michael Miloro

Introduction

The field of dentistry continues to evolve as it adopts developing new technologies. Within dentistry, oral and maxillofacial surgery has found applications for these innovations throughout its subspecialty areas. Digital and computer-aided methods have changed approaches to data collection and assessment as well as delivery of patient care and interim follow-up. The digitization of three-dimensional imaging has improved communication among practitioners and has enhanced team-based approaches to surgical planning. Online webinars have become virtual operating rooms during treatment planning where surgical simulations and telesurgery can now be performed remotely using robotic surgeries.

Of the recent technological advances, imaging has played the biggest role in changing patient care. Within oral and maxillofacial surgeries, facial reconstruction is a rapidly progressing field. Reconstruction may be required for oncologic, congenital, dentoalveolar, and traumatic defects in addition to temporomandibular joint pathology and esthetic facial enhancement. Digital imaging in combination with CAD/CAM technologies has

remained at the vanguard of surgical innovation, particularly for reconstruction.

As these technologies are adopted, their efficacies must constantly be reassessed in relation to traditional methods. Outcome analysis needs to consider drawbacks such as increased cost, treatment time, and adverse patient effects such as increased radiation exposure.

Imaging

Plain films versus digital films

For the oral and maxillofacial surgeon, the advantages of digital radiography are congruent to those in other fields of dentistry. Digital radiography generally allows for a dose-dependent reduction in radiation. This reduction varies between 0% and 50% depending on the unit and film speed used. A comparison of digital versus conventional panoramic radiography revealed a dosage of 5–14 microSv and 16–21 microSv, respectively (Sabarudin and Tiau, 2013). Using digital imaging, image acquisition is easier and faster allowing for a more rapid and accurate diagnosis. Furthermore,

Clinical Applications of Digital Dental Technology, First Edition. Edited by Radi Masri and Carl F. Driscoll.
© 2015 John Wiley & Sons, Inc. Published 2015 by John Wiley & Sons, Inc.

the use of digital imaging eliminates the need for a dark room and regular maintenance of chemical fixation and developing solutions. Storage and transfer of images is streamlined allowing for more efficient communication between the dentist and patient or consulting and referral sources. Most importantly, various image analysis and enhancement tools may allow for better interpretation of images (Szalma et al., 2012). Image processing tools allow for manipulation of brightness, contrast, density, magnification, sharpness, noise filters, and inversion (Raitz et al., 2012).

For the oral and maxillofacial surgeon, imaging plays an important role in risk assessment prior to third molar extractions. Risk factors predictive of higher rates of inferior alveolar nerve paresthesia include interruption, narrowing, or diversion of the cortical canal wall and deflection or darkening of the third molar roots. Despite the aforementioned advantages of digital radiography, no statistically significant differences were seen in a comparison of digital versus conventional panoramic radiography with regard to predicting inferior alveolar nerve (IAN) paresthesia (Szalma et al., 2012). Qualitative assessment using a four-point grading scale demonstrated improved density and contrast of digital rather than conventional panoramic images (Sabarudin and Tiau, 2013). This was improved further with post-processing enhancement.

Other comparisons between digital and conventional panoramic radiography have been studied. A comparison between the two methods with regard to diagnostic accuracy of unilocular lesions also failed to show a statistically significant difference (Raitz et al., 2006).

Cone-beam CT

Of the digital imaging modalities, the cone-beam CT scan has proven to be the most valuable asset to the oral and maxillofacial surgeon.

CBCT differs from conventional CT scans in several ways. Most importantly it exposes the patient to less radiation which, depending on the type of scanner, has been reported to be up to a 20% reduction (Quereshy et al., 2008). The CBCT uses a cone-shaped X-ray beam rather than a fan-shaped beam and only makes a single

rotation around the head of the patient. Various scanners are available with small, medium, and larger fields of view, each demonstrating an indirect relationship between field of view and resolution (Friedland et al., 2012). With improved accessibility and decreased cost, the CBCT has become the gold standard for three-dimensional imaging of hard tissues. Furthermore, less scatter from various objects such as dental implants and metallic restorations allows for improved visualization and image interpretation. For a better understanding of soft tissue, conventional CT and MRI remain better options, although advances in soft tissue imaging modalities continue.

In comparison to plain films (e.g., panoramic and cephalographs), cone-beam imaging offers several advantages (Figure 11.1a–c). Most importantly, CBCT imaging allows for a better understanding of anatomical regions by limiting superimposition of structures. As a three-dimensional analysis, it provides a better understanding of interrelationships between various landmarks. With CBCT, the variability of magnification and distortion of panoramic radiography are eliminated. A greater field of view is possible with the additional capability of creating two-dimensional views as needed.

Dentoalveolar surgery

For the oral and maxillofacial surgeon, CBCT imaging is obtained most commonly for dentoalveolar indications (Figure 11.2). Of these, the advantages of this imaging prior to implant placement are most obvious (Figure 11.3a, b). Assessment of bone quality and quantity are possible in addition to measurement of distances from adjacent vital structures (e.g., maxillary sinus and inferior alveolar canal).

The use of CBCT scans for evaluation of impacted teeth has been valuable especially for the localization of deeply impacted maxillary canine or other impacted non-third molar teeth (Figure 11.4a, b). For third molar impactions the literature does not support the routine use of CBCT imaging (Guerrero et al., 2014) (Figure 11.5). Randomized trials comparing panoramic radiography to cone-beam CT failed to demonstrate a

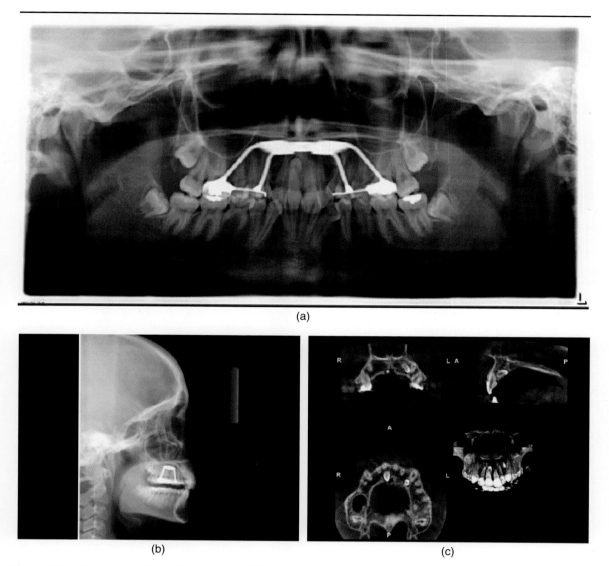

Figure 11.1 (a) Panoramic radiograph depicting maxillary supernumerary teeth. The two-dimensional film limits buccal/lingual localization. (b) Lateral cephalogram of the above patient. Superimposition limits the precise localization of the impacted supernumeraries. (c) Cone-beam CT scan with coronal, sagittal, axial, and three-dimensional views allowing for improved localization of the impacted supernumerary maxillary teeth.

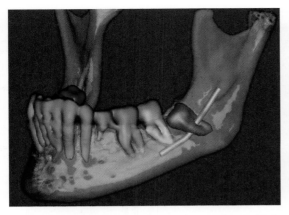

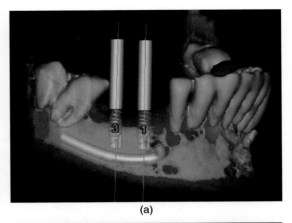

(a)

Figure 11.2 Three-dimensional view of a cone-beam CT: the relationship of the inferior alveolar nerve and impacted third molar are clearly depicted.

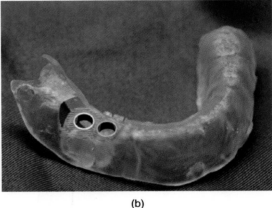

(b)

Figure 11.3 (a) 3D virtual planning of implants to ensure avoidance of the inferior alveolar nerve. (b) Fabrication of a surgical guide to guide the placement of implants as planned.

difference with regard to prediction of postoperative complications prior to third molar removal (Guerrero *et al.*, 2014).

For impacted supernumerary teeth, three-dimensional imaging with CBCT allows for a better understanding of the relationships of the teeth with adjacent structures over plain film imaging (Figure 11.6a, b). It allows for assessment of adjacent root resorption and prediction of the bone support remaining following surgical access (Figure 11.7a–c). In the pediatric population, localization eliminates the compliance needed to tolerate multiple periapical films required for the "SLOB" (same lingual-opposite buccal) rule (Tiwana and Kushner, 2005).

Maxillofacial pathology

For benign tumors and cysts, three-dimensional assessment may enhance the understanding of the internal composition of lesions such as calcifications or root or nerve proximity (Figure 11.8).

Associated cortical expansion can be visualized without the need for obtaining additional films (Figure 11.9a, b). Postoperatively, cone-beam imaging may be more helpful for surveillance of recurrent lesions (Ahmad *et al.*, 2012). The role of CBCT for evaluation of malignant lesions

is somewhat restricted by the relative soft tissue limitations. Conventional CT and in some instances MRI represent better alternatives for lesions with soft tissue components.

For inflammatory diseases of the bone such as osteomyelitis, three-dimensional imaging has helped delineate the bony regions of involvement including cortical destruction, periosteal reaction, and sequestrum (Figure 11.10). A comparison of various imaging modalities (panoramic vs MRI vs CT) for detection of Bisphosphonates-Related Osteonecrosis of the Jaw (BRONJ) demonstrated higher correlations of actual disease involvement with CT imaging (Stockmann *et al.*, 2010).

In regard to salivary gland pathology, and specifically sialolithiasis, multiple imaging

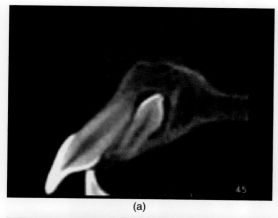

(a)

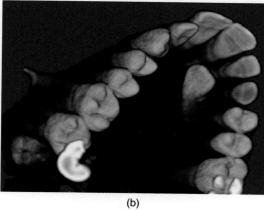

(b)

Figure 11.4 (a) Cone-beam CT scan, sagittal view depicting an impacted mesiodens. This view demonstrates the close apposition of the impacted tooth along the palatal aspect of the central incisor. Given the close apposition, there is a potential for loss of bone support after extraction of the impacted mesiodens. (b) Three-dimensional imaging allows for localization and orientation of impacted teeth.

options exist (Figure 11.11). For palpable stones associated with the distal aspects of Warthin's duct, occlusal films may be sufficient. Sialendoscopy not only provides diagnostic information regarding ductal obstructions, but when coupled with the appropriate instrumentation, it can be used for retrieval of calculi or dilation of the duct (Figure 11.12). This method uses miniature endoscopes approximately 1–3 mm wide to enter the duct system allowing for visualization and treatment of obstructions. This provides access to more proximally located obstructions that

might otherwise have resulted in gland removal. CT virtual Sialendoscopy is another diagnostic technology available. After injecting 1.5–2 cc of contrast intraductally, a CT scan is obtained and then processed to provide a three-dimensional view of the entire ductal system. As a diagnostic modality, virtual CT endoscopy overcomes several drawbacks of sialendoscopy. The rigidity of endoscopes makes it hard to navigate the entire ductal system and in doing so damage to the orifice and ductal walls may introduce scarring and resultant stenosis. In addition, with traditional endoscopy, the ductal system proximal to the obstruction cannot be viewed until its removal (Su *et al.*, 2009).

For analysis of maxillary sinus pathology, CT scan images are clearly superior to panoramic radiography. In patients with radiographic maxillary sinus pathology on CT scans (categorized as mucosal thickening, mucous cyst or occupation of the entire sinus) panoramic radiography was concordant only 4.3% of the time (Maestre-Ferrin *et al.*, 2011).

For the temporo-mandibular joint, multiple imaging options are available. Plain films (transmaxillary, Reverse Towne's, transpharyngeal, etc.) are limited once again by superimposition. They do not provide information regarding nonmineralized tissues and bony changes may not be seen until significant destruction has occurred. The panoramic radiograph is commonly used as an initial screen to rule out gross bony pathology. CBCT is more sensitive for identification of bony changes such as erosions, sclerosis, osteophytes, and condylar hyperplasia. Bone scans are helpful in ruling out an active metabolic process in the setting of condylar hyperplasia. MRI's greatest advantage is in providing information regarding the nonmineralized components of the joint. T1 weighted images provide anatomical detail of the osseous as well as discal tissues whereas T2 provides information regarding effusions and inflammation. MRI has supplanted arthrography for identification of disk perforation. More importantly, MRI remains represents the best modality for identification of internal derangement (Lewis *et al.*, 2008).

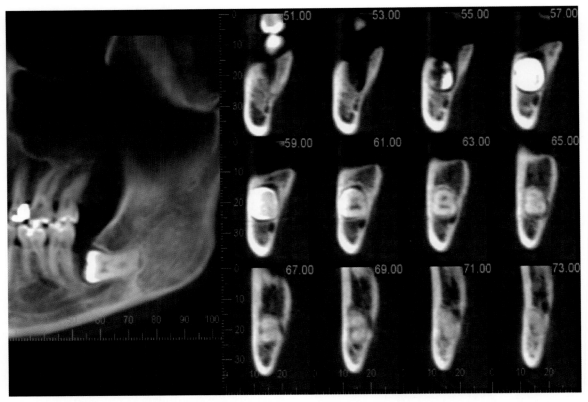

Figure 11.5 Improved resolution allows visualization of the relationship of the third molar to the inferior alveolar canal.

Orthognathic surgery

Imaging is very important to the preoperative planning for orthognathic surgery as it allows for cephalometric analysis. Three-dimensional images can enhance the localization of key landmarks that may otherwise be difficult on plain film radiography (see Chapter 10). Analyses of 2D images are limited by superimposition of landmarks, magnification of objects closer to the X-ray source, and the inherent difficulty of facial asymmetry. Various studies which have compared conventional, digital, and CT-derived cephalograms have demonstrated statistically significant differences in landmark localization (Ghoneima *et al.*, 2012). A comparison of two dimensional digital cephalograms with 3D CBCT derived images demonstrated a greater mean error of landmark identification for 2D images and overall 3D imaging results in better interobserver

and intraobserver reliability in the majority of landmarks (Chien *et al.*, 2009).

Despite the improvements gained from 3D images obtained via CBCT, limitations exist. The goal is to digitally represent all three tissue groups (skin/soft tissues of the face, bony skeleton, and dentition) of the craniofacial region in three dimensions (Plooij *et al.*, 2011). When different modalities are used for each unit, an image fusion process is necessary to synthesize the data into a virtual representation of the craniofacial complex and allow planning of maxillary and mandibular orthognathic surgical procedures (Plooij *et al.*, 2011) (Figure 11.13). When imaging the dentition, CBCT is limited by streak artifact from restorations and appliances.

Digital impressions using intraoral scanning devices have the advantage of eliminating the work involved with traditional dental impressions and cast fabrication. More commonly, laser scans

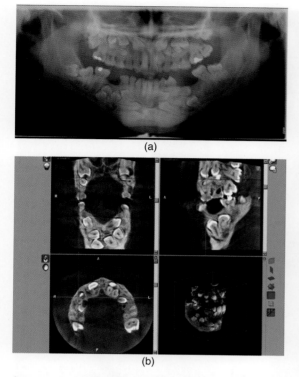

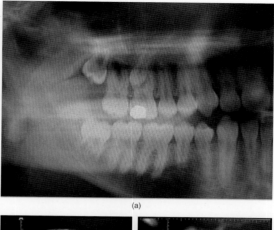

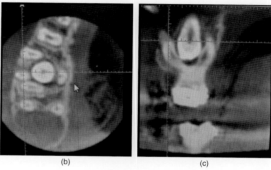

Figure 11.6 In patients with multiple supernumerary impactions, a cone-beam CT is more efficient for localization than taking multiple periapical films. Example 1(a) and Example 2(b).

Figure 11.7 (a) Two-dimensional imaging is limited in providing information regarding the relationships of superimposed structures such as impacted teeth. (b) An axial slice from the CBCT demonstrates the inter-radicular location of the impacted tooth. (c) Coronal view corroborating the location.

are obtained of dental casts (Plooij *et al.*, 2011). With regard to the soft tissue envelope, there are several modalities with advantages over CBCT: 2D photography, MRI, 3D ultrasonography, 3D surface laser scanning, and 3D photography/stereo photogrammetry (Plooij *et al.*, 2011) (Figure 11.14). Cost, time needed for data acquisition, and risks of laser damage to the eye represent some of the limitations of these modalities (Plooij *et al.*, 2011). Three-dimensional photography provides accurate textured surfaces efficiently and without the need for ionizing radiation (Plooij *et al.*, 2011). Three-dimensional photography works by using multiple cameras (at least two) placed at different known distances with respect to a reference point (Naudi *et al.*, 2013). A landmark on the object must be captured by each camera. The distance of the landmark from a reference point is compared with each image and the differences are used

to determine the position of the object in the third dimension (z axis). Fusion of the stereo photograph with the CBCT is performed using software, which uses iterative algorithms to match the surfaces (Naudi *et al.*, 2013).

Protocols, which allow for the simultaneous capture of the CBCT and stereo photograph, have been shown to have improved accuracy (Naudi *et al.*, 2013). As these technologies become more popularized, the 3D data obtained pre- and postoperatively can be utilized to enhance surgical predictions. A 3D orthognathic surgery planning program known as Maxilim (Medicim Medical Image Computing) was developed in order to predict the soft tissue response to surgery. Using data obtained from CBCT scans, one obtained immediately pre-op and a second obtained 6–12

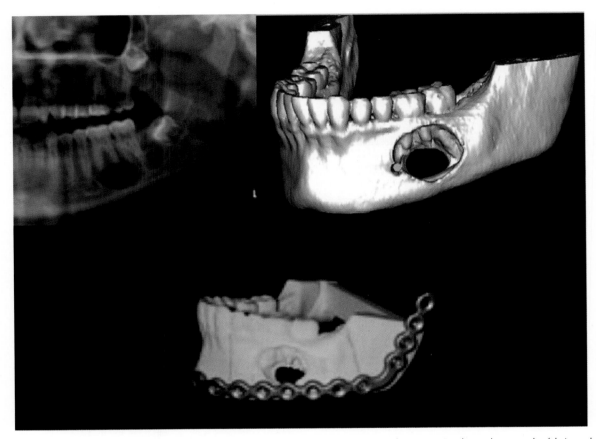

Figure 11.8 Unicystic ameloblastoma represented on panorex and three-dimensional imaging. Pre-bent plates can be fabricated using the DICOM data.

months post-op, the accuracy of soft tissue predictions using Maxilim was studied. The results indicated accuracy within 3mm for all areas of the face except for the upper lip which as larger then 3mm (Shafi *et al.*, 2013). Studies using other prediction software have demonstrated similar difficulty of predicting the postsurgical location of the upper lip region (Figure 11.15).

Obstructive sleep apnea syndrome (OSAS)

Three-dimensional images obtained from CBCT scans have been applied to treatment of obstructive sleep apnea. Cross-sectional imaging of airway has been a helpful adjunct in the identification of regions that may predispose a patient to airway obstruction (Figure 11.16a–c). Compared with 2D cephalometric analysis, 3D CBCT data allows for both cross-sectional and volumetric analysis of the entire airway. The airway volumes of patients with OSAS tend to be smaller and narrow laterally (Strauss and Wang, 2012). Using this data, correlations between the shape and the orientation of the airway and compliance and OSAS have been studied (Strauss and Wang, 2012). It is important to understand; however, that dimensions of the airway are dynamic. Changes occur during the sleep phase and with positioning. Even though the CBCT is limited to a static dimension, it is still possible to study correlations between the data and to see how surgeries used in treatment affect these volumes. The goal of surgical intervention, specifically maxillomandibular advancement, is to decrease airway resistance by

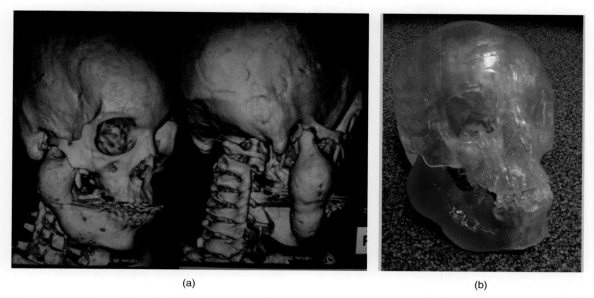

(a)   (b)

Figure 11.9 (a) Fibrous dysplasia of the mandible. Three-dimensional imaging allows for an assessment of buccal – lingual expansion. (b) A stereolithographic model has been constructed using the DICOM data from the CBCT.

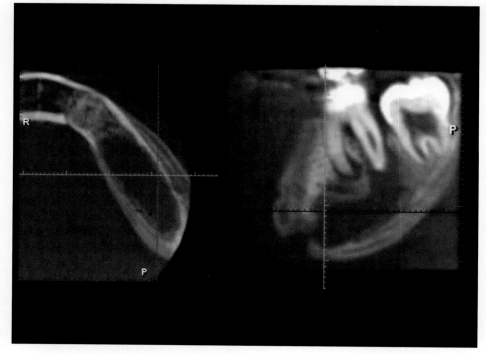

Figure 11.10 Garre's osteomyelitis with periosteal thickening.

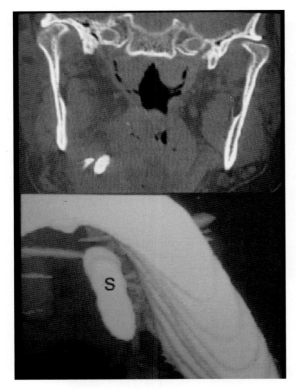

Figure 11.11 Sialolith (S) identified with CT scan imaging.

widening the airway. Studies that combined maxillomandibular and genial tubercle advancement have demonstrated an enlargement of the airway in both sagittal and transverse dimensions and shortened vertically (Abramson *et al.*, 2011). These changes were correlated with a 60% decrease in the RDI (Abramson *et al.*, 2011). With time, the collection of normative data may allow for better predictions.

Maxillofacial trauma

Imaging is one of the most important adjuncts to the physical examination in the diagnosis of facial trauma, particularly with nondisplaced fractures or in patients with limited consciousness. Diagnosis is limited with two-dimensional imaging in the same manner as discussed in previous sections (Figure 11.17a, b). For complex pan facial trauma, three-dimensional reformats of CT scan data can be helpful in surgical planning. A comparison

of two-dimensional and three-dimensional scans for the diagnosis of maxillofacial trauma was performed. Two-dimensional analysis was more accurate for orbital floor/medial wall and frontal sinus fractures (Jarrahy *et al.*, 2011). Review of 3D data was more accurate for the diagnosis of Le Fort I fractures and palatal fractures. No significant difference existed between the diagnostic accuracy of 2D and 3D analyses for zygomatico-maxillary complex fractures (Jarrahy *et al.*, 2011). In general, two-dimensional CT scans took an average of 2.3 times longer than 3D CT scans of diagnosis. Intraoperative imaging is commonly used for assessment of fracture reduction during orthopedic surgery. For maxillofacial trauma, intraoperative CBCT/CT scans are used more commonly for treatment of zygomatico-maxillary complex fractures, orbital floor fractures and in some cases retrieval of foreign bodies. The combination of intra-operative CT scans, navigation, and endoscopes have improved the esthetic outcomes of repositioned segments as well as have allowed for minimally invasive access. For example, traditional repair of the anterior table of the frontal sinus requires a large coronal incision with resultant scar through the hairline. Using intraoperative CT scans, smaller incisions can be used for instrumentation and the reduction is then verified radiographically. Subsequent fixation is performed with endoscopic visualization (Bui *et al.*, 2012).

CAD/CAM technology applications

CAD/CAM technology allows for the creation of customized tools to be used to assist with or plan for surgery in an efficient manner. These surgical tools include the following: customized anatomical replicas, cutting guides for osteotomy design, implant placement guides. Anatomical replicas and templates may be used in the pre-operative bending of reconstruction plates, design of customized bone appliances (distraction devices), or fabrication of customized implants (Figure 11.18). The initial step in customized design involves patient imaging. The digital images are converted into a 3D format known as a .stl file. Software is used to deconstruct the volume into thin slices. During manufacturing, each of these slices is

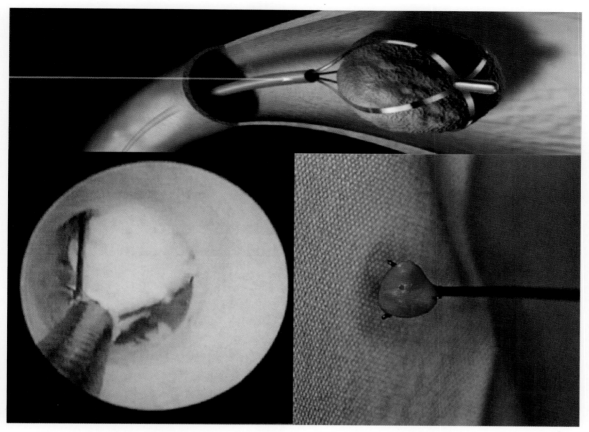

Figure 11.12 Various endoscopic retrieval devices used in conjunction with sialendoscopy for retrieval of salivary gland stones.

recombined layer by layer to recreate the object. The manufacturing varies greatly particularly with the type of material used. Both liquid and solid based materials are used and both additive and subtractive methods can be employed (Abboud and Orentlicher, 2012). With stereolithography, photosensitive plastic monomers react with a laser to induce selective solidification in layers (Abboud and Orentlicher, 2012).

CAD/CAM in maxillofacial pathology and reconstruction

Microvascular tissue transfer allows for the reconstruction of large and complex ablative defects. Microvascular surgical techniques continue to

evolve as they become more widespread in their use. CAD/CAM technologies applied to reconstruction allow for more efficient use of intraoperative time by pre-planning osteotomies and segment positioning. The goal is to reduce both intraoperative time as well as ischemic time to the flap following ligation of the vascular pedicle. In addition, better positioning and contour of the reconstructed segment is anticipated. After uploading the imaging data, the surgery is performed virtually beginning first with the planned resection. Margins are drawn, the interval of bone is removed, and an image of the bone used for reconstruction (e.g., fibula) is adjusted to the defect using virtual osteotomies (Figure 11.19a–d). The data from the surgical plan

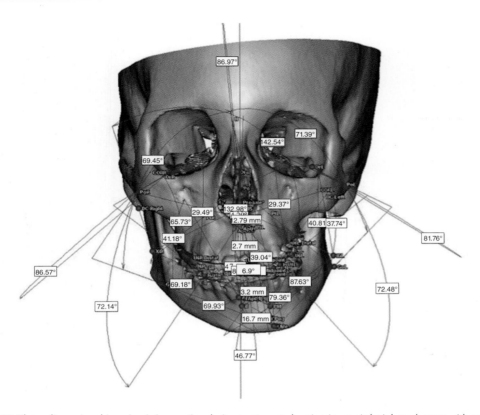

Figure 11.13 Three-dimensional imaging is imperative during treatment planning in craniofacial syndromes with asymmetries.

is then used for fabrication of cutting guides. The guides are designed with slots that allow entry of surgical cutting blades for osteotomy of the bone at a pre-determined angle. The guides commonly have holes to allow them to be secured to the bone during instrumentation. In instances where postoperative radiation is not anticipated, guides may also be used for simultaneous placement of implants. Most importantly, the osteotomies, implant placement, and attachment of the reconstruction plate to the bone flap can be performed prior to transection of the pedicle.

CAD/CAM in temporomandibular joint disorders

The prostheses used for total joint reconstruction have continued to evolve. CAD/CAM technologies have played a role in the development of customized TMJ prostheses (Figure 11.20). Using a custom prosthesis theoretically decreases operative time by decreasing the amount of adjustment and bony re-contouring required to fit the unit. This can be especially difficult in the end stage joint which has been operated on multiple times resulting in a complex anatomy which does not allow easy adaptation of stock prostheses. Most importantly, because of the superior fit of custom prostheses, micro movement is reduced (Sidebottom and Gruber, 2013). This improved stability may improve the long-term success.

CAD/CAM in orthognathic surgery

Three-dimensional imaging and CAD/CAM technologies have greatly influenced the approach to orthognathic surgery. These modalities have

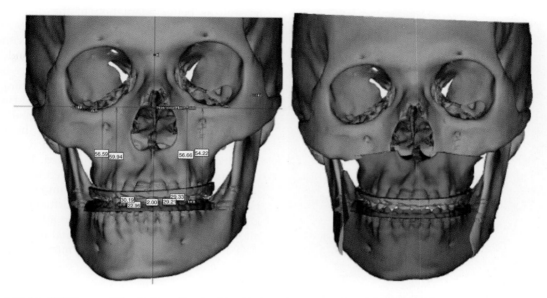

Figure 11.14 CBCT image of the skeleton. The dentition has been laser scanned and fused to the CBCT image of the remaining hard tissue. The surgical plan (LeFort I osteotomy and bilateral sagittal split osteotomies (BSSO)) is represented on the right.

allowed for improvements at each step of the process from treatment planning, intra-operatively, and during postsurgical analysis.

The presurgical evaluation involves a considerable amount of data acquisition. This appointment includes the following: clinical examination, dental-facial measurements, photographs, dental impressions, bite registration, cone-beam CT scan and a virtual facebow.

The bite registration is performed using an acrylic resin jig with attached fiducial markers (Figure 11.21). A virtual facebow is then performed by attaching this bite jig to a gyroscope, which provides a numerical value for pitch, yaw and roll in natural head position (Gelesko et al., 2012). The CT scan is performed with the bite jig in place. Using the data obtained from the gyroscope, the CT image can be re-oriented to the patient's natural resting head position. Next the dental casts are sent for processing. For better accuracy, digital imaging of the dentition is performed via a laser surface scan of the dental casts. This data is then integrated with the CT scan.

The DICOM files from the CT scan may be used for both 3D and 2D assessment (panorex, lateral/PA ceph etc.). A cephalometric analysis is performed using traditional landmarks in order to quantify the dental and skeletal relationships. The addition of three-dimensional analysis is most helpful for identifying and quantifying facial asymmetries.

Traditionally, cast surgery is performed after data collection and cephalometric analysis. This can be a time consuming process and the accuracy of planning for complex movements can be challenging particularly for patients with asymmetries. Virtual surgery using the available digital images allows for a 3D assessment of the dental-skeletal relationships obtained in real time during various virtual surgical movements. In addition, this allows for identification of various skeletal interferences that may arise, especially with mandibular set backs.

After conformation of the surgical plan, CAD/CAM technology allows for fabrication of occlusal splints that allow for repositioning of the maxilla and mandible in relation to each other (Figure 11.22). Finally, 3D imaging allows for an enhanced understanding of the postsurgical change during recall. Using stable skeletal landmarks in regions that were not changed by surgery, the pre- and postoperative CT images

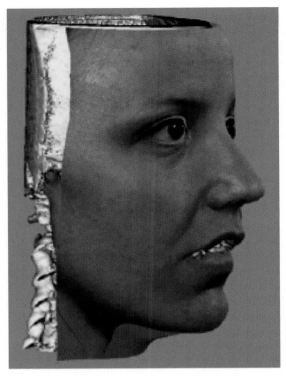

Figure 11.15 Our ability to image the soft tissues even with computer planning is less than ideal. Superimposition of 2D photos with the volume-rendered CBCT is represented above.

can be superimposed to demonstrate the final outcome.

Esthetic facial surgery

CAD/CAM technologies can be used for fabrication of custom facial implants (Figure 11.23). Esthetic enhancement of deficiencies in facial contour can be performed with implants. While stock implants exist, they commonly require modification prior to placement in order to minimize contour irregularities. This prolongs operative time and minor irregularities may persist. Pre-operative assessment using 3D CT scan imaging allows for a better assessment of the hypoplastic regions while CAD/CAM technology allows for the fabrication of a custom implant with more predictable improvements of enhancement

as well as better adaptation to the underlying skeletal contour.

In the past, custom implants made without digital technologies required patients to undergo facial impressions. This required compliance from the patient and the impressions did not accurately capture the underlying bony anatomy (Goldsmith et al., 2012). Custom implants using digital data can be produced in a variety of ways. In some instances, a stereo lithographic model is created first and a modeling putty is provided. The modeling material is adapted and molded to the area of interest. This is then sent to a manufacturer for fabrication of the final implant. Virtual planning is available as well which has the advantage of allowing for mirroring of the digital image. This aids in correction of facial asymmetries when there is a unilateral defect.

Maxillofacial prosthetics

Despite advances in microvascular reconstruction, some maxillofacial defects may be better served esthetically using a prosthetic approach (Figure 11.24). One of the major challenges in prosthetic reconstruction is retention of the unit. Various options exist including tissue adhesives, carriers such as attached eyeglasses, and osseointegrated implants (Bedrossian and Branemark, 2012). Three-dimensional digital technologies have had the biggest impact in planning for implant associated maxillofacial prosthesis. As with intraoral implants, extra oral implants require accurate 3D placement. Improper spacing, depth and angulation render the implants nonfunctional. Instead a philosophy of reverse engineering understands that it should be the final form of the prosthesis which dictates the specifications of implant placement (Bedrossian and Branemark, 2012). Three-dimensional imaging allows for assessment of residual bone available as well as identification of the distances from vital anatomical structures. In addition, the digitization of data images allows for enhanced communication among the reconstructive team members which may include a maxillofacial prosthodontist, surgeon, and anaplastologist. The variability of overlying soft tissue thickness poses another challenge to extraoral implant retained prostheses.

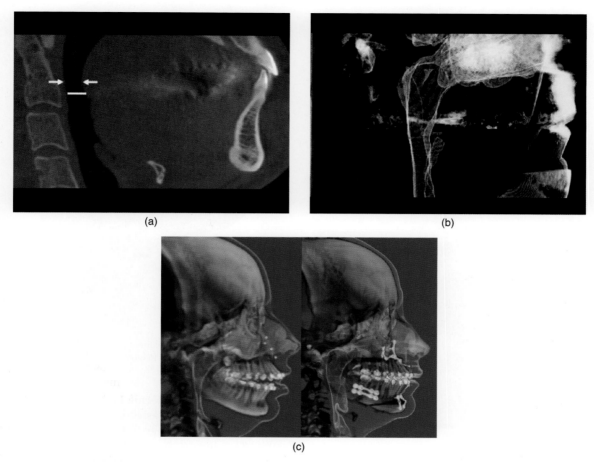

(a)

(b)

(c)

Figure 11.16 (a) Sagittal view from a CBCT used to identify potential regions of airway resistance. (b) Three-dimensional imaging allows for an assessment of the cross-sectional area and volume of the airway in OSA patients. This helps during treatment planning when deciding between surgical and nonsurgical alternatives. (c) Airway volumes can be assessed pre- and post-op following bimaxillary advancement and genioplasty.

However with 3D imaging, a soft tissue reformat can be superimposed over the skeletal structures for pre-operative analysis and planning.

Navigation in oral and maxillofacial surgery

Computer assisted surgery includes template guided approaches (obtained via CAD/CAM technology) as well as surgical navigation (Figure 11.25a–f). Navigation utilizes data obtained from 3D imaging to provide directional and spatial assistance to surgeons intraoperatively. Most importantly, the image guidance is provided

in real time. Prior to surgical navigation, imaging is obtained. MRI data has been associated with volumetric deformation and therefore CT scans are most commonly used. To ensure accuracy, image slices around 1mm are required. This data is then uploaded to the computer module. Next various anatomical landmarks are registered on the patient and correlated with the same regions on the uploaded imaging. These landmarks may either be surface landmarks, screws placed and secured to bony prominences, or using landmarks attached to a mask secured to the patient. The registration is performed using a stylus, which is recognized by camera linked to the imaging

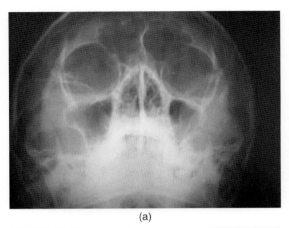

(a)

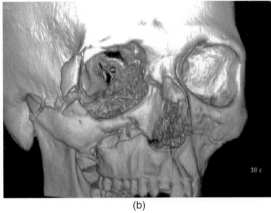

(b)

Figure 11.17 (a) Water's view: Superimposition limits eval-uation of plain films. This is particularly difficult with pan-facial trauma involving the midface. (b) Panfacial trauma with comminution may be understood better with 3D reformats.

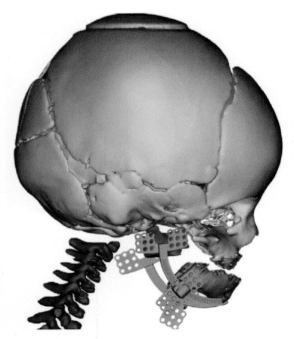

Figure 11.18 Treatment planning for custom distraction devices used in mandibular lengthening.

display module. Each landmark is confirmed between the display image and the patient. The camera links to the registered stylus using either infrared, electromagnetic, or ultrasound data transfer (Kaduk *et al.*, 2013; Edwards, 2010). Surgical instruments may be registered in addition to the stylus. The literature reports that accuracy of anatomical localization is approximately 1mm. During surgery, it is important to verify the previously registered landmarks. In some instances, error may be introduced from movement of surface tissues or following surgical manipulation.

The goal of this technology is to decrease morbidity, reduce invasiveness, and assist with teaching through image guided localization of surgical landmarks. Access is a common limitation of most surgeries; the adequacy of visualization is restricted by anatomical structural limitations as well as cosmetic demands. Regions such as the deep orbit are particularly challenging and image guidance is helpful to avoid vital structures here such as the optic nerve. Commonly, normative reference values are used to determine safe dissection distances from the intraorbital rim to each structure. With extensive comminution of the rim these reference values are immaterial.

Comminution also complicates proper reduction and subsequent esthetic outcome of traumatic bony defects. With the loss of bony landmarks, verification of reduction is lost. As a result, the accuracy in projection of the involved bone is challenged. For example, failure to reposition the zygoma appropriately may result in malar hypoplasia and a compromised facial esthetic result. If the defect is unilateral, surgical navigation software can help restore facial symmetry

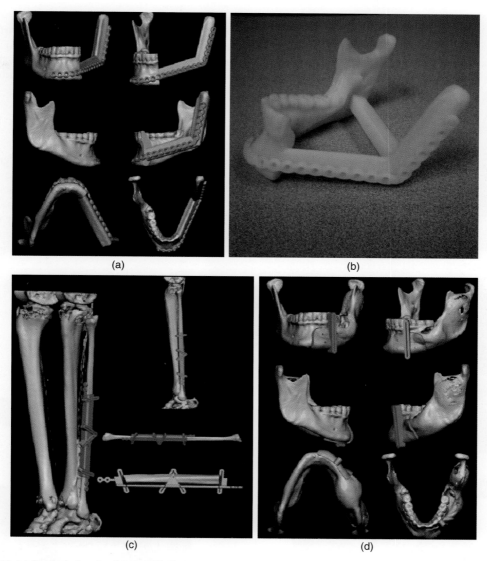

Figure 11.19 (a) Surgical planning for mandibular reconstruction using a free fibula flap. (b) A stereolithographic model of the planned reconstruction can be fabricated for bending the reconstruction plate pre-operatively. (c) Operative cutting guides are fabricated to assist with the osteotomies of the fibula used in reconstruction of the mandible. (d) Cutting guides are also made to ensure accuracy of the osteotomies used in the resection.

through the use of mirroring. The image of the uninjured side is replicated, a mirror image is created and superimposed to the injured side. The malpositioned bone is then repositioned three dimensionally until an adequate projection is obtained and verified using the navigation module (Bui *et al.*, 2012). Fixation is then applied.

Navigation requires time for operative set up, especially during landmark registration. Furthermore, as this technology is still new it requires training of residents and staff prior to use. Careful case selection is required in order for the benefits of this technology to be useful.

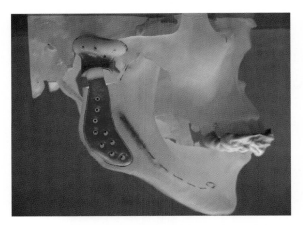

Figure 11.20 Stereolithographic models may be used during the planning of custom temporomandibular joint prostheses.

Future directions may improve this modality in its use for treatment of pathology; particularly with the incorporation of PET/CT data to aid with resection margins, staging, or in vessel localization during microvascular reconstruction (Kaduk *et al.*, 2013).

Robotic maxillofacial surgery

Endoscopic technology has played a large role in the development of minimally invasive surgery, allowing for smaller incisions, decreased blood loss, decreased pain/analgesic use, and faster patient recovery from surgery. Minimally invasive surgery has evolved to include robotic or computer assisted surgery. Instead of manipulating

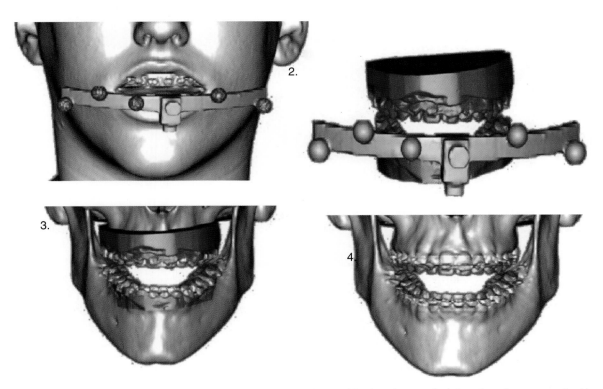

Figure 11.21 Fiducial markers attached to the bite jig are used for fusion of the dental casts (which have been laser scanned) with the CT scan.

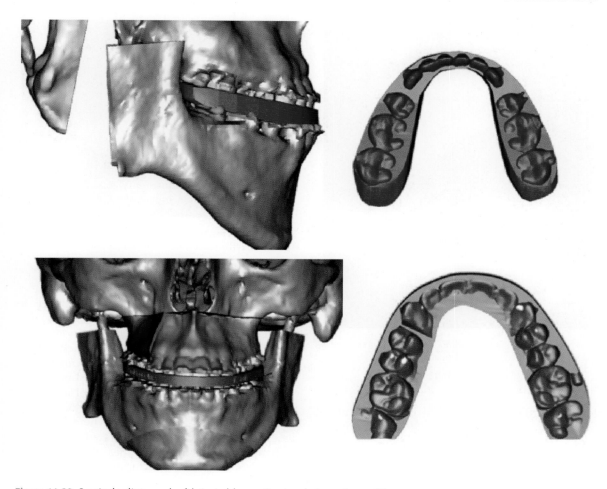

Figure 11.22 Surgical splints can be fabricated for positioning during orthognathic surgery.

instruments directly, the surgeon controls the movement of various robotic arms distantly from a console. This technology was initially developed to allow surgeons to perform procedures from remote locations. Compared with laparoscopic instruments, the robotic arms allow for more degrees of movement and visualization is improved. The components involved include the surgeon's console, robotic arms with attached instruments, and a hi-definition camera, which transmits images to the console. At the console, the surgeon's finger movements are translated into scaled down micro movements of the remote robotic arms. It has played a role in cardiac, obstetric, and urological procedures. Recently, the FDA has cleared the use of this technology for treatment of T1/T2 tumors involving the head and neck (Balasundaram *et al.*, 2012). This technology, known as TORS (transoral robotic surgery), has reportedly eliminated the need

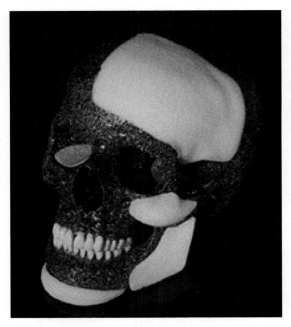

Figure 11.23 Examples of various custom implants (porous polyethelene) which may be fabricated.

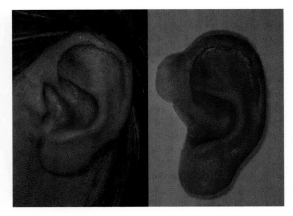

Figure 11.24 Prosthetic ear replacement may be esthetically superior to other reconstructive techniques in some instances.

for mandibulotomy in several instances, during treatment of poorly accessible oropharyngeal tumors (Figure 11.26). While the initial cost of this technology may be prohibitive, the decrease in health care expenditure associated with decreased inpatient time may offset this. Other drawbacks include the time required for training of staff and the duration of time required for pre-operative set up.

Summary

Technological developments will continue to transform the health care industry. We must apply these technologies carefully and with a comparative perspective considering increased cost, adverse effects and time. As a tool, these technologies are an adjunct to care and in regard to assessment, they are not intended to replace the assessment gained from a thorough physical examination and history. Furthermore, we cannot lose sight of traditional methods. For example, while imaging may allow for a closed or limited

access approach during surgery, the ability to perform open approach may be necessary as a result of equipment failure or complication.

While there may be some drawbacks, these technologies have enhanced our learning, provided better understandings of the anatomical limitations unique to each patient and have helped us predict outcomes better/choose alternative therapies. In instances where outcome assessment has not demonstrated significant difference among the modalities, the benefits of these technologies as an educational tool are still evident.

Reconstruction, either following trauma or pathologic resection, continues to be an area with challenging functional and esthetic demands. Digital and computer assisted technologies have been particularly helpful in reconstruction by offering a more tailored end product with less intra-operative effort. More of the surgical decision making can be performed in the virtual operating room rather than the OR or dental laboratory. Through digitization, our surgical intentions can be quantitized and applied more accurately.

Finally, the digitization of patient data can be used for generation of 3D normative data sets to be used for surgical predictions. Predicting the soft tissue response to skeletal manipulation has both functional (bimaxillary advancement) as well as esthetic (orthognathic surgery) implications.

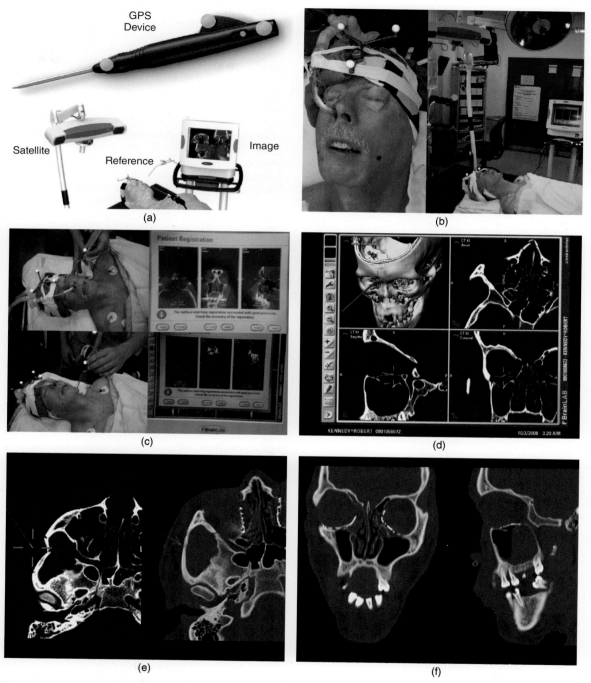

Figure 11.25 (a) Depiction of the components used in navigation. A satellite identifies the location of the stylus in relation to reference points on the patient. The images are depicted on a module in axial, sagittal, and coronal views. (b) Stable landmarks affixed to a mask to be used as landmarks during navigation. (c) Registration of various landmarks (medial canthus, pogonion) prior to navigation guided surgery. The selected points on the patient are correlated with the CT scan data visualized on the module. (d) Screen shot of the computer module used during navigation guided trauma surgery. The positioning of implants for reconstruction of the orbital floor can be verified in relation to the pre-op CT scan. This is most helpful in confirming the posterior location of the implant, which is difficult to visualize. (e) Pre- and post-reduction of zygomatic arch fractures. (f) Repair of orbital fractures, coronal and sagittal views.

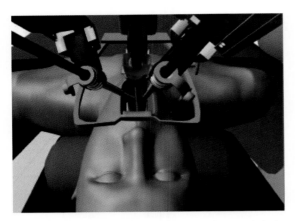

Figure 11.26 Depiction of the instrumentation used during robotic surgery.

References

Abboud, M. & Orentlicher, G. (2012) Computer-aided manufacturing in medicine. *Atlas of the Oral and Maxillofacial Surgery Clinics of North America*, **20**, 19–36.

Abramson, Z., *et al.* (2011) Three-dimensional computed tomographic airway analysis of patients with obstructive sleep apnea treated by maxillomandibular advancement. *Journal of Oral and Maxillofacial Surgery*, **69**, 677–686.

Ahmad, M., Jenny, J., & Downie, M. (2012) Application of cone beam computed tomography in oral and maxillofacial surgery. *Australian Dental Journal*, **57**(Suppl. 1), 82–94.

Balasundaram, I., Al-Hadad, I., & Parmar, S. (2012) Recent advances in reconstructive oral and maxillofacial surgery. *British Journal of Oral and Maxillofacial Surgery*, **50**, 695–705.

Bedrossian, E. & Branemark, P.I. (2012) Systematic treatment planning protocol for patients with maxillofacial defects: avoiding living a life of seclusion and depression. *Atlas of the Oral and Maxillofacial Surgery Clinics of North America*, **20**, 135–158.

Bui, T.G., Bell, R.B., & Dierks, E.J. (2012) Technological advances in the treatment of facial trauma. *Atlas of the Oral and Maxillofacial Surgery Clinics of North America*, **20**, 81–94.

Chien, P.C., *et al.* (2009) Comparison of reliability in anatomical landmark identification using two-dimensional digital cephalometrics and three-dimensional cone beam computed tomography in vivo. *Dento Maxillo Facial Radiology*, **38**, 262–273.

Edwards, S.P. (2010) Computer-assisted craniomaxillofacial surgery. *Oral and Maxillofacial Surgery Clinics of North America*, **22**, 117–134.

Friedland, B., Donoff, B., & Chenin, D. (2012) Virtual technologies in dentoalveolar evaluation and surgery. *Atlas of the Oral and Maxillofacial Surgery Clinics of North America*, **20**, 37–52.

Gelesko, S., *et al.* (2012) Computer-aided orthognathic surgery. *Atlas of the Oral and Maxillofacial Surgery Clinics of North America*, **20**, 107–118.

Ghoneima, A., *et al.* (2012) Measurements from conventional, digital and CT-derived cephalograms: a comparative study. *Australian Orthodontic Journal*, **28**, 232–239.

Goldsmith, D., Horowitz, A., & Orentlicher, G. (2012) Facial skeletal augmentation using custom facial implants. *Atlas of the Oral and Maxillofacial Surgery Clinics of North America*, **20**, 119–134.

Guerrero, M.E., *et al.* (2014) Can preoperative imaging help to predict postoperative outcome after wisdom tooth removal? A randomized controlled trial using panoramic radiography versus cone-beam CT. *Clinical Oral Investigations*, **18**, 335–342.

Jarrahy, R., *et al.* (2011) Diagnostic accuracy of maxillofacial trauma two-dimensional and three-dimensional computed tomographic scans: comparison of oral surgeons, head and neck surgeons, plastic surgeons, and neuroradiologists. *Plastic and Reconstructive Surgery*, **127**, 2432–2440.

Kaduk, W.M., Podmelle, F., & Louis, P.J. (2013) Surgical navigation in reconstruction. *Oral and Maxillofacial Surgery Clinics of North America*, **25**, 313–333.

Lewis, E.L., *et al.* (2008) Contemporary imaging of the temporomandibular joint. *Dental Clinics of North America*, **52**, 875–890, viii.

Maestre-Ferrin, L., *et al.* (2011) Radiographic findings in the maxillary sinus: comparison of panoramic radiography with computed tomography. *International Journal of Oral and Maxillofacial Implants*, **26**, 341–346.

Naudi, K.B., *et al.* (2013) The virtual human face: superimposing the simultaneously captured 3D photorealistic skin surface of the face on the untextured skin image of the CBCT scan. *International Journal of Oral and Maxillofacial Surgery*, **42**, 393–400.

Plooij, J.M., *et al.* (2011) Digital three-dimensional image fusion processes for planning and evaluating orthodontics and orthognathic surgery. A systematic review. *International Journal of Oral and Maxillofacial Surgery*, **40**, 341–352.

Quereshy, F.A., Savell, T.A., & Palomo, J.M. (2008) Applications of cone beam computed tomography in the practice of oral and maxillofacial surgery. *Journal of Oral and Maxillofacial Surgery*, **66**, 791–796.

Raitz, R., *et al.* (2006) Conventional and indirect digital radiographic interpretation of oral unilocular radiolucent lesions. *Dento Maxillo Facial Radiology*, **35**, 165–169.

Raitz, R., *et al.* (2012) Assessment of using digital manipulation tools for diagnosing mandibular radiolucent lesions. *Dento Maxillo Facial Radiology*, **41**, 203–210.

Sabarudin, A. & Tiau, Y.J. (2013) Image quality assessment in panoramic dental radiography: a comparative study between conventional and digital systems. *Quantitative Imaging in Medicine and Surgery*, **3**, 43–48.

Shafi, M.I., *et al.* (2013) The accuracy of three-dimensional prediction planning for the surgical correction of facial deformities using Maxilim. *International Journal of Oral and Maxillofacial Surgery*, **42**, 801–806.

Sidebottom, A.J. & Gruber, E. (2013) One-year prospective outcome analysis and complications following total replacement of the temporomandibular joint with the TMJ Concepts system. *British Journal of Oral and Maxillofacial Surgery*, **51**, 620–624.

Stockmann, P., *et al.* (2010) Panoramic radiograph, computed tomography or magnetic resonance imaging. Which imaging technique should be preferred in bisphosphonate-associated osteonecrosis of the jaw? A prospective clinical study. *Clinical Oral Investigations*, **14**, 311–317.

Strauss, R.A. & Wang, N. (2012) Cone beam computed tomography and obstructive sleep apnoea. *Australian Dental Journal*, **57**(Suppl. 1), 61–71.

Su, Y.X., *et al.* (2009) CT virtual sialendoscopy versus conventional sialendoscopy in the visualization of salivary ductal lumen: an in vitro study. *Laryngoscope*, **119**, 1339–1343.

Szalma, J., *et al.* (2012) Digital versus conventional panoramic radiography in predicting inferior alveolar nerve injury after mandibular third molar removal. *Journal of Craniofacial Surgery*, **23**, e155–e158.

Tiwana, P.S. & Kushner, G.M. (2005) Management of impacted teeth in children. *Oral and Maxillofacial Surgery Clinics of North America*, **17**, 365–373.

12 The Virtual Patient

Alexandra Patzelt and Sebastian B. M. Patzelt

Introduction

With the invention of the first computer by Konrad Zuse in the late 1930s, the basis for a new age, the "digital" age, was accomplished. Today, a daily life without computers is almost inconceivable, and in nearly every aspect, there is a need for digital support: from phone calls to delivery chains. As collecting, processing, and connecting information to people is also crucial in medicine, it was a logical consequence that medicine began implementing those technologies as well. One of the milestones in medicine might be considered the introduction of three-dimensional (3D) radiological techniques, for example, computer tomography. In 1998, Mozzo et al. (1998) adapted this technology for dental purposes by reducing the radiation dose, acquisition costs, and device size. Meanwhile, further 3D technologies became available. Mormann announced the first commercially available intraoral computer-aided impressioning (CAI) system in 1987, the CEREC system, for digitization of dental hard tissue and to manufacture computer-aided (CAM) dental restorations chair-side (Lutz et al., 1987; Mormann and Brandestini, 1987; Mormann et al., 1987). Three-dimensional implant planning is already

a wide-spread and acknowledged procedure in implant dentistry. In addition to 3D face scans, digital shade selection data, computer-based caries detection, and dental findings, it seems to be obvious to utilize this amount of digital data to create a virtual portrayal of a patient. Most patient data is already collected via special programs to facilitate data availability, data storage, and billing. Some of those programs are also capable of creating special computer simulated patient casts out of collected data, the so-called "virtual patients." Virtual patients can be considered digital simulations of real human beings (Ellaway et al., 2008) and related medical findings. They can be helpful in education, research, treatment planning, and patient enlightenment.

This chapter will provide the reader with information about the definition of a virtual patient, the different types of virtual patients, their purpose, what the state-of-the-art in dentistry is, and what one can expect in the future focusing on the dental application of virtual patients. It is not the purpose of this chapter to enmesh in details and principles of informatics knowledge, rather it is designed to give an overview of the increasingly used term virtual patient (also referred to as the digital patient or the artificial patient). For more information about

Clinical Applications of Digital Dental Technology, First Edition. Edited by Radi Masri and Carl F. Driscoll.
© 2015 John Wiley & Sons, Inc. Published 2015 by John Wiley & Sons, Inc.

the background of the described technologies, the authors would like to refer to pertinent literature of informatics, health informatics, and physics.

What is a virtual patient?

The basic idea of a virtual patient can be divided into three main parts. One part is the idea of creating a database containing patient related information to get an overview of the patient's medical and dental history. Results of such personalized data collections are Electronic Health Records (EHRs). The second part is the concept of digitally connecting particular diseases with symptoms, EHRs, and therapies. Thus, on the one hand electronic case scenarios can be created for training purposes and on the other hand this information can represent a useful source for research. A 3D computer-based reconstruction of human body parts, for example, limbs, organs, head, and neck, or even the entire human body represents the third part. Obviously, 3D reconstructions have the advantage over 2D paper-based illustrations of being vivid and multidimensional and so in most cases easier to interpret.

From a dental point of view, 3D visualization of the head, especially the orofacial region, is of high importance. Such a digital portrayal is based on and is limited to previously captured findings, for example, dental findings, functional findings, and digital data such as 3D radiographs (cone-beam computer tomography), facial 3D scans, and 3D tooth scanning. Putting these data together is the challenge of the creation of a virtual, informative, and above all a useful reconstruction of the patient. The basis for a digital assembly of a variety of information is the presence of ordinary analog (nondigital) information transformed to digital information. A vivid example is the utilization of a common computer keyboard: typing in a letter, one translates analog information, the letter on a paper, into digital information, the letter on the screen. All devices incorporated in a digital workflow have some kind of analog–digital conversation (A/D-converter, Figure 12.1). Furthermore, after the digitization inter-compatible data formats are necessary to gather acquired information in one model. Common formats are the DICOM-Format (Digital Imaging and

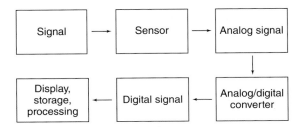

Figure 12.1 Schematic illustration of the transformation workflow of signals.

Communication in Medicine), mainly used for the exchange of radiographic imaging data, the Extensible Markup Language (XML) and Health Level 7 (HL7) format used for the exchange of clinical data, and the STL-format (Surface Tessellation Language, Standard Triangulation Language, Standard Tesselation Language), a common file format for 3D surface data. A specially developed software is applied to bring these data together and to create a digital simulation of a patient – a virtual patient.

Types of virtual patients

The aforementioned thoughts offer the possibility of creating different types of virtual patients. Generally, two basic types can be distinguished based on the purpose of simulation: virtual patients in educational simulation and in simulation of patient-related issues.

Virtual patients in medical education

Diagnostic errors represent a significant source of harm throughout the health-care profession (Newman-Toker and Pronovost, 2009). They can lead to wrong or unnecessary therapies, loss of patients' trust, and in the worst case scenario to the death of a patient. Therefore, it is important to improve the education of future health-care professionals by optimizing their cognitive and practical skills. In times of high expectations on health care but decreasing time for education (Reed et al., 2007), this goal seems to be a real challenge. One attempt to improve the health-care education system is the implementation of virtual patient models into the educational process offering students and practitioners the opportunity of learning in a safe environment while avoiding potential harm to real patients.

A considerable number of virtual patient programs are already part of medical education worldwide; however, because the development of such programs is cost intensive, not each university is able to afford creating its own (Huang et al., 2007). Therefore, different companies and institutions have started to develop programs that could be accessible to a larger community all over the world.

One example of such software is the Virtual Patient Project (University of Southern California Institute for Creative Technologies, Los Angeles, CA), which allows for the incorporation of different scenarios to simulate patients by implementing a virtual standardized life-like avatars. Others have a more quiz-like character that combines case-scenarios with various types of short questionnaires (Virtual Patients Application, Imperial College London, United Kingdom). A more hands-on approach is offered with manikin-based and virtual reality simulations (Johns Hopkins Medicine Simulation Center, Baltimore, MD, USA). Common to most of these programs is that they employ a case-based digital scenario as a feature in combination with textual and multimedia components such as audio, graphics, or animations, the so-called game-based elements. Although the increasing number of virtual patient concepts seems to be indicative for a positive influence on health-care education, one cannot say which concept seems to be the most effective so far and what might be the most promising way to implement this new educational approach (Cook et al., 2010).

Virtual patients in diagnostics, treatment planning, and execution

Besides the utilization in education, the application of digital simulations prior to treatment is already implemented in several medical disciplines, such as reconstructive facial or cardiovascular surgery. For centuries, medicine was based on a do-and-test approach because there were no tools available to predict any treatment outcomes. Now with the inclusion of high-performing computer models, more

and more opportunities to a better predictable treatment outcome can be established. There are numerous examples in dentistry where computer assisted planning and navigation is used as a successful strategy of controlling treatment quality and preventing unnecessary procedures. Preoperative planning and intraoperative navigation are already described as a useful tool not only in complex facial reconstructive cases (Schramm and Wilde, 2011) and corrective jaw surgery but also in total face transplant simulation (Brown et al., 2012). In this case, it could be shown that precise surgical accomplishment supported by computer-assisted planning and navigated surgery ensured a good donor-recipient match, which is a crucial factor of such highly sensitive procedures.

There are also approaches in medicine using computer models for a better accessibility of physiological parameters and risk factors in certain diseases such as atherosclerosis. With new computer models, researchers already tried to predict the 10-year mortality rate in cases of common artherosclerotic risk factors (Ogata et al., 2013). They were able to estimate these rates with a high accuracy. Another research group used a real-time simulation model of hemodynamics and oxygen transport to improve the understanding for the pathology of cardiovascular diseases and to predict specific treatment outcomes (Broome et al., 2013). This model could already improve understanding the qualitative influence of physiological parameters in health or disease, but it is not capable of predicting patient-specific outcomes yet.

Nevertheless, it is noteworthy that complex mathematical models can also help in evaluating strategies for control and prevention of pandemic events. This might not guarantee a certain outcome of the event but it could help in accelerating important decision processes.

Virtual patients: state-of-the-Art in dentistry

Virtual patients in dental education

For years, dental education was restricted to unrealistic phantom heads and artificial teeth

Table 12.1 Dental simulation units.

Product Name	Company/Developer/Inventor
DentSim	Image Navigation Ltd., New York NY, USA
Forsslund System	Forsslund Systems AB, Solna, Sweden
HAP-DENT	Department of Oromaxillofacial Regeneration, Department of Periodontology Osaka University; Technical Group Laboratory Inc., Osaka; Department of Computer Science, Osaka Electro-Communication University; Bionic, Co. Ltd., Osaka, Japan
HapTel	King's College, London and University of Reading, United Kingdom
Iowa Dental Surgical Simulator	College of Dentistry, University of Iowa, USA
MOOG Simodont Dental Trainer	MOOG, East Aurora, NY, USA
	ACTA, Amsterdam, Netherlands
PerioSim®	College of Dentistry, University of Illinois at Chicago, USA (C. J. Luciano)
VirDenT System	Faculty of Dental Medicine, University of Constanta Medical School, Romania
Virteasy Simulator	DIDHAPTIC, Laval cedex, France
Virtual Dental Patient	AIIA Laboratory Computer Vision and Image Processing Group, Department of Informatics, Aristotle University of Thessaloniki, Greece
Virtual Reality Dental Training System	Novint Technologies, Washington, PA, USA
VOXEL-MAN	University Medical Center Hamburg-Epperndorf, Hamburg, Germany

mimicking patient scenarios. Nowadays, digital 3D simulators are available. These devices are designed to help students grow and advance their manual skills in a representative virtual environment (Rees *et al.*, 2007; Gottlieb *et al.*, 2005). This virtual environment is comprised at least of one visual display on which a mouth or even an entire patient's head is projected. These displays can be integrated in eyewear to increase the perception of reality and haptic input devices can be utilized to provide the user with the opportunity to receive feedback in terms of tactile sensations and to provide additional dimensions to the virtual reality (sounds, vital signs, and even emergency scenarios).

The term virtual reality sounds very modern and established in recent years. Unknown to most, Morton L. Heilig patented a device more than 40 years ago (1962) that was used to incorporate virtual reality in film-making experience (Heilig, 1962). This device, Sensorama, enabled the user to not only watch and hear a movie in the common way, but also to watch it in 3D (stereo vision). This allowed the individuals to feel vibrations and smell artificial odors that enriched the movie-going experience. This could be considered the prototype of simulators nowadays, for example, every airline trains their pilots and staff using virtual reality simulators.

In the field of dentistry, approximately 12 virtual reality simulators are currently available (Table 12.1). Some are still prototypes, and some are already available commercially. Probably by the release of this book, some will not be available anymore and some newly developed systems will be on the market. To give the reader an overview of the current technologies, three systems of different technologies and their application will be considered.

One of the first computerized dental training simulators is the *DentSim* system (Welk *et al.*, 2004; Lackey, 2004). This system contains a common physical phantom head, a handpiece, and an optical tracking camera (LTD, 2013). Hereby, it is feasible to transfer and visualize the movements made in the phantom head to a computer display. The actual tooth preparations on the phantom head and the entire process of preparing a tooth – handpiece positioning, depth, wall angle, retention, and outline – can be evaluated immediately and superimposed to preexisting reference preparations providing students and faculty with immediate on-screen feedback (Buchanan, 2004;

Welk *et al.*, 2008; Gottlieb *et al.*, 2011; Hollis *et al.*, 2011) (Figure 12.2).

In contrast, the *MOOG Simodont Dental Trainer* is a simulation unit with no need for a physical phantom head. The system consists of a display projecting the mouth and teeth of a virtual patient as a stereo image on a mirror right above a haptic handpiece. A haptic device (Greek: πτικός pertaining to the sense of touch) generates a tactile feedback to the user by vibrating or generating a counterforce to the actual movements; thus simulating a real sensual experience of a virtual illusion. By wearing stereoscopic glasses, spatial illusions are created that enable the user to apply a physical drill handle as typically done on real patients, thus creating the illusion of a real dental experience. The drill handle is designed to provide different haptic feedbacks depending on the material being prepared virtually (e.g., enamel, dentin, or pulp)

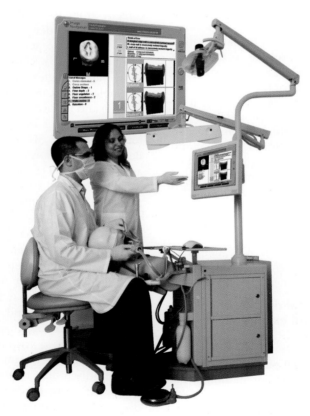

Figure 12.2 Illustration of the *DentSemi* simulation unit in a preclinical educational setting.

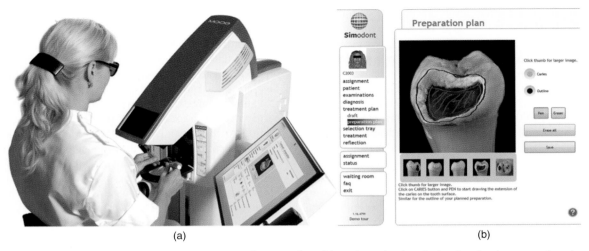

(a)   (b)

Figure 12.3 (a) *MOOG Simodont Dental Trainer* unit. (b) Screenshot of the units evaluation display showing the preparation plan for the training session.

(de Boer *et al.*; 2012; ACTA, 2013; MOOG, 2013; Vervoorn and Wesselink, 2013). The simulator is connected to a courseware computer that displays data of the virtual patient. This enables training on diagnostic reasoning and systematic patient approach and treatment, resulting in a comprehensive treatment plan before actually treating the virtual patient in the simulator (Figure 12.3).

Another systems, the *PerioSim©* haptics, is a virtual reality dental simulator that provides the ability to train students and practitioners on periodontal procedures. Visualizing a virtual human mouth including teeth and surrounding gingival soft tissue, the user is taught to develop abilities of how to examine subgingival surfaces, handle gingival tissue, or perform scaling and root planing. Central to the PerioSim system are the advanced haptic components, the high-performance PC and graphics card, and stereo glasses for the 3D visualization (Steinberg, 2004; Kolesnikov *et al.*, 2008).

Virtual patients in dental diagnostics, treatment planning, and execution in dentistry

In contrast to educational purposes, a virtual patient in diagnostics, treatment planning, and execution has to represent exactly the real patient in a digital environment. A digital copy of a patient only makes sense if it provides more

information; information that can be used to improve the treatment outcome, than one can get directly from the patient. For the purpose of a virtual patient, dental medicine is still far away from a realistic, practical, and wide-spread implementation into the clinical practice. Nevertheless, some technologies are already commercially available and in use. Fusion of radiological data (CBCT) and intraoral surface scans can be used to simulate patient's intraoral soft and hard tissues for prospective 3D implant planning (Sirona, Bensheim, Germany). The first CBCT system with an integrated 3D facial photo acquisition unit was established by Planmeca (Oy, Helsinki, Finnland) and presented at the 35th International Dental Show (Cologne, Germany) in 2011. This device enables the user to receive a 3D model of the face and maxillo-facial hard tissue. Kau *et al.* used an advanced commercially available software (3dMDvulutus, 3dMD, Atlanta, GA, USA) to fuse different datasets of a human being including facial surface scan and CBCT data to generate digital study models based on CBCT data (Kau *et al.*, 2011). These virtual patients can be used to simulate possible treatment options, for planning of multidisciplinary treatment approaches (e.g., orthognatic surgery) (Schendel *et al.*, 2013), or even during the execution of a surgery for real-time navigation purposes (Suenaga *et al.*, 2013).

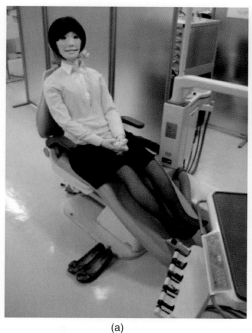 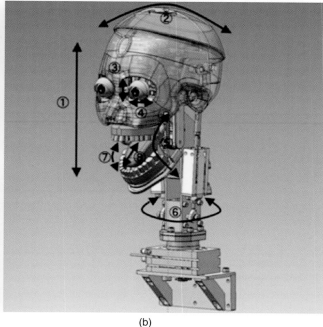

(a)   (b)

Figure 12.4 (a) Robot patient on a dent chair mimicking a real patient. (b) Technical drawing of the robot's head illustrating the range of motion. 1/2/6 possible movements of the head, 3/4 – possible movements of the eyes, 5/7/8 – possible movements of the mandible. (Source: Tanzawa *et al.* 2011, figure 1 and 2, page 196. Reproduced with permission of John Wiley & Sons, Inc.)

Virtual patients – what to expect in the future?

It is always challenging to predict what is going to happen in the future, nevertheless, it looms that dental education, diagnostic, planning, and treatment will more and more implement the available digital technologies in a more comprehensive way than today. Improvements and further developments are still necessary to make those technologies practicable for the wide-spread use in daily practice.

From an educational point of view, simulation units mimicking not only individual parts of a patient will be implemented in dental curricula combining physical models and virtual simulation. Tanzawa *et al.* describe a robot patient for dental education designed as a full-body replica, capable of secreting saliva and capable of communicating with users (Tanzawa *et al.*, 2012) (Figure 12.4). Combined with virtual evaluation instruments such a device could be the ultimate teaching tool. Future developments will more and more bring the actual technology closer to the real world.

Another aspect is, of course, the integration of augmented reality in which virtual data is superimposed on living objects (e.g., on an arm or even an entire body), thus empowering a doctor to look "inside" a patient (Figure 12.5). Such a technology would be extremely beneficial in dentistry and can be used to delineate, for example, the position of critical anatomical structures (nerves) to reduce potential nerve injury during surgical procedures (implant placement). These technologies are only beginning to be integrated in dental medicine and it can be expected they will lead to a more reliable and predictable patient treatment and reduce the cost of the treatment. Digital technologies will move together and it will be possible to integrate all obtained data in one virtual patient model. Three input information can be distinguished: Clinical findings, such as dental, prosthodontic, periodontal, orthodontic, and radiological findings; 3D data, such as facial and intraoral surface data, 3D

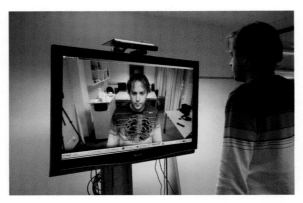

Figure 12.5 Illustration of augmented reality. On the screen a radiological image is superimposed to a real-time capturing of a person

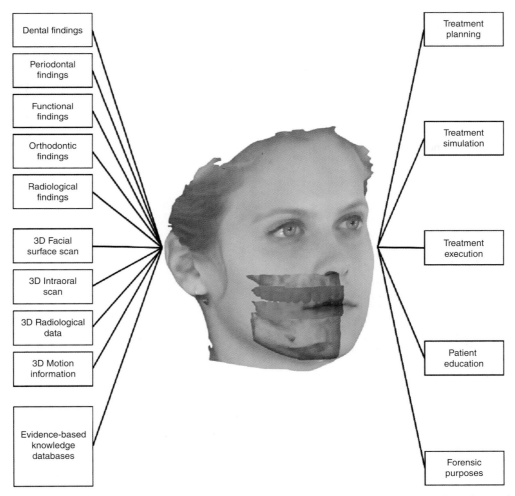

Figure 12.6 Illustration of the input information, the virtual patient and the output applications of a virtual simulation of different datasets.

radiological data, and 3D motion information; and evidence-based knowledge, for example, data from online databases or facility-based resources. Integrated in a comprehensive virtual model, those data provide the possibility of treatment planning, treatment simulation, and treatment execution on an evidence-based background in a virtual simulation (Figure 12.6).

References

ACTA (2013) *Simodont* [Online]. VU University Amsterdam. Available: http://www.acta.nl/en/studying-at-acta/student-services/simodont/index.asp [Accessed November 9, 2014].

Broome, M., Maksuti, E., Bjallmark, A., Frenckner, B., & Janerot-Sjoberg, B. (2013) Closed-loop real-time simulation model of hemodynamics and oxygen transport in the cardiovascular system. *Biomedical Engineering Online*, **12**, 69.

Brown, E.N., Dorafshar, A.H., Bojovic, B., *et al.* (2012) Total face, double jaw, and tongue transplant simulation: a cadaveric study using computer-assisted techniques. *Plastic and Reconstructive Surgery*, **130**, 815–823.

Buchanan, J.A. (2004) Experience with virtual reality-based technology in teaching restorative dental procedures. *Journal of Dental Education*, **68**, 1258–1265.

Cook, D.A., Erwin, P.J., & Triola, M.M. (2010) Computerized virtual patients in health professions education: a systematic review and meta-analysis. *Academic Medicine*, **85**, 1589–1602.

De Boer, I.R., Bakker, D.R., Wesselink, P.R., & Vervoorn, J.M. (2012) The Simodont in dental education. *Nederlands Tijdschrift voor Tandheelkunde*, **119**, 294–300.

Ellaway, R., Poulton, T., Fors, U., Mcgee, J.B., & Albright, S. (2008) Building a virtual patient commons. *Medical Teacher*, **30**, 170–174.

Gottlieb, R., Buchanan, J.A., Berthold, P., & Maggio, M.P. (2005) Preclinical dental student's perception of t he implementation of VR-based technology. *Journal of Dental Education*, **69**, 109–162.

Gottlieb, R., Lanning, S.K., Gunsolley, J.C., & Buchanan, J.A. (2011) Faculty impressions of dental students' performance with and without virtual reality simulation. *Journal of Dental Education*, **75**, 1443–1451.

Heilig, M. L. (1962) Sensorama Simulator. USA patent application.

Hollis, W., Darnell, L.A., & Hottel, T.L. (2011) Computer assisted learning: a new paradigm in dental education. *The Journal of the Tennessee Dental Association*, **91**, 14–18. quiz 18–9

Huang, G., Reynolds, R., & Candler, C. (2007) Virtual patient simulation at US and Canadian medical schools. *Academic Medicine*, **82**, 446–451.

Kau, C.H., Olim, S., & Nguyen, J.T. (2011) The Future of Orthodontic Diagnostic Records. *Seminars in Orthodontics*, **17**, 39–45.

Kolesnikov, M., Steinberg, A.D., Zefran, M., & Drummond, J.L. (2008) PerioSim: Haptics-based virtual reality dental simulator. *Digital Dental News*, **331**, 6–12.

Lackey, M.A. (2004) One year's experience with virtual reality preclinical laboratory simulation at the University of Tennessee. *International Journal of Computerized Dentistry*, **7**, 131–141.

LTD. (2013). *DentSim Technology* [Online]. Available: http://www.denx.com/DentSim/technology.html. [Accessed November 9, 2014].

Lutz, F., Krejci, I., & Mormann, W. (1987) Tooth-colored posterior restoration. *Phillip Journal für Restaurative Zahnmedizin*, **4**, 127–137.

MOOG. (2013) *Haptic Technology in the Moog Simodont Dental Trainer* [Online]. MOOG Inc. Available: http://www.moog.com/markets/medical-dental-simulation/haptic-technology-in-the-moog-simodont-dental-trainer/ [Accessed November 9, 2014].

Mormann, W.H. & Brandestini, M. (1987) Cerec-System: computerized inlays, onlays and shell veneers. *Zahnärztliche Mitteilungen*, **77**, 2400–2405.

Mormann, W.H., Brandestini, M., & Lutz, F. (1987) The Cerec system: computer-assisted preparation of direct ceramic inlays in 1 setting. *Quintessenz der zahnärztlichen Literatur*, **38**, 457–470.

Mozzo, P., Procacci, C., Tacconi, A., Martini, P.T., & Andreis, I.A. (1998) A new volumetric CT machine for dental imaging based on the cone-beam technique: preliminary results. *European Radiology*, **8**, 1558–1564.

Newman-Toker, D.E. & Pronovost, P.J. (2009) Diagnostic errors--the next frontier for patient safety. *JAMA*, **301**, 1060–1062.

Ogata, K., Miyamoto, T., Adachi, H., *et al.* (2013) New computer model for prediction of individual 10-year mortality on the basis of conventional atherosclerotic risk factors. *Atherosclerosis*, **227**, 159–164.

Reed, D.A., Levine, R.B., Miller, R.G., *et al.* (2007) Effect of residency duty-hour limits: views of key clinical faculty. *Archives of Internal Medicine*, **167**, 1487–1492.

Rees, J.S., Jenkins, S.M., James, T., *et al.* (2007) An initial evaluation of virtual reality simulation in teaching pre-clinical operative dentistry in a UK setting. *The European Journal of Prosthodontics and Restorative Dentistry*, **15**, 89–92.

Schendel, S.A., Jacobson, R., & Khalessi, S. (2013) 3-Dimensional Facial Simulation in Orthognathic Surgery: Is It Accurate? *Journal of Oral and Maxillofacial Surgery*, **71**, 1406–1414.

Schramm, A. & Wilde, F. (2011) Computer-assisted reconstruction of the facial skeleton. *HNO*, **59**, 800–806.

Steinberg, A. (2004) *UIC Periodontal Procedures Training Simulator (PerioSim)* [Online]. Available: http://www.uic.edu/classes/dadm/dadm396/ADSreserch/Contents.htm [Accessed November 9, 2014].

Suenaga, H., Hoang Tran, H., Liao, H., *et al.* (2013) Real-time in situ three-dimensional integral videography and surgical navigation using augmented reality: a pilot study. *International Journal of Oral Science*, **5**, 98–102.

Tanzawa, T., Futaki, K., Tani, C., *et al.* (2012) Introduction of a robot patient into dental education. *European Journal of Dental Education*, **16**, e195–e199.

Vervoorn, J.M. & Wesselink, P.R. (2013) Abstract. In: The perception of the level of realism of a dental training simulator (Simodont). Academic Center for Dentistry Amesterdam, Amsterdam, The Netherlands.

Welk, A., Maggio, M.P., Simon, J.F., *et al.* (2008) Computer-assisted learning and simulation lab with 40 DentSim units. *International Journal of Computerized Dentistry*, **11**, 17–40.

Welk, A., Splieth, C., Rosin, M., Kordass, B., & Meyer, G. (2004) DentSim - a future teaching option for dentists. *International Journal of Computerized Dentistry*, **7**, 123–130.

Index

Clinical Applications of Digital Dental Technology, First Edition. Edited by Radi Masri and Carl F. Driscoll.
© 2015 John Wiley & Sons, Inc. Published 2015 by John Wiley & Sons, Inc.

radiometry, 12, 23
radiopaque, 66, 140, 147, 155, 158, 162
radius, 91
random, 67
randomized, 63, 68–69, 162, 165, 182–183, 188–190, 208, 228
randomly, 2
range, 3–5, 7, 12, 14–15, 28–29, 38, 44, 47–49, 67, 71, 83, 98–100, 102, 148, 151, 164, 183, 202, 237
rapid, 39, 46, 49, 52–53, 55, 62, 108, 137–138, 140, 144, 148, 164–165, 197, 205–206, 207
rate, 6–7, 10, 49–50, 67–70, 96–98, 130, 154, 177, 182, 188, 190, 204, 208, 233
rather, 4–5, 51, 58, 60, 65, 67, 75, 82–83, 96, 99, 151, 154, 171–172, 177, 179, 183, 208, 226, 231
ratio, 10, 13, 21
reach, 2, 10, 13–14, 90
reaction, 11, 138, 162, 210
read, 6, 49, 143–144
reader, 188, 190, 204, 231, 235
reading, 11, 234
real, 28–29, 35, 37, 59, 99, 143, 151, 181–182, 188, 202, 219, 221, 231–233, 235–240
reality, 5, 96, 162, 204, 233–234, 236–240
reason, 2, 8, 15, 59, 142–143, 158, 183
reasonably, 5, 178, 184
receive, 7, 18, 30, 51, 92, 99, 101, 144, 234, 236
recementation, 85
recent, 15, 38, 71, 79, 98, 108, 149–150, 153–154, 178–179, 181–183, 187, 207, 234
recently, 2, 12, 18, 51, 53, 65–67, 79, 89, 91, 107, 109–110, 132, 139, 142, 147, 178, 182–183, 185, 187, 193, 225
receptor, 1, 3–6, 14, 25
recess, 108, 113–116, 128
reciprocating, 184–185
reciprocation, 185
recommendation, 5–6, 15, 22–24, 89, 91–92, 104
reconstruct, 12, 108, 143, 201
reconstructed, 12–13, 194, 196, 198, 202, 206, 217
reconstruction, 12, 18, 41, 54–55, 85, 140, 142, 145, 158, 161, 194–196, 198–199, 201, 207, 216–218, 220, 223–224, 226–228, 232, 240
reconstructive, 163, 220, 226, 228, 233, 239
record, 3, 33, 57–60, 67, 98, 108–110, 112, 119, 124, 127–129, 131, 232, 239
recorded, 31, 57–60, 68–69, 99, 109, 113, 127–128, 190, 193, 201–202
recording, 58–59, 63, 71, 114, 116, 119
rectangular, 5–6, 8, 151
RedCam, 28, 33
reduce, 6, 29, 38, 77, 79, 85, 87, 91, 93, 95, 98–100, 110, 153–154, 182, 187, 201, 217, 222, 237
reduced, 2, 28, 54, 66, 68, 90, 96, 108, 133, 142, 148, 153, 179, 182–183, 185, 218
reduction, 12, 22, 25, 49, 58, 92–96, 100–101, 103, 109–110, 153, 173, 185, 196, 207–208, 216, 222, 227
refer, 1, 3–4, 78, 85, 147, 232
refine, 63, 139
reflection, 178–179
reformat, 216, 221–222
refraction, 11
refractory, 82, 133, 138

regardless, 58, 94, 96, 120
regeneration, 153–154, 234
regenerative, 153
region, 6, 10–11, 14–15, 51, 81, 83, 88–89, 91, 93, 96–97, 99–103, 142, 164, 179, 193–194, 196–198, 205, 208, 210, 212, 214, 219–222, 232
registration, 111, 115, 118, 151, 163, 170, 175, 219, 221, 223, 227
regulations, 5, 24
rehabilitated, 151
rehabilitation, 104, 137, 162–163, 165, 206
rehabilitative, 202
reinforced, 34, 65–66, 69–70, 78–80, 86, 90, 96, 102
reinforcement, 46
related, 15, 24, 29, 49, 59, 140, 142–143, 150–152, 162–165, 175–176, 179, 188, 206, 231–232
relation, 4, 14, 18, 37, 110, 112, 115, 119, 149, 207, 219, 227
relationship, 15, 24, 60, 108, 115, 162, 196, 198, 208, 210, 212–213, 219
reliability, 3, 7, 11, 24, 71, 163, 175, 178, 204, 212
relief, 134
relined, 87, 113
rely, 8–9, 11–12, 15, 57–58, 63, 66, 140, 143, 150–151, 178–179, 183, 185
RelyX, 68–69, 73
remain, 38, 44, 141, 173, 193–194, 204, 208, 211
remake, 30, 38, 60
remineralization, 24
remineralize, 10
remote, 225
remotely, 207
removable, 35, 48, 54, 85, 107–109, 111, 113, 115, 117, 119, 121, 123, 125, 127, 129–133, 135, 137–138, 161, 167
removal, 44–46, 48, 51, 59, 86, 97, 137, 179, 183, 210–211, 228–229
rent, 183, 205
repair, 85, 190, 202, 206, 216, 227
repaired, 204
replace, 37, 41, 226
replaced, 14, 27–28, 85, 128, 179
replacement, 67, 109, 226, 229
replacing, 5
replica, 57, 59, 62–63, 65, 98, 176, 216, 237
report, 2, 5–6, 22, 24–25, 39, 41, 55, 62, 67–68, 72, 96, 104, 132–133, 137–138, 151, 155, 162, 164–165, 189, 222
reported, 20, 36, 52, 60, 63, 65, 67–70, 91, 94, 96–99, 102, 108, 133, 142, 149, 153–154, 182, 185, 208
represent, 18, 65, 79, 88, 154–155, 179, 186, 210–213, 232, 236
representation, 29, 87, 144, 195, 212
reproduce, 60, 140, 145, 178
reproduced, 33–36, 152, 181, 237
reproducibility, 24, 142
reproducible, 147, 153
require, 3–6, 8, 10, 12, 14, 21, 32, 36, 45, 50–52, 58–59, 78, 80–82, 84–86, 88, 92–95, 101, 103, 109, 144, 147, 153–155, 162, 178, 193, 197–198, 202, 216, 220, 223
research, 8–9, 11, 15, 22–26, 29, 37, 39, 62, 65, 67, 71–72, 98, 104, 109, 137–138, 162–165, 175–176, 186, 188, 193, 206, 231–233

reservoir, 48
residual, 49, 51–52, 55, 87, 108–110, 142, 187, 220
resilience, 149
resin, 31, 34, 47, 51–52, 62, 64–66, 69–71, 73, 76–79, 86–87, 104, 107–111, 114–116, 122, 124–126, 128, 131–132, 135–136, 138, 139, 144, 146, 161, 219
resistance, 2, 24, 76, 78, 86, 88, 90, 92, 104, 132, 138, 168, 214, 221
resonance, 14, 20, 22–23, 25, 179, 229
resonant, 179
resorption, 16, 18, 179, 184, 188–189, 195–196, 201, 204–206, 210
resource, 148, 239
respond, 7, 177
response, 6–7, 177–179, 190, 213, 226
rest, 27, 51, 95, 101, 115, 132, 135, 193
restoration, 10, 12, 14, 21, 28–30, 32, 33, 35–39, 41–42, 45, 54, 57–60, 62–73, 75–80, 82–105, 139, 142, 155, 157–162, 167–173, 175, 177–179, 181, 184, 187–188, 208, 212, 231, 239
restorative, 11, 38, 44, 54, 58, 63, 65–66, 68, 71, 77, 99, 105, 138, 158, 162, 164, 168, 170, 174–175, 239
restoratively, 95
restore, 36, 100, 130, 222
restored, 7, 10, 86, 88, 104, 145, 154, 173, 188
restoring, 9, 37–38, 71
result, 5, 7, 9–13, 18, 21, 24–25, 28, 49, 55, 60, 67–69, 72, 86, 95–96, 98, 103–105, 110, 120, 142, 146–147, 149–153, 178–179, 183, 186, 190, 195–197, 206, 212, 214, 222, 226, 232, 239
retain, 168, 171
retained, 160, 167–169, 172–174, 220
retaining, 168, 173
retention, 66–67, 70, 88, 130, 134, 138, 168, 220, 235
retracted, 59
retracting, 36
retraction, 36, 59, 71
retreatment, 177, 180, 183–184, 187
retrievability, 3
retrievable, 164
retrieval, 42, 211, 216–217
retromolar, 111
revascularization, 189
reverse, 211, 220
review, 3, 5–6, 11, 20, 22–25, 38–39, 67, 72–73, 98, 104–105, 138, 143, 149–150, 162–165, 170, 189, 193, 205, 216, 228, 239
revolution, 41, 139
ridge, 14–15, 96, 109, 111–113, 118, 126–127, 129, 159
rim, 109, 116, 222
risk, 2, 5–8, 12–13, 16, 24–25, 29, 42, 137, 142–143, 177, 208, 213, 233, 239
robocast, 175
robot, 237, 240
robotic, 162, 175, 207, 224–225, 228
role, 3, 5, 24, 151, 187, 207–208, 210, 218, 224–225
roll, 14, 37, 178, 219
room, 30, 179, 207–208, 226
root, 9, 15–16, 20, 59, 70, 86, 159, 177, 179–191, 194–196, 201, 204–206, 208, 210, 236
rotary, 27, 80, 97, 184–185, 188–191
rotate, 44, 141–142